Parkinson's Disease in the Older Patient

Edited by
Jeremy R. Playfer MD FRCP
Consultant Physician in Geriatric Medicine,
Royal Liverpool University Hospital, Liverpool

and

John V. Hindle FRCP MRCPsych
Consultant Physician in Geriatric Medicine,
Llandudno Hospital, Wales

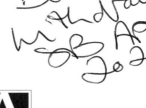

ARNOLD

A member of the Hodder Headline Group
LONDON

First published in Great Britain in 2001
This impression printed in 2002 by
Arnold, a member of the Hodder Headline Group,
338 Euston Road, London NW1 3BH

http://www.arnoldpublishers.com

Distributed in the United States of America by
Oxford University Press Inc.,
198 Madison Avenue, New York, NY10016
Oxford is a registered trademark of Oxford University Press

© 2001 Arnold

British Library Cataloguing in Publication Data
A catalogue record for this book is available from the British Library

Library of Congress Cataloguing-in-Publication Data
A catalog record for this book is available from the Library of Congress

ISBN 0 340 75914 3

3 4 5 6 7 8 9 10

Publisher: Georgina Bentliff
Project Manager: Paula O'Connell
Production Editor: Lauren McAllister
Production Controller: Martin Kerans

Typeset in 10pt Palatino
Printed and bound in Great Britain

What do you think about this book? Or any other Arnold title?
Please send your comments to feedback.arnold@hodder.co.uk

To our patients who suffer from Parkinson's disease, who have been our teachers and our guides

Contents

Contributors

Dr L. Allcock,
Registrar in Geriatric Medicine,
Royal Victoria Infirmary,
Newcastle upon Tyne,
UK

Ana Aragon
Senior I Occupational Therapist
Bath & West Community NHS Trust

Mary G. Baker MBE,
Chief Executive ,
Parkinson's Disease Society,
London,
UK

Dr Richard G. Brown,
Reader in Cognitive Neuroscience,
Institute of Psychiatry,
King's College London,
UK

Dr Colin Chandler,
Reader,
University of Northumbria at Newcastle,
Newcastle upon Tyne,
UK

Dr Rosanna Cousins,
Lecturer in Psychology,
Edge Hill College,
Ormskirk,
UK

Ann D.M. Davies
Senior Lecturer in Psychology,
University of Liverpool,
Liverpool,
UK

Dr Janice Fiske,
Guy's Hospital,
London,
UK

Dr Duncan R. Forsyth,
Consultant Geriatrician,
Dept of Medicine for the Elderly,
Addenbrooke's NHS Trust Hospital,
Cambridge,
UK

Dr C.M. Hindle,
General Practitioner,
Cadwgan Surgery,
Old Colwyn,
Conwy,
UK

Dr John Hindle,
Dept for Care of the Elderly,
Llandudno General Hospital,
Gwynedd,
UK

Dr Karen M. Hyland,
Senior Dietician,
Nutrition and Dietetic Services,
Colindale Hospital,
London,
UK

Diana Jones,
Research Fellow,
Institute of Rehabilitation,
University of Northumbria at Newcastle
UK

Professor R.A. Kenny,
Professor of Cardiovascular Research,
Dept of Geriatric Medicine,
Royal Victoria Infirmary,
Newcastle upon Tyne,
UK

Dr C. Lien,
Specialist Registrar,
Medicine for the Elderly,
Royal Victoria Hospital,
Dundee,
UK

Dr D. MacMahon,
Consultant Geriatrician,
Barncoose Hospital,
Cornwall,
UK

Dr G.J.A. Macphee,
Consultant Physician,
Dept of Medicine for the Elderly,
Southern General Hospital NHS Trust,
Glasgow,
UK

Lizzy Marks,
Principal Speech and Language Therapist,
The Middlesex Hospital,
London
UK

Dr R.J. Meara,
Academic Unit,
Dept of Health Care - Elderly,
Glan Clwyd Hospital,
Clwyd,
UK

Gay Moore,
Superintendent IV Physiotherapist,
Bath & West Community NHS Trust,
UK

Maralyn Moran,
Parkinson's Disease Research Centre,
Morriston Hospital,
Swansea,
UK

Elizabeth Morgan,
Parkinson's Disease Nurse Specialist,
Rookwood Hospital,
Cardiff,
UK

Dr W.J. Mutch,
Consultant Physician,
Medicine for the Elderly,
Parkinson's Clinic,
Ashludie Hospital,
Dundee
UK

Dr Desmond O'Neill ,
Senior Lecturer in Medical Gerontology,
Trinity Centre for Health Sciences,
Adelaide and Meath Hospital,
Dublin,
Ireland,

Dr P.W. Overstall,
Consultant in Geriatric Medicine,
Hereford Hospitals NHS Trust,
The General Hospital,
Hereford,
UK

Prof. Rowena Plant,
Professor of Rehabilitation/Therapy,
Institute of Rehabilitaion,
University of Northumbria at Newcastle,
UK

Dr Jeremy R. Playfer,
Dept of Geriatric Medicine,
The Royal Liverpool University Hospital,
Liverpool,
UK

Dr Dorothy Robertson,
Consultant in Geriatric Medicine,
Royal United Hospital,
Bath,
UK

Dr J.C. Sharma,
Consultant Physician,
Mansfield Community Hospital,
Nottingham,
UK, and Newark & Mansfield Parkinson's Disease Service,
Notts,
UK

Dr David A. Stewart,
Consultant Physician,
Medicine for the Elderly,
Parkinson's Clinic,
Victoria Infirmary,
Glasgow,
UK

Christopher J. Turnbull,
Consultant Geriatrician,
Wirral Hospitals NHS Trust,
Wirral,
UK

Mr T.R.K. Varma,
Consultant Neurosurgeon,
The Walton Centre for Neurology and Neurosurgery,
Liverpool,
UK

Liz Whelan,
Parkinson's Disease Specialist Nurse,
Bath & West Community NHS Trust,
UK

Foreword

I am honoured to have been asked to write the Foreword for *Parkinson's Disease in the Older Patient'*, which has been prepared by many healthcare professionals who specialize in the management of this chronic and debilitating neurological condition.

During the past three decades, several changes to society have had implications for people and their families living with Parkinson's disease which include:

- The change in the role of voluntary organizations highlighting the importance of listening to the needs of the customers.
- Demographic changes resulting in the increase in the number of elderly, frail people.
- The change in the roles of women within our society through education and career structure.
- The decrease in the availability of informal carers due to a falling birth rate and a change in family structure.
- The need to focus more sharply on the needs of the ageing population in order to meet appropriately the needs of the elderly, the customers.

Demographic changes mean that Parkinson's disease is set to become more common with the rise in the number of elderly, putting even more pressure on carers. There is an urgent need to focus more sharply on families affected by neurological disorders so that their needs can be met appropriately. People want to participate in the management of their illness.

We need to combine the knowledge and clinical observations of the healthcare professionals with the experiences of those people living with, and impacted by, chronic neurological illnesses on a daily basis. It is only then that it will be possible to achieve an integrated picture of the challenges of managing a chronic neurological illness such as Parkinson's disease.

Parkinson's Disease in the Older Patient concentrates upon the holistic care of people impacted by Parkinson's disease, and stresses the importance of improving standards of care which will improve participation in life.

On behalf of the Parkinson's Disease Society of the United Kingdom, I would like to thank all who have contributed their time and expertise in producing such a valuable resource.

Mary G. Baker, MBE
Chief Executive
Parkinson's Disease Society

Preface

Parkinson's disease (PD) is a chronic progressive neuropsychiatric disorder, which is the second most common cause of chronic neurological disability in the UK. Although PD does occur in younger people, it is predominantly a condition of the elderly.

It is increasingly recognized that PD is not simply a movement disorder, but is a multisystem neurological disorder which affects cognitive processes, emotion and autonomic function. The recent Global Parkinson's Disease Survey found that quality of life depended not only on the stage of disease and medication but also on the level of depression, satisfaction and optimism.[1] At the Sixth International Congress of Parkinson's Disease and Movement Disorders, held in Barcelona in June 2000, many presenters confirmed that the effects of treatment on quality of life are dependent upon factors other than the quality of movement. Depression, disability, postural instability and cognitive impairment have the greatest influence on quality of life in PD.[2] PD has a marked effect on quality of life at all stages of the disease, and at all ages. Impaired quality of life and carer strain increase with advancing disease and age, and parallel increasing costs.[3] The economic effects of PD vary according to the stage of the condition. The total costs of the condition increase with advancing age and advancing disease stage. In younger patients the greatest costs are for the drugs and loss of earnings, while in older patients the largest costs are social and long-term institutional care. These cost burdens fall on patients, carers, health and social care agencies.[4]

Neurological services have increasingly recognized the importance of interdisciplinary working in the management of PD. Interdisciplinary working has always been at the centre of the speciality of geriatric medicine, and the importance of the involvement of physiotherapists, occupational therapists, speech therapists and other disciplines in the management of PD is well recognized. The Cochrane Systematic review has, however, identified the requirement for more rigorous study of physiotherapy, occupational therapy and speech and language therapy in the treatment of PD.[5] The efficacy of the PD nurse specialist in moderate disease severity has been shown in one randomized trial,[6] and the role of these nurses in primary care is expanding.

In the UK there is a relatively small number of neurologists, but there is a large and well-developed geriatric service based on interdisciplinary teams. Geriatricians have always recognized the importance of cognition and depression in the management of many disorders, and this approach is now the focus of neurological practice in the management of PD. In the UK, the majority of patients with PD are cared for through geriatric PD services. Specialists in geriatric medicine have developed a large expertise in the management of

PD, focusing particularly on the needs of elderly patients. In this book we have brought together many of the leading experts in the management of PD in the elderly in the UK. The specialist expertise of the contributors to this book is widely recognized through participation at national and international conferences, and the publication of research on aspects of PD in the elderly. In this book we provide a unique insight into the management of elderly patients suffering from PD.

Acknowledgements

In bringing together this book we acknowledge the help and support of the British Geriatrics Society Special Interest Group in Parkinson's Disease and the Parkinson's Disease Society of the United Kingdom. We would like to thank Orion Pharma for an unrestricted educational grant and for the personal interest and drive of Steve Hughes and Steve Flatt who helped initiate the project. We are very grateful for the help and support given to us by the editorial and production staff at Arnold Publishers. We thank all the patients and staff at the Llandudno and Liverpool Parkinson's disease clinics for their help and encouragement. We thank especially our secretaries Mrs Pauline Doran and Mrs Christine Ellis for their patience. Finally we would like to thank our families for allowing us space and time, particularly our wives Dr Catherine Hindle and Mrs Elizabeth Playfer for their tolerance.

Dr J. V. Hindle, Dr J.R. Playfer
February 2001

References

1. The Global Parkinson's disease Survey – An insight into quality of life with Parkinson's disease. Available from: The Parkinson's Disease Society, 215 Vauxhall Bridge Road, London SW1V 1EJ, UK.
2. Schrag A, Jahanshahi M, Quinn N. What contributes to quality of life in patients with Parkinson's disease? *Movement Disord.* 2000; 15 (suppl. 3): 840.
3. Findley L, Pugner K, Holmes J, Baker M, MacMahon DG. The impact of Parkinson's disease on quality of life: results of a research survey in the UK. *Movement Disord.* 2000; 15 (suppl. 3): 862.
4. MacMahon DG, Findley L, Holmes J, Pugner K. The true economic impact of PD: a research survey in the UK. *Movement Disord.* 2000; 15 (suppl. 3): 861.
5. Deane KHO, Ellis-Hill ED, Playford Y, et al. Cochrane reviews of occupational therapy, speech and language therapy and physiotherapy for Parkinson's disease. *Movement Disord.* 2000; 15 (suppl. 3): 827-829.
6. Jarman B, Hurwitz B, Cook A. Parkinson's disease specialist nurses in primary care, a randomised controlled trial. *Movement Disord.* 2000; 15 (suppl. 3): 860.

Part 1: Background to Parkinson's disease

A history of Parkinson's disease

J.V. Hindle

Symptoms suggestive of Parkinson's disease have been described for many centuries, having been found in Egyptian papyrus and Sanskrit texts and other documents in ancient times. Parkinson's disease was first distinguished from other causes of tremor and weakness by Dr James Parkinson in his famous paper of 1817 entitled *An Essay on the Shaking Palsy*. In this, he defined the condition as 'involuntary tremulous motion, with lessened muscular power, in parts not in action and even when supported; with a propensity to bend the trunk forwards, and to pass from a walking to a running pace: the senses and intellect being uninjured'.[1]

The influence of Galen

It is difficult to understand this contribution by James Parkinson and the subsequent evolution of his ideas without awareness of the concepts of neurological disorder used at the time. Parkinson called his disease the shaking palsy, or paralysis agitans, and at that time the use of the term palsy or paralysis was very wide, and included the loss of motion and sensation.[2] In his treatise, Parkinson concentrated mainly on the tremor and gait disturbance, because the concepts of rigidity and akinesia had not yet been defined. Parkinson's understanding of tremor was based on the developments of the concepts of Galen. These concepts were the most important influences on the development of ideas on tremor over a period of more than 1500 years. Galen of Pergamum was a Greek physician who founded experimental physiology and was one of the most distinguished physicians of antiquity. Galen's influence on medical theory and practice was dominant in Europe throughout the middle ages, and particularly during the renaissance. Galen learned much of his practical knowledge of medicine through the medical school attached to the shrine of the healing god Asclepius. Here he was also attached as chief physician to the Gladiators, and gained practical knowledge of anatomy and tested remedies for treating wounds. Galen became particularly renowned as a physician in Rome where he treated the Co-Emperor and the heir to the throne.[3] Between AD 169 and 180, Galen wrote a short text, 'De Tremore' in which he distinguished *voluntary* motion (due to impulse and mediated by nerves and muscles) from *vital* motion (activated through arteries and the heart). Galen described tremor as occurring on intended motions and caused by weakness of the force that supports and moves the body. Shaking at rest was described as palpitation, and was thought to be due to unnatural expansion and collapse of heart and arteries.[4]

The theories of Galen were refined through the sixteenth to eighteenth centuries, particularly by Dutch physicians. The term palpitation gradually came to be applied to pathology of the heart and arterial pulsations. The distinction between action and rest tremor was further clarified, notably through the writings of the German chemist and physician Junker (1679–1759), the French physician Boissier De La Croix Sauvages (1706–1767) and the Dutch physicians Sylvius de la Boe (1614–1672) and Van Swieten (1700–1772).[4] In his essay, Parkinson refers to Junker and Sylvius De Le Boe, and reviews the previous definitions of tremor.[5] James Parkinson complained that 'tremor has been adopted, as a genus, by almost every nosologist; but always unmarked, in their definitions, by such characters as would embrace this disease'.[1] He then went on to describe the natural history of the tremor of his own disease. It is unclear whether Parkinson had read the Latin texts by these previous authors prior to collecting his case histories, or whether he came across them in his search for literature after his interest was aroused by a stimulus closer to home.

James Parkinson

James Parkinson was born in 1755 as a son of a physician in Hoxton, a suburb in the Shoreditch area of London. Following the death of his father in 1784, James Parkinson took over the practice at Hoxton Square. He became a distinguished physician and the first recipient of the honorary gold medal of the Royal College of Surgeons in 1822. He was also a very committed family man, was married in 1781, and had six children.[1,6,7]

James Parkinson was a man of eclectic interests. By the age of 25 he was well established as a formidable political writer and a prominent member of the London Corresponding Society. He published, under the *nom de plume* of 'Old Hubert', many pamphlets promoting the reform of the House of

Commons and universal suffrage. He wrote on the iniquities of taxation, child abuse, the elderly, the lot of lunatics, and many other matters. His political writings ceased suddenly in 1794, probably following a subpoena to give evidence to a special court of inquiry in which he was cross-examined by William Pitt the younger, who was then Prime Minister. By that time he had also produced many medical texts, including a report of the first case of appendicitis found in English medical literature and an influential book on medical education entitled *The Hospital Pupil*. Following cessation of his political writings he took a great interest in chemistry and scientific palaeontology. He wrote several books on geology and was a founder member of the Geological Society.[1,6,7]

At the time of Parkinson's early medical career John Hunter was becoming established as an influential teacher at one of London's anatomy schools. He became famous for his anatomical dissection and as a lecturer attracted many students from around the British Isles. He held night courses, giving the prestigious Croonian lectures over a period of several years. At the age of 30 James Parkinson attended these lectures and took detailed notes, which were published posthumously in 1833, edited by his son. Much earlier, in 1776 at the age of 21, as an apprentice to his father who was an anatomical warden of the Surgeons Company, James Parkinson may have attended a lecture by John Hunter on muscular motion. In this Hunter described a case of Lord L, whose hands were 'almost perpetually in motion and he never feels the sensation in them of being tired. When he is asleep his hands are perfectly at rest; but when he wakes in a little time they begin to move'.[5] This condition sounds very much like Parkinson's disease. James Parkinson's famous essay was published in 1817 towards the end of his career, and presumably it must have taken him a long time to collect the six cases he presented. At this time neurology was a descriptive subject, and this is why Parkinson characterized the cases, even from a distance, but did not examine patients in detail. Some have suggested that it was John Hunter who inspired Parkinson to write his famous essay.[5] Parkinson's essay did break new ground and was extensively quoted. His conjecture that the illness was related to a diseased state of the higher cervical cord, extending into the medulla, was quite remarkable. Despite receiving many awards, mainly for palaeontology, the fellowship of the Royal Society still eluded James Parkinson by the time of his death in 1824.[6]

Parkinsonism: clinical features

Unfortunately, over the next 45 years, Parkinson's treatise on the shaking palsy received little attention in England. During this period, however, Wilhelm Von Humboldt, in his letters from 1828 until his death in 1835, gave one of the clearest clinical descriptions of the condition by a patient. He described a resting tremor, akinesia, and was the first to describe micrographia. He called the problems in writing a 'special clumsiness', which he attributed to a disturbance in executing rapid complex movements. He described 'internal tremor not visible by others, which causes a distortion of the continuity of my movements'. He insisted that he was not suffering from a disease, but the effects of accelerated aging.[9]

It was not until the 1860s that Parkinson's treatise really came to light, when the French neurologists Trousseau and then Charcot and Vulpian, working at the Salpetriere in Paris, further elucidated the clinical features of the condition.[8] Trousseau described the use of the term paralysis agitans as inappropriate since 'there is no paralysis at the commencement of this strange form of chorea'. He confirmed the absence of weakness, described rigidity and proposed explanations for the festinant gait. His description of the condition as 'a strange form of chorea' was however wide of the mark.[10] It was Charcot's descriptions which first allowed physicians really to differentiate Parkinson's disease from other neurological disorders. Whilst acknowledging James Parkinson's original description, it is impossible to overestimate Jean-Martin Charcot's contribution to further clarifying the nature of Parkinson's disease. Charcot had difficulty acquiring a copy of Parkinson's *Essay on the Shaking Palsy*, and had his students translate it into French. Charcot referred to Parkinson's essay and stated that 'this is a descriptive and vivid definition that is correct for many cases, most in fact, and will always have the advantage over others of having been the first, but it errs by being too general'. Charcot described tremor by the frequency of movement and action associated with the tremors' greatest intensity, much as in modern neurology. He undertook many famous experiments in his lecture theatre, including one to prove that the head tremor in Parkinson's was only secondary to limb and trunk tremor, in which he tied feathers on rods to patients' heads. He clarified the observation that movement, or support, diminishes limb tremor, clearly demonstrating that he realized the importance of movement in the control of Parkinsonian tremor. He also described abnormalities of bradykinesia, stance, posture and gait. Parkinson did not describe rigidity, but Charcot identified it as an important sign and differentiated it from spasticity. This emphasis on the absence of pyramidal weakness was an important advance. Charcot discarded the term 'shaking palsy', realising that there was no paralysis involved, and generously coined the term 'Parkinson's disease'.[11] Paul Richer, who was a student of Charcot's and later the head of the laboratory at the Salpetriere, drew many famous pictures of Charcot's cases (see Figure 1.1). He later became the Professor of Creative Anatomy at the school of fine arts, and it is through his work that we can clearly see the accuracy of Charcot's clinical descriptions.[10]

Psychological symptoms

Psychological symptoms were described by Charcot and British neurologists, but were thought not to be an integral part of the disorder (see Chapter 8). Benjamin Ball, the first Professor of the new speciality of psychiatry, in Paris, compared the mental slowing in Parkinson's disease to melancholic depression. He stated in 1882 that, 'The psychiatric complication takes the form of

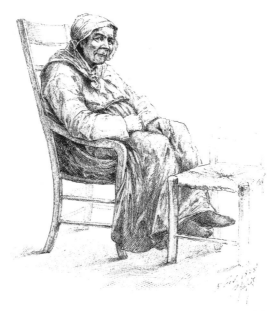

Fig. 1.1 'Maladie de Parkinson' by Paul Richer. Illustration © AP-HP/Phototheque, reproduced with permission.

depression ... accompanied by suicidal behaviour, hallucinations and stupor'.[2] Psychiatric phenomena were, however, not accepted as a part of the disorder until the early twentieth century.

Parkinsonism and neurotransmission

The cause of Parkinson's disease was still unclear, but another student of Charcots', Edouard Brissaud, favoured the 'locus niger' as a site for the condition, based on cases in the literature and other pathological findings. In 1912 Frederick H. Lewy described inclusion bodies in the cells of the striatum and globus pallidus. A world-wide epidemic began in 1916, with some people being struck down by an illness that resembled Parkinson's disease. Constantine Von Economo, who named the disease encephalitis lethargica, recognized this condition to be caused by a virus. In 1919, Tretiakoff further confirmed abnormalities of the substantia nigra by demonstrating inflammatory lesions in encephalitis lethargica. Despite this momentous finding a hundred years after the original description, the site of Parkinson's disease was not universally accepted.[2,12]

The father of British neurology, William Gowers, working in London in 1888 published his standard text of neurology, *A Manual of Diseases of the Nervous System*. He described the symptoms of Parkinson's disease and recommended some interventions, including rest and avoidance of stress. He also recommended the use of morphia and Indian hemp, which helped the symptoms for quite a while, though it was unclear at the time why these chemicals helped.[2,12] Around the same time, in 1887, the Spanish scientist Cajal, carrying on from the work of the Italian scientist Golgi, developed a theory of interconnections between nerves cells functioning across minute spaces, which he later called synapses. Much later, in 1920, a married couple of German pioneers Cecile and Oscar Vogt, proposed a theory of chemical connections between the striatum and other parts of the brain. In the 1930s, the German pharmacologist Otto Loewi linked these theories by developing a theory of neurotransmission, and this was supported by the British physiologist and pharmacologist Henry Dale, who observed that acetycholine produced responses in the parasymphathetic nervous system.[12]

Pharmacotherapy: dopa and levodopa

In 1912, Funk discovered dihydroxyphenylalanine (dopa) while synthesizing adrenaline. Over many years the full chain of reactions and formation of adrenaline from tyrosine, dopa, dopamine and noradrenaline was elucidated. Hornykiewicz, working in Vienna in 1959, discovered the importance of dopamine in the basal ganglia, and described a lack of dopamine in the striatum. Working with another Viennese doctor, Walther Birkmayer, Hornykiewicz began a series of investigations into the clinical use of levodopa as a medication for parkinsonism. Together, they realized the importance of levodopa as a precursor to dopamine, and also ascertained the need for the administration of this precursor in order to penetrate through the blood–brain barrier into the brain. In 1961, they described the stunning effects of intravenous administration of levodopa on parkinsonian patients, producing a complete abolition of akinesia. Bedridden patients who were previously unable to sit up could suddenly perform all activities with ease. Difficulties were experienced in establishing correct dosage regimes. Eventually Dr George S. Cotzias, a senior scientist in Brookhaven Laboratory, in the USA, opted for gradually increasing dosages, after acclimatization, to avoid nausea and other side effects. After reporting, in 1968, moderate to dramatic results of 26 patients, Dr Cotzias was snowed under with appeals for help.[12]

Following publication of the efficacy of levodopa, Dr Oliver Sacks, who was a staff physician at Mount Carmel Hospital in New York, utilized this drug in the treatment of patients with encephalitis lethargica, and in his book *Awakenings*, he tells the moving story of the results of treatment.[13] With increasing use of levodopa it soon became clear that the effects of treatment were not long-lasting, and problems of abnormal involuntary movements developed. Strategies to combat these difficulties included development of drugs to block the breakdown of levodopa in the blood and the use of Benserazide and Carbidopa combined with levodopa. Subsequent developments have tried to improve on the 'gold standard' effect of levodopa and to minimize the consequence of long-term levodopa treatment.

Neurosurgery

In parallel to all the development in drug therapy, there was increasing interest in functional neurosurgery for Parkinson's disease. The first approach was open functional surgery, which included lesioning of the cortical spinal tracts and transventricular surgery of the basal ganglia, but these procedures were abandoned because of high mortality.[14]

In 1888, Dr Robert H. Clark, who was a graduate from Cambridge and studied medicine at St George's Hospital, and Victor Horsley from the University College in London, developed pioneering aseptic procedures and a stereotactic apparatus for investigation of cat cerebellum. This apparatus enabled a small probe to reach with absolute precision, by the shortest path, predetermined points within the cranium.[12] Much later in 1947, Wycis and Spiegel developed a stereotactic apparatus based on Clarke's earlier machine. They used their stereo-encephalotome to produce lesions by electrodes. It became clear that most effective lesions for the treatment of Parkinson's disease symptoms were in the thalamus and globus pallidus portion of the basal ganglia. These were replaced at the end of the 1950s by lesions in the venterolateral thalamus. A few surgeons had pioneered lesions of the subthalamic area, with favourable results, and by 1969 the results of more than 37 000 stereotactic operations had been published. Clear criteria for techniques and selection were described, and stereotactic atlases were published. At this time, levodopa became generally available and stereotactic operations declined dramatically. As a result of the shortcomings of levodopa therapy in long-term treatment, thalamotomy gradually regained its place with the reintroduction of pallidotomy by Laitinen in 1992, and then thalamic stimulation for pharmacotherapy resistant tremor by Benabid and collaborators in 1991.[14]

Modelling the condition

In conjunction with the advances in the drug and surgical treatment of Parkinson's disease, there were major developments in modelling of the functions of the basal ganglia. Hughlings Jackson in 1868, claimed that instability of activities of the striatum led to choreoform, or overactive, movements. Theories of the interaction between the basal ganglia and production of movement disorders were further developed by many workers, including Ramsay Hunt in the 1920-30s and Denny Brown in the 1960-70s. These led to the theory of the striatum being a clearing-house for the neurological mechanisms of voluntary movements. It became clear that the basal ganglia have an important role in control of posture and locomotion, and a major role in cognition. The single most important development in the study of models of Parkinson's disease, was the discovery that methyl-phenyl-tetrahydro-pyridine (MPTP), was a specific neurotoxin for the basal ganglia. This substance was produced as a by-product of manufacture of illegal 'designer' drugs, and led to the presentation of typical parkinsonism in drug abusers.[15]

This discovery led to the ability to model Parkinson's disease in animals and study movement and cognition and the effects of treatment.[15]

From the historical perspective, it is clear that much of the understanding of tremor and movement up until the nineteenth century was based on modifications of Galenic theory. James Parkinson's classical observation that his condition did not fit with this previous framework, followed by the amphitheatre teaching sessions at the Salpetriere Hospital under Charcot's direction, together laid the foundations of our modern clinical understanding of the entity of Parkinson's disease.

References

1. Parkinson J. *An Essay on the Shaking Palsy.* First published London: Sherwood, Neely and Jones, 1817. Modern edition: London: Macmillan Magazines and Parkinson's Disease Society of the United Kingdom, 1992.
2. Berrios GE. *The History of Mental Symptoms – Descriptive Psycho-pathology since the 19th Century.* Cambridge: Cambridge University Press, 1996.
3. *The New Encyclopedia Britannica.* 15th edition. Micropaedia, vol. 5. Chicago, Encyclopaedia Britannica inc., 1988.
4. Koehler PJ, Keyser A. Historical review of tremor in Latin texts of Dutch physicians: 16th to 18th centuries. *Movement Disord.* 1997; **12**(5):798–806.
5. Curier RD. Did John Hunter give James Parkinson an idea? *Arch. Neurol.* 1996; **53**: 377–8.
6. Jefferson M. James Parkinson 1775–1824. *Br. Med. J.* 1973; **2**(866): 601–3.
7. Yahr MD. A physician for all seasons. James Parkinson 1755–1824. *Arch. Neurol.* 1978; **35**(4): 185–8.
8. Louis ED. The shaking Palsy, the first 45 years: a journey through the British literature. *Movement Disord.* 1997; **12**(6): 1068–72.
9. Horowski R, Horowski L, Vogel S, Poewe W, Kielhorn F W. An essay on Wilhelm Von Humboldt and the shaking palsy; first comprehensive description of Parkinson's disease by a patient. *Neurology* 1995; **45**: 565–8.
10. Tyler KL. A history of Parkinson's disease. In: Koller WC (ed.). *Handbook of Parkinson's Disease.* New York: Marcel Dekker, 1987.
11. Goetz C G. Charcot on Parkinson's Disease. *Movement Disord.* 1986; **1**(1): 27–32.
12. Dauphin S. *Parkinson's Disease: The Search and the Promise.* Florida: Pixel Press, 1992.
13. Sacks O. *Awakenings.* New York: Doubleday & Company, 1974.
14. Speelman JD, Bosch DA. Resurgence of functional neurosurgery for Parkinson's disease: a historical perspective. *Movement Disord.* 1998; **13**(3): 582–8.
15. Tetrud JW, Langston W. MPTP-induced parkinsonism as a model for Parkinson's disease. *Acta Neurol. Scand.* 1989; **126**: 35–40.

Pathology, aetiology and pathogenesis

D.A. Stewart

Introduction

Despite intensive research activity over many years, the cause of Parkinson's disease (PD) remains unknown. Major advances have been made, however, in our understanding of the mechanisms involved in neural degeneration, in neurotransmitter biology, and in the role of genetic factors. It has been suggested that different presentation and progression of disease in young-onset and elderly patients might indicate that these are different conditions. Apart from the possibility that genetic factors might be of more relevance in young-onset patients, there is no evidence to suggest that the underlying pathology and pathophysiology differ with age of presentation. This chapter is a review of the current state of our knowledge of the pathology, pathophysiology and aetiology of PD as it relates to our understanding of the clinical presentation and management of the condition.

Neurochemistry

Depletion of the neurotransmitter dopamine is the main neurochemical abnormality in PD. Other neurotransmitters affected include noradrenaline, serotonin and acetylcholine, but the role of these substances is uncertain.

Almost 80 per cent of brain dopamine is found in the striatonigral complex comprising the putamen, caudate and substantia nigra pars compacta (SNc). The SNc is the principal source of dopaminergic neurones. These project mainly to the putamen and caudate.[1] The extent of dopamine depletion in these structures correlates with neuronal loss in the SNc. In PD dopamine depletion is more evident in the putamen than caudate.[2]

In the brain, dopamine is synthesized from the amino acid tyrosine. The first step is conversion of tyrosine to L-3,4-dihydroxyphenylalanine (L-dopa, levodopa), catalysed by the enzyme tyrosine hydroxylase. This is the rate-limiting step in dopamine production. Levels of tyrosine hydroxylase are low in PD, which explains why tyrosine is ineffective as therapy. Levodopa is converted to dopamine by dopa decarboxylase (aromatic amine decarboxylase), and the dopamine is stored in vesicles and released by a calcium-dependent mechanism. After release, dopamine is removed from the synaptic cleft by an active re-uptake mechanism, following which it is available again for vesicular storage. Dopamine is metabolized enzymatically by both intracellular monoamine oxidase (principally MAO-B) and extracellular catechol-O-methyl transferase (COMT).[3] Homovanillic acid is the main metabolite.

Dopamine receptors

Two families of dopamine receptor have been identified: the D1 family which includes D1 and D5 receptors, and the D2 family which includes D2, D3 and D4 receptors. After binding to D1 type receptors dopamine acts via an increase in cyclic AMP, whereas the effect on D2 type receptors is to decrease cyclic AMP.[4] D2 receptors are thought to be important mediators of the therapeutic effects of pharmacological agents, while the role of D1 receptors is less clear.

Physiology of basal ganglia motor control

The defect in PD causes disruption to the dopaminergic nigrostriatal projections and interferes with function of the motor circuit of the basal ganglia. This circuit is involved in the control of both voluntary and involuntary movements. The function of the motor circuit is very complicated, and several subcircuits which interact in a complex manner (and are still poorly understood) are involved.[5] These include the interaction between the globus pallidus externa (GPe) and the subthalamic nucleus (STN), which is thought to be of particular importance. The following is a simplified version of current understanding of how motor activity is influenced by this circuit and how this function is altered in PD.

The key to understanding the function of the basal ganglia in controlling movement is the appreciation of the roles of the globus pallidus interna (GPi) and the venterolateral thalamus (VL). The VL has an excitatory output to the motor cortex and thus facilitates movement. The GPi, along with the substantia nigra pars reticulata (SNr), has an inhibitory output to VL and therefore acts as a 'brake'. This means that the effect of increased output from the GPi/SNr is to inhibit movement.

GPi receives input from the putamen via two pathways – direct and indirect. The direct pathway runs monosynaptically from putamen to GPi and its effects are inhibitory, i.e. to release the brake on movement exerted by GPi. The indirect pathway runs from the putamen via GPe and STN. STN has an excitatory effect on GPi, mediated by glutamate.[6] The effect of the indirect pathway is therefore to increase the braking on movement from GPi.

Normal dopamine release from the SNc acts on both these pathways, direct and indirect. By acting on dopamine D1 receptors, the direct pathway is stimulated to decrease the braking effect on movement from GPi. By acting on dopamine D2 receptors, the indirect pathway is inhibited, decreasing the stimulus for GPi to exert a braking effect.[7] Normal SNc function therefore results in a low braking effect from GPi to VL and thus allows VL to facilitate movement via its excitatory effects on the motor cortex.

In PD, decreased dopamine release from SNc disrupts this mechanism. Understimulation of the direct pathway and underinhibition of the indirect pathway result in an increased inhibitory ('braking') output from GPi to VL. Thus, the excitatory effects of VL on the motor cortex are diminished and movement inhibited (Fig. 2.1). The important consequences of abnormal increased activity of GPi and STN on motor function are the reason these areas are important target sites for neurosurgery whether by ablation or high-frequency stimulation.

Pathology

The pathological changes of PD include cell loss in a specific distribution, the presence of Lewy bodies in surviving cells, and an undamaged striatum (comprising putamen and caudate).

CELL LOSS

The main area of cell loss is in the substantia nigra (SN), although cell loss also occurs outwith the SN in a widespread but specific pattern. Other areas affected include the noradrenergic locus coeruleus, the thalamus, the hypothalamus, the cholinergic nucleus basilis of Meynert, dopaminergic neurones of the ventral tegmentum, the serotonergic raphe nuclei, the limbic cortex and cerebral neocortex, and the autonomic nervous system (including sympathetic and parasympathetic ganglia and the myenteric plexus in the walls of the oesophagus and colon).[8,9]

The SN is divided into the pars reticulata and the pars compacta (SNc), the latter portion being affected predominantly. Cell loss in excess of 50 per cent of normal levels is required for clinical symptoms to develop.[10] The SNc can be further subdivided into ventral and dorsal tiers. Cells in the dorsal

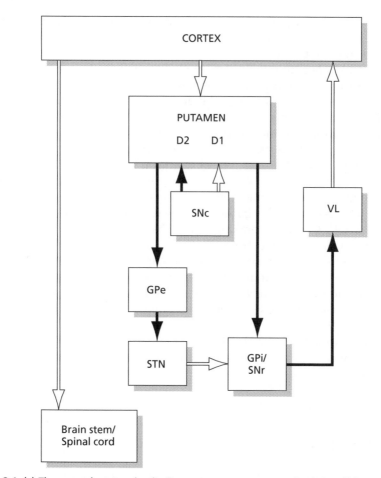

Fig. 2.1 (a) The normal motor circuit. Open arrows represent excitation; solid arrows indicate inhibition. Key: SNc = substantia nigra pars compacta; GPe = globus pallidus externa; STN = subthalamic nucleus; GPi = globus pallidus interna; SNr = substantia nigra pars reticulata; VL = venterolateral thalamus.

tier contain more neuromelanin compared with the ventral tier. Neuromelanin is derived from the auto-oxidation of dopamine and accumulates throughout life. The increase in neuromelanin in the dorsal tier probably represents more active dopamine turnover compared with the paler ventral cells.[11]

Cell loss in the SNc in PD preferentially affects the ventral tier.[12] By death, about 23 per cent of cells in the SNc remain compared with normal, but the surviving cells are mainly in the dorsal tier.[9] This is in contrast with normal ageing where the dorsal tier is mainly affected, the SNc showing an approximately 5 per cent neuronal loss per decade after the age of 40 years. The loss is greater in the dorsal tier by a ratio of over 3:1.[10] This is evidence that PD is not simply an exaggeration of the ageing process.

The pathological changes seen in PD are more active that those seen in ageing. An increase is seen in neuronal fragmentation, extraneuronal melanin

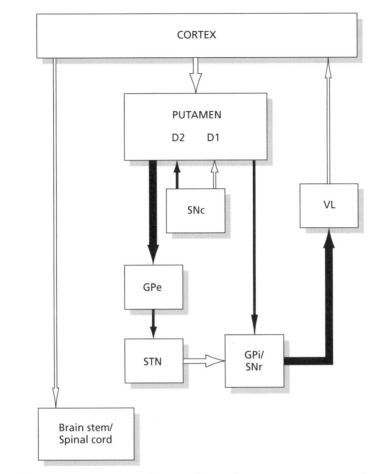

Fig. 2.1 (b) The motor circuit in Parkinson's disease. Open arrows represent excitation; solid arrows indicate inhibition. Key: SNc = substantia nigra pars compacta; GPe = globus pallidus externa; STN = subthalamic nucleus; GPi = globus pallidus interna; SNr = substantia nigra pars reticulata; VL = venterolateral thalamus.

and gliosis over and above that seen age in age-matched controls. Six times as many neurones are being actively phagocytosed compared with controls.[13]

The functional consequence of nigral cell loss is the loss of normal nigros-triatal innervation and the clinical features of PD. As much as 80 per cent of dopamine may be lost in the striatum by the time that clinical symptoms emerge. By death, dopamine levels are reduced to 2 per cent of normal in the putamen, and to 16 per cent of normal in the caudate.[9]

The consequences of cell death in other affected areas are less well under-stood. It is thought that damage in the cerebral cortex, nucleus basilis of Meynert, and the ventral tegmentum is associated with cognitive dysfunction. Although damage to the autonomic system can be linked to clinical features of autonomic failure, other factors (including antiparkinsonian medication) are relevant. The consequence of damage in other areas including the thalamus, locus coeruleus and raphe nuclei is unknown.

Despite the consequences of abnormal innervation from the SN, it is likely that no cell loss occurs in the striatum. This is in contrast to the marked striatal degeneration seen in other conditions such as multiple system atrophy (striatonigral degeneration), progressive supranuclear palsy, corticobasal degeneration and Huntington's disease.[14]

Lewy bodies

Lewy bodies are neuronal inclusions found in PD, and occur in all areas of neuronal degeneration, including the cortex. They consist of a central core which stains densely with haemotoxylin and eosin. This is surrounded by an area staining less densely, and a peripheral halo staining lightly or not at all.[8] Lewy bodies contain neurofilament proteins along with several other proteins involved in proteolysis, including ubiquitin and proteases.[15] Other constituents include tubulin and α-synuclein.[16] It has been suggested that the function of Lewy bodies is to eliminate damaged proteins from cells as part of a protective response to stress.[17] It is not known whether this is ever successful, or whether the presence of a Lewy body indicates that the cell is doomed.

Lewy bodies are not unique to PD; other conditions in which they may be seen in degenerating neurones include corticobasal degeneration, progressive supranuclear palsy, motor neurone disease, ataxia telangectasia and Hallevorden-Spatz disease.[18] Parkinson's disease, however, is the only condition in which Lewy bodies are invariably found, their occurrence being identified in only a proportion of these other conditions.

Another cellular inclusion – the 'pale body' – is frequently (but not always) found in PD. These consist of round, vacuolated granular areas within cell bodies.[19] They also stain positively for ubiquitin and neurofilament proteins, and it has been suggested that they are a precursor to the Lewy body. Pale bodies have been described only in PD.[14]

Incidental Lewy body disease

Lewy bodies and neuronal loss in the characteristic pattern of that found in PD can be demonstrated at post-mortem examination in subjects with no clinical evidence of PD during life. This condition has been termed incidental Lewy body disease (ILBD), the prevalence being ~1 per cent of the non-parkinsonian population dying in their fifth decade, rising to 10 per cent of those dying in their eighth decade.[18] Cell loss is found in the ventral tier of the SNc to a degree intermediate between that found in PD and in normal ageing. As well as typical pathology, ILBD shows low levels of reduced glutathione in the substantia nigra, indicating oxidative stress (see Pathophysiology, p. 23). These findings are not a feature of normal ageing, and ILBD is therefore regarded as preclinical PD.

Rate of progression of PD

There is no evidence to suggest that the rate of progression of PD is affected by age of onset.[8] The fact that 50–60 per cent of pigmented nigral cells are lost at the onset of symptoms, yet this decreases to only 20 per cent of normal after a disease duration of 25 years, suggests that cell loss is slow.[10] A 1 per cent prevalence of ILBD at ages 50–59 years corresponds to a 1 per cent prevalence of PD at ages 80–89, suggesting that there is a 30-year delay before symptoms emerge.[18] Other evidence, however, from serial positron emission tomography (PET) scans[20] and from post-mortem cell counts in different disease durations have suggested a shorter preclinical phase of 5–10 years.[10]

Overlap pathologies

Parkinson's disease shares some clinical and pathological features with a number of other neurodegenerative conditions, in particular dementia with Lewy bodies (DLB) and Alzheimer's disease (AD). The precise relationship between these conditions is unclear and remains controversial.

DLB is the preferred term for a condition previously described as Lewy body dementia, the Lewy body variant of AD, senile dementia of Lewy body type or diffuse Lewy body disease.[21] The range of nomenclature reflects different interpretations depending on the range of clinical and pathological findings in cases studied. The condition is thought by some to be the second most common cause of dementia after AD.[15] Pathologically, DLB is characterized by the presence of cortical Lewy bodies; these are less well-defined and differ from those seen in subcortical regions.[17] Lewy bodies are also seen in subcortical structures, including the substantia nigra. These subcortical changes are identical to those found in PD, but can be mild. Most cases of DLB also have pathology which overlaps that of AD including plaques and neurofibrillary tangles.[22] There are however some differences in morphology and distribution of these features compared with AD. It is also the case that patients with PD who are cognitively intact invariably have a number of cortical Lewy bodies. These can be of a number and distribution which overlaps that seen in DLB.[15]

There is also evidence of some overlap between PD and AD. Dementia is common in PD, occurring in one-quarter to one-third of patients.[23,24] Likewise, parkinsonism – principally bradykinesia and rigidity – is common in AD, again with rates of 33 per cent and more being reported.[25] It is possible that these figures are an underestimate due to poor recognition of cognitive deficit by movement disorders specialists and of extrapyramidal features by psychiatrists. In both these conditions there is a progressive loss of specific neurones and the occurrence of intraneuronal inclusions. Plaques and neurofibrillary tangles are found in the brains of PD patients at post-mortem examination up to six times more frequently than in controls, and in all cases of PD with severe dementia.[26,27] Conversely, between 20 per cent and 40 per cent of AD patients show changes in the substantia nigra at post-mortem, consistent with a diagnosis of PD.[28,29] Cases of clinically typical, levodopa-responsive PD have been described showing neurofibrillary tangles in the substantia nigra, but no Lewy bodies.[30]

There is therefore considerable pathological overlap between these conditions, including the presence of Lewy bodies, plaques and neurofibrillary tangles. It has been suggested that there is a spectrum of Lewy body disorders, with PD at one extreme and DLB at the other. Some have gone further, suggesting a broader spectrum of disease ranging from PD to AD with DLB as an intermediate condition.[22] Other possible interpretations are that these are distinct conditions sharing final common pathological pathways or that the coincidence of pathology represents common genetic risk factors for these conditions.

Aetiology

A major problem in defining aetiological factors in PD is the presence of a large amount of preclinical disease. The overall age-adjusted prevalence of ILBD is 5.6 per cent compared with a typical prevalence of clinical PD of 0.2 per cent.[31] ILBD is therefore many times more common than clinical disease. Most individuals with ILBD will never go on to manifest clinical PD, perhaps because they do not live long enough for this to become apparent.[18] It has been postulated that clinical PD represents the youngest 5–10 per cent of a virtual bell-shaped distribution curve of incidence that has a maximum at an age approaching 175 years.[31] Thus, only a small percentage of individuals with PD pathology are open to study in a search for aetiological factors. Furthermore, there might be important differences in these subjects with respect to risk factors compared with the majority with ILBD.

Ageing

Advancing age is the single most important risk factor for developing PD. Prevalence rates for PD in epidemiological studies typically show an exponential increase from 1 per 1000 in the general population to as much as 2 per cent in those over 80 years of age.[32] It is difficult to define what 'normal' ageing of the central nervous system (CNS) is. It is unclear to what extent the changes seen are physiological or represent the accumulated effects of pathological processes. Nonetheless, a number of changes are recognized to occur with ageing. These include a decrease in the numbers of pigmented neurones in the substantia nigra,[33] a decrease in striatal dopamine,[34] a decrease in striatal tyrosine hydroxylase (involved in dopamine synthesis),[35] and a decrease in dopamine receptor density.[36] As previously discussed, however, the distribution of neuronal loss within the substantia nigra is different from that seen in PD. The exact role of ageing in pathogenesis is not clear, but it does not appear that PD is caused by an exaggeration of normal ageing processes. It is likely that age-related changes combine with other pathological mechanisms to produce the clinical syndrome.[37]

Genetics

Genetic studies are difficult to carry out in PD. Evidence for a genetic role in the aetiology of PD has come from a number of sources including twin, family, case-control and epidemiological studies. Each has its problems, mainly due to the absence of a good marker for the condition and the subsequent difficulty in case ascertainment.

Genetic disease can be either single gene and Mendelian or due to a complex interaction of multiple genes in a non-Mendelian manner. The latter almost certainly accounts for the majority of genetic influence on PD, but a number of major advances have taken place in recent years in describing the role of single gene defects in causing familial PD.

FAMILY STUDIES

Most patients with PD do not have a family history, and it is highly likely that non-genetic factors are important in aetiology. Nonetheless, family history is the next most important risk factor for PD after age. A positive family history can be obtained in 20–30 per cent of patients with PD.[38] This rises to a positive history in 43 per cent versus 9 per cent of controls if a history of tremor alone is included.[39] In case-control studies the relative risk for a first-degree relative of developing PD is around 3.5.[40] This evidence provides strong support for the role of genetic factors on the development of PD.

TWIN STUDIES

Early twin studies in PD failed to demonstrate a significantly increased concordance rate in monozygotic compared with dizygotic twins, and were interpreted as evidence that genetic factors were not relevant. The studies were potentially flawed due to the fact that PD could only be identified if it had become clinically apparent in a sibling and a failure to recognize atypical presentation, e.g. isolated tremor as a *forme fruste* of PD. Later, however, the use of PET scans has demonstrated abnormal flurodopa uptake in apparently unaffected siblings. Concordance rates of 45 per cent in monozygotic versus 29 per cent in dizygotic twins have been reported,[41] but the results were inconclusive. A recent study, again using flurodopa PET scanning to identify asymptomatic disease, has shown concordance rates rising to 75 per cent in monozygotic twins compared with 22 per cent in dizygotic twins over a seven-year follow-up period. Such evidence suggests a significant role for inheritance in the development of sporadic PD.[42]

EPIDEMIOLOGY

Epidemiological studies have shown that the prevalence of PD is not uniform throughout the world. A number of studies have shown that populations moving from a low prevalence area to one in which there is a higher prevalence of PD, gradually acquire the same prevalence as the 'host' country. For example, the prevalence of PD in Nigeria is much lower than among African-Americans in the USA, despite a fairly homogeneous genotype.[43] This is good evidence for an environmental factor in the causation of PD, but such studies must be interpreted with some caution. There are a number of possible sources of error. It is difficult to be sure of the true prevalence in the country of origin, particularly if it has poorly developed medical services. Cases of PD may not be reliably diagnosed, giving a falsely low prevalence. It is also possible that, in some cases, migrants are not typical of the population at large and do not share the same predilection to develop PD.

SINGLE GENE DEFECTS AS A CAUSE OF PD

In 1990, the pedigree of an Italian American family was described in which parkinsonism was inherited as an autosomal dominant condition.[44] Clinically, the disease was consistent with idiopathic PD, but there was a tendency for an earlier age of onset and a rather more aggressive course than usual. Post- mortem studies have confirmed the presence of typical pathology with Lewy bodies. Subsequent investigations showed that the problem lay in a mutation of the α-synuclein gene on chromosome 4.[45] The same mutation has subsequently been identified in three Greek families,[46] and a second mutation in a German family.[46] The biological role of α-synuclein is unknown; it is a protein found in the cell nuclei and nerve terminals (hence the name) of a wide range of species. It is known to be expressed in young birds while learning to sing, and it has therefore been suggested that it has role in neuronal plasticity.[47] It is interesting to note that Lewy bodies in idiopathic PD (without the α-synuclein mutation) stain more positively for α-synuclein than for ubiquitin.[16] α-Synuclein is now the best marker for Lewy bodies, but the role of the protein in pathogenesis is unknown. It has been postulated that the mutation results in an abnormality in folding of the protein, causing it to accumulate.[48]

Since the report of this gene mutation a number of groups have searched for its occurrence in kindred with familial PD. No other cases have been found in either a large European study of familial PD[49] or in a British study of sporadic PD,[50] and it is clear that the α-synuclein mutation is a very rare cause of PD.

More recently, another single gene defect causing parkinsonism has been described – the 'parkin' gene. Although clinically similar to idiopathic PD, Lewy bodies are not seen at post-mortem examination. This gene defect was first described by a group of Japanese workers as a cause of juvenile parkinsonism inherited as an autosomal recessive.[51] The gene has been found in a number of other kindred in Europe and elsewhere, and may be a relatively common cause of familial parkinsonism presenting before the age of 58.[52] The protein product of the parkin gene has a homology to ubiquitin and is present in brain and substantia nigra. The mechanism whereby loss of this protein relates to neurodegeneration is unknown.

Other single gene defects are under investigation, but an emerging pattern is of younger-onset disease than in sporadic PD.

'CANDIDATE' GENE STUDIES

The developments in describing single defects as a cause of PD have been exciting and valuable in providing clues to pathophysiology. These single gene defects, however, do not account for the majority of sporadic cases of PD since inheritance is likely to be determined by a number of genes interacting in a complex manner. Rather than search randomly in the genome for genes associated with PD, a more rapid approach may be to use our knowledge of the pathology and factors involved in pathophysiology of PD and to target genes known to have a biological action which might be relevant – so-called 'candidate' studies. Genes involved in dopamine metabolism, oxidation reactions and in detoxification have been examined. Results have been inconsistent and no clear linkage with PD has been demonstrated. Recently, it has been found that the slow acetylator genotype for N-acetyltransferase-2 is more common in familial PD.[53] This has prompted the hypothesis that there may be an impaired ability to handle neurotoxic substances.

Environmental factors

A great deal of effort has been made to identify environmental factors causing PD. Toxic substances have been found which cause a parkinsonian syndrome that is similar, but not identical, to idiopathic PD. A number of factors that appear to be associated with an increased risk of PD have also been described. Evidence for the important role of environmental factors comes for the USA Veteran Twin Study.[54] In this study the ratio of PD in monozygotic twins was 1.06 in those with disease onset greater than 50 years of age. This implies that genetic factors are unlikely to be important. In contrast, for those with disease onset under 50 years the ratio was 6.00 in favour of the monozygotic twin, implying a more important role for genetic factors. It is therefore likely that environmental factors are important in the development of PD and become more important with increasing age of disease onset. It is likely that the less 'genetic' the susceptibility to PD, the more age and environment need to contribute to the development of disease.[55]

SPECIFIC TOXINS

Manganese causes an akinetic rigid syndrome in man, predominantly due to a toxic effect on the globus pallidus and striatum. The mechanism of this toxic action is unknown. There are clear clinical differences, however, from PD.[56] Other metals (including copper and iron) have been shown to be increased in the substantia nigra, but this is probable a secondary phenomenon and not the primary cause of PD.[38] In survivors of poisoning, carbon monoxide causes parkinsonism to develop after a few days or weeks by necrosis of the globus pallidus.[57]

The discovery that the 'designer drug' contaminant 1-methyl-4-phenyl 1,2,3,6- tetrahydropyridine (MPTP) could cause an acute parkinsonian syndrome has proven to be an extremely valuable clue as to the pathogenesis of

PD.[58] A number of individuals who repeatedly injected themselves with this agent developed an akinetic rigid syndrome within days, the clinical syndrome being very similar to idiopathic PD. There is a response to levodopa and typical complications of therapy (including fluctuations and dyskinesias) develop.[59] Lewy body pathology is not seen, however, and the syndrome cannot therefore be regarded as identical to idiopathic disease. MPTP is a protoxin; it is converted to the toxic metabolite 1-methyl-4-phenylpyridium ion (MPP$^+$). This compound is actively taken up by the dopamine re-uptake system and concentrated in dopaminergic neurones. Once in the cells, MPP$^+$ interferes with mitochondrial function and thus cellular energy production. The specific site of action is Complex 1 of the mitochondrial respiratory chain. MPP$^+$ is also a generator of free radicals – another mechanism for neurotoxicity.[57] MPTP causes acute parkinsonism in other primates, and has permitted the development of animal models for PD.

The discovery of MPTP stimulated a search for other toxic substances in the environment as possible causes of idiopathic disease. High on the list of suspects have been pesticides and herbicides, particularly as MPP$^+$ is chemically related to paraquat, a previously commonly used herbicide. This hypothesis would fit well with a reported increase in PD in association with rural living (see below). Against this, however, is the fact that the prevalence of PD has not risen since the widespread introduction of these chemicals.[38]

OTHER RISK FACTORS

A number of studies have described a relationship between rural living and the development of PD.[60,61] The evidence is contradictory, however, with other studies showing no such association.[62] A number of factors have been suggested to explain this, including well-water drinking and exposure to agricultural chemicals.

The possibility that oxidative mechanisms are relevant for the pathogenesis of PD (see below) has prompted examination of dietary factors, and an association with increased animal fat consumption has been described.[63] The role of antioxidants including vitamins E and C have been examined for a potentially protective role, but no clear consensus has emerged. Vitamin E supplementation is likely to have no effect on the progression of PD.[64]

Cigarette smoking has been shown repeatedly to be associated with a decreased risk of developing PD,[38] with non-smokers having generally been shown to be twice as likely to develop the disease. This effect remains even after allowing for differences in mortality. Suggested mechanisms include the fact that nicotine causes dopamine release and up-regulation of dopamine receptors, potentially masking signs of early or mild disease. Cigarette smoke contains a monoamine oxidase B (MAO-B) inhibitor.[65] This might be relevant for a number of reasons: MAO-B inhibition decreases dopamine breakdown and could therefore boost levels in the brain. Reduced free radical production associated with this action on dopamine could also protect against oxidative stress. Finally, MPTP- induced parkinsonism may be ameliorated by MAO-B inhibition by preventing conversion to MPP$^+$.[66]

Not all studies have confirmed the protective effect of smoking. There is some doubt as to whether there is a true dose–response relationship; indeed, it has been suggested that the relationship may be the other way round, i.e. that PD might reduce smoking, perhaps due to psychological factors.[39]

Pathogenesis

Apoptosis

Whatever the cause or causes of PD, it is likely that nigral cell loss occurs via a common pathophysiological pathway, leading to apoptosis (programmed cell death). Cells can die either by necrosis or apoptosis. In necrosis, an external insult is responsible for death, whereas in apoptosis cell death occurs as a result of an intracellular process regulated by genes. Apoptosis is well documented as a normal physiological process in the development of the nervous system.[67] More recently, its pathological role in neurodegenerative disorders has been recognized. The identification of apoptosis depends on finding specific morphological changes, including chromatin clumping.[68] This is technically difficult and there some controversy remains over whether apoptosis is important in PD.[69,70] There is, however, a developing consensus that changes of apoptosis can be identified in the SNc at post-mortem examination. The number of apoptotic nuclei in the SNc in PD at 2 per cent is approximately 10-fold that seen in normal ageing.[55]

A number of processes interact to cause apoptotic cell death in the SNc in PD, including oxidative stress, mitochondrial dysfunction and excitotoxicity.

OXIDATIVE STRESS

The cells of the SNc are particularly vulnerable to oxidative damage due to the presence of dopamine, neuromelanin, and high levels of iron.[55,57] Dopamine undergoes oxidative deamination (mediated by monoamine oxidase); in addition, dopamine is prone to auto-oxidation. These processes yield metabolites including hydrogen peroxide. Neuromelanin binds ferric iron, and can reduce it to its reactive ferrous form – a process which facilitates the conversion of hydrogen peroxide to oxyradicals, including the highly toxic hydroxyl radical. Other products of dopamine auto-oxidation include the superoxide radical (Fig. 2.2).

Increased iron levels also occur in other neurodegenerative diseases including multiple system atrophy and progressive supranuclear palsy. These conditions are also associated with cell loss in the basal ganglia. Increased iron is not seen in ILBD; it is probable therefore that this is a secondary and late phenomenon. Nonetheless, it is might still be of importance as it could form part of the cascade leading to cell death.[57,71]

In normal cells there are a number of defence mechanisms to protect against oxidative damage, including the scavenger enzymes catalase and peroxidase. Important in this process is the presence of reduced glutathione

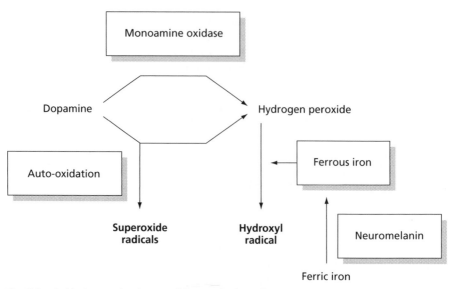

Fig. 2.2   Oxidative mechanisms and free radical production.

(GSH), levels of which have been shown to be low in the substantia nigra in PD, suggesting increased free radical generation. Low nigral glutathione levels are also found in ILBD but not in other parts of the brain or in other neurodegenerative diseases. It is possible therefore that this is an important mechanism early in the development of PD.[57,71]

There is direct evidence for oxidative damage in the substantia nigra in PD. Levels of malondialdehyde are increased, indicating increased lipid peroxidation.[72] In addition, 8-hydroxy-2-deoxyguanosine is increased, indicating oxidative damage to DNA.[73]

MITOCHONDRIAL DYSFUNCTION

Mitochondria play a crucial role in cellular energy production by generating ATP in the process of oxidative phosphorylation. The mitochondrial respiratory chain consists of five protein complexes. Complex 1 is deficient in the substantia nigra in PD by approximately 35 per cent.[57] The deficiency is specific to Complex 1, with other proteins in the respiratory chain being unaffected. The deficiency is also site- and disease-specific; other parts of the brain appear to be unaffected and the deficiency is not found in other degenerative diseases such as multiple system atrophy which show a similar nigral cell loss.[55] A modest (20–25 per cent) reduction in Complex 1 activity can also be demonstrated in the platelets of patients with PD,[74] though this is not sufficiently sensitive to be used as a biological marker for the condition.

It has been suggested recently that mitochondria may have a critical role in the sequence of events leading to apoptosis. A decrease in mitochondrial membrane potential and increased intramitochondrial calcium appear to be important early events in this process. These lead to the opening of a mito-chondrial pore and the release of apoptosis-initiating factors.[55]

Mitochondrial dysfunction and oxidative stress may interact to reinforce the toxic effects of each. It is postulated that Complex 1 deficiency is associated with superoxide ion generation, increasing oxidative stress. This in turn might worsen the Complex 1 defect in a vicious spiral of toxicity.[57]

EXCITOTOXICITY

The striatum contains widespread glutaminergic projections acting on N-methyl-D-aspartate (NMDA) receptors. Glutamate is an excitatory neuro-transmitter with the potential to cause cell damage via excitotoxicity. Glutaminergic stimulation is mediated by an influx of calcium ions into the cell. If excessive, this can cause toxicity via activation of a variety of enzyme systems.[75] Normally, excessive calcium influx is blocked by magne-sium ions within the receptor ion channel, this blockade being dependent on the ability of the cell to maintain a normal membrane electrical poten-tial. This in turn is dependent on mitochondrial ATP production. Thus, mitochondrial dysfunction in PD may lead to decreased magnesium block-ade and expose the nigral cells to excitotoxicity from excessive calcium influx.[76] In PD, physiological levels of glutamate stimulating the NMDA receptors might be toxic, further increasing mitochondrial damage and oxidative stress[55] (Fig. 2.3).

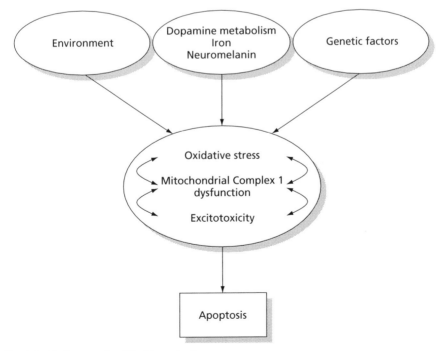

Fig. 2.3 Pathogenesis of Parkinson's disease.

Conclusion

Ageing is an important aetiological factor which interacts with a genetic predisposition, environmental factors and pathological processes to increase a persons liability to develop PD.

References

1. Graybiel AM, Hirsch EC, Agid Y. The nigrostriatal system in Parkinson's disease. *Adv. Neurol.* 1990; **53**: 17–29.
2. Agid Y, Cervera P, Hirsch E, *et al.* Biochemistry of Parkinson's disease 28 years later: a critical review. *Movement Disord.* 1989; **4**: 126–44.
3. Goldstein M, Lieberman A. The role of the regulatory enzymes of catecholamine synthesis in Parkinson's disease. *Neurology* 1992; **42**: 8–12.
4. Calne DB. Treatment of Parkinson's disease. *N. Engl. J. Med.* 1993; **329**: 1021–7.
5. Wichmann T. Physiology of the basal ganglia and pathophysiology of movement disorders of basal ganglia origin. In: Watts RL, Koller WC (eds). *Movement Disorders – Neurological Principles and Practice.* New York: McGraw-Hill, 1997; 87–97.
6. Greenberg DA. Glutamate and Parkinson's disease. *Ann. Neurol.* 1994; **35**: 639.
7. Gerfen CR, Engber TM, Mahan LC, *et al.* D1 and D2 dopamine receptor-regulated gene expression of striatonigral and striatopallidal neurons. *Science* 1990; **250**: 1429–32.
8. Gibb WRG, Lees AJ. Pathological clues to the cause of Parkinson's disease. In: Marsden CD, Fahn S (eds). *Movement Disorders.* Oxford: Butterworth-Heinemann, 1994; 147–66.
9. Gibb WRG. Functional neuropathology in Parkinson's disease. *Eur. Neurol.* 1997; **38**: 21–5.
10. Fearnley JM, Lees AJ. Aging and Parkinson's disease: substantia nigra regional selectivity. *Brain* 1991; **114**: 2283–301.
11. Gibb WRG. Neuropathology of the substantia nigra. *Eur. Neurol.* 1991; **31**: 48–59.
12. Gibb WRG, Lees AJ. Anatomy, pigmentation, ventral and dorsal subpopulations of the substantia nigra, and differential cell death in Parkinson's disease. *J. Neurol. Neurosurg. Psychiatry* 1991; **54**: 388–96.
13. McGeer PL, Itgaki S, Akiyama H, McGeer EG. Rate of cell death in parkinsonism indicates active neuropathological process. *Ann. Neurol.* 1988; **24**: 574–6.
14. Oertel WH, Hartmann A. The pathology of Parkinson's disease and its differentiation from other parkinsonian disorders. In: LeWitt PA, Oertel WH (eds). *Parkinson's Disease. The Treatment Options.* London: Martin Dunitz, 1999; 11–20.
15. Lennox GG, Lowe JS. Dementia with Lewy bodies. In: Quinn NP (ed.). *Bailliere's Clinical Neurology.* London: Bailliere Tindall, 1997; 147–66.
16. Spillantini MG, Crowther RA, Jakes R, Hasegawa M, Goedert M. alpha-Synuclein in filamentous inclusions of Lewy bodies and Lewy neurites from Parkinson's disease and dementia with Lewy bodies. *Proc. Natl Acad. Sci. USA* 1998; **95**: 6469–73.
17. Lowe JS. Lewy bodies. In: Calne DB (ed.). *Neurodegenerative Diseases.* Philadelphia: WB Saunders, 1994; 51–69.
18. Gibb WRG, Lees AJ. The relevance of the Lewy body to the pathogenesis of idiopathic Parkinson's disease. *J. Neurol. Neurosurg. Psychiatry* 1988; **51**: 745–52.
19. Gibb WRG, Scott T, Lees AJ. Neuronal inclusions of Parkinson's disease. *Movement Disord.* 1991; **6**: 2–11.

20. Morrish PK, Sawle GV, Brooks DJ. An [^{18}F]dopa-PET and clinical study of the rate of progression in Parkinson's disease. *Brain* 1996; **119**: 585–91.

21. McKeith IG, Galasko D, Kosaka K, *et al*. Consensus guidelines for the clinical and pathologic diagnosis of dementia with Lewy bodies (DLB): report of the consortium on DLB international workshop. *Neurology* 1996; **47**: 1113–24.

22. Perl DP, Olanow CW, Calne DB. Alzheimer's disease and Parkinson's disease; distinct entities or extremes of a spectrum of neurodegeneration? *Ann. Neurol.* 1998; **44**: S19–31

23. Aarsland D, Tandberg E, Larsen JP, Cummings JL. Frequency of dementia in Parkinson's disease. *Arch. Neurol.* 1996; **53**: 538–42.

24. Lieberman A, Dziatolowsky M, Kupersmith M, *et al*. Dementia in Parkinson disease. *Ann. Neurol.* 1979; **6**: 335–9.

25. Molsa PK, Martilla RJ, Rinne UK. Extrapyramidal signs in Alzheimer's disease. *Neurology* 1984; **34**: 1114–16.

26. Boller F, Mizutani T, Roessmann U, Gambetti P. Parkinson disease, dementia and Alzheimer disease: clinicopathological correlations. *Ann. Neurol.* 1980; **7**: 335.

27. Hakim AM, Mathieson G. Dementia in Parkinson disease: a neuropathologic study. *Neurology* 1979; **29**: 1209–14.

28. Hulette C, Mirra S, Wilkinson W, Heyman A, Fillenbaum G, Clark C. The consortium to establish a registry for Alzheimer's disease (CERAD). Part IX. A prospective cliniconeuropathologic study of Parkinson's features in Alzheimer's disease. *Neurology* 1995; **45**: 1991–5.

29. Leverenz J, Sumi SM. Parkinson's disease in patients with Alzheimer's disease. *Arch. Neurol.* 1986; **43**: 662–4.

30. Rajput AH, Uitti RJ, Sudhakar S, Rozdilsky B. Parkinsonism and neurofibrillary tangle pathology in pigmented nuclei. *Ann. Neurol.* 1989; **25**: 602–6.

31. Golbe LI. The epidemiology of Parkinson's disease. In: LeWitt PA, Oertel WH (eds). *Parkinson's Disease. The Treatment Options*. London: Martin Dunitz, 1999; 63–78.

32. Mutch WJ, Dingwall-Fordyce I, Downie AW, Paterson JG, Roy SK. Parkinson's disease in a Scottish city. *Br. Med. J.* 1986; **292**: 534–6.

33. McGeer PL, McGeer EG, Suzuki JS. Aging and extrapyramidal function. *Arch. Neurol.* 1977; **34**: 33–5.

34. Kish SJ, Shannak K, Rajput A, Deck JH, Hornykiewicz O. Aging produces a specific pattern of striatal dopamine loss: implications for the etiology of idiopathic Parkinson's disease. *J. Neurochem.* 1992; **58**: 642–8.

35. Cote LJ, Kremzner LT. Biochemical changes in normal aging in human brain. In: Mayeux R, Rosen WG (eds). *The Dementias. Advances in Neurology, Vol. 38*. New York: Raven Press, 1983; 19–30.

36. Wagner HN. Quantitative imaging of neuroreceptors in the living human brain. *Semin. Nucl. Med.* 1986; **16**: 51–62.

37. Samii A, Calne DB. Research into the etiology of Parkinson's disease. In: LeWitt PA, Oertel WH (eds). *Parkinson's Disease. The Treatment Options*. London: Martin Dunitz, 1999; 229–43.

38. Veldman BAJ, Wijn AM, Knoers N, Praamstra P, Horstink MWIM. Genetic and environmental risk factors in Parkinson's disease. *Clin. Neurol. Neurosurg.* 1998; **100**: 15–26.

39. Bonifati V, Fabrizio E, Vanacore N, De Mari M, Meco G. Familial Parkinson's disease: a clinical genetic analysis. *Can. J. Neurol. Sci.* 1995; **22**: 272–9.

40. Wood N. Genetic aspects of parkinsonism. In: Quinn NP (ed.). *Bailliere's Clinical Neurology*. London: Bailliere Tindall, 1997; 37–53.

41. Burn DJ, Mark MH, Playford ED, *et al.* Parkinson's disease in twins studied with ^{18}F-DOPA and positron emission tomography. *Neurology* 1992; **42**: 1894–900.
42. Piccini P, Burn DJ, Ceravolo R, Maraganore D, Brooks DJ. The role of inheritance in sporadic Parkinson's disease: evidence from a longitudinal study of dopaminergic function in twins. *Ann. Neurol.* 1999; **45**: 577–82.
43. Schoenberg BS, Osuntokun BO, Adeuja AO, *et al.* Comparison of the prevalence of Parkinson's disease in black populations in the rural United States and in rural Nigeria: door-to-door community studies. *Neurology* 1988; **38**: 645–6.
44. Golbe LI, Di Lorio G, Bonavita V, Miller DC, Duvoisin RC. A large kindred with autosomal dominant Parkinson's disease. *Ann. Neurol.* 1990; **27**: 276–82.
45. Polymeropoulis MH, Lavedan C, Leroy E, *et al.* Mutation in the α-synuclein gene identified in families with Parkinson's disease. *Science* 1997; **276**: 2045–7.
46. Krüger R, Kuhn W, Müller T, *et al.* Ala30Pro mutation in the gene encoding α-synuclein in Parkinson's disease. *Nature Genet.* 1998; **18**: 106–8.
47. Clayton DF, George JM. The synucleins: a family of proteins involved in synaptic function, plasticity, neurodegeneration and disease. *Trends Neurosci.* 1998; **21**: 249–54.
48. Spillantini MG, Schmidt ML, Lee VM-Y, Trojanowski JQ, Jakes R, Goedert M. α-Synuclein in Lewy bodies. *Nature* 1997; **388**: 839–40.
49. Vaughan J, Durr A, Tassin J, *et al.* The alpha-synuclein Ala53Thr mutation is not a common cause of familial Parkinson's disease: a study of 230 European cases. European Consortium on Genetic Susceptibility in Parkinson's Disease. *Ann. Neurol.* 1998; **44**: 270–3.
50. Warner TT, Schapira AHV. The role of the α-synuclein gene mutation in patients with sporadic Parkinson's disease in the United Kingdom. *J. Neurol. Neurosurg. Psychiatry* 1998; **65**: 378–9.
51. Kitada T, Asakawa S, Hattori N, *et al.* Mutations in the parkin gene cause autosomal recessive juvenile parkinsonism. *Nature* 1998; **392**: 605–8.
52. Jarman P, Wood N. Parkinson's disease genetics comes of age. *Br. Med. J.* 1999; **318**: 1641–2.
53. Bandmann O, Vaughan J, Holmans P, Marsden CD, Wood NW. Association of slow acetylator genotype for *N*-acetyl transferase 2 with familial Parkinson's disease. *Lancet* 1997; **350**: 1136–9.
54. Langston JW. Epidemiology versus genetics in Parkinson's disease: progress in resolving an age-old debate. *Ann. Neurol.* 1998; **44**: S89–98
55. Marsden CD, Olanow CW. The causes of Parkinson's disease are being unraveled and rational neuroprotective therapy is close to reality. *Ann. Neurol.* 1998; **44**: S189–96
56. Calne DB, Chu NS, Huang CC, Lu CS, Olanow CW. Manganism and idiopathic Parkinsonism: similarities and differences. *Neurology* 1994; **44**: 1583–6.
57. Schapira AHV. Pathogenesis of Parkinson's disease. In: Quinn NP (ed.). *Bailliere's Clinical Neurology*. London: Bailliere Tindall, 1997; 15–36.
58. Langston JW, Ballard P, Tetud JW, Irwin I. Chronic parkinsonism in humans due to a product of meperidine analog synthesis. *Science* 1983; **219**: 979–80.
59. Langston JW, Ballard P. Parkinsonism induced by 1-methyl-4-phenyl 1,2,3,6 tetrahydropyridine: implications for treatment and the pathophysiology of Parkinson's disease. *Can. J. Neurol. Sci.* 1999; **11**: 160–5.
60. Rajput AH, Uitti RJ, Stern W, *et al.* Geography, drinking water, chemistry, pesticides and herbicides and the etiology of Parkinson's disease. *Can. J. Neurol. Sci.* 1987; **14**: 414–18.

61. Svenson LW, Platt GH, Woodhead SE. Geographic variations in the prevalence rates of Parkinson's disease in Alberta. *Can. J. Neurol. Sci.* 1993; **20**: 307–11.
62. Jimenez-Jimenez FJ, Mateo D, Gimenez-Roldan S. Exposure to well water and pesticides in Parkinson's disease: a case control study in the Madrid area. *Movement Disord.* 1992; **7**: 149–52.
63. Logroscino G, Marder K, Cote L, Tang MX, Shea S, Mayeux R. Dietary lipids and antioxidants in Parkinson's disease: a population-based case-control study. *Ann. Neurol.* 1996; **39**: 89–94.
64. Parkinson Study Group. Effects of tocopherol and deprenyl on the progression of disability in early Parkinson's disease. *N. Engl. J. Med.* 1993; **328**: 176–83.
65. Baron JA. Cigarette smoking and Parkinson's disease. *Neurology* 1986; **36**: 1490–6.
66. Yong VW, Perry TL. Monoamine oxidase B, smoking and Parkinson's disease. *J. Neurol. Sci.* 1986; **72**: 265–72.
67. Raff MC, Barres BA, Burne JF, Coles HS, Ishizaki Y, Jacobson MD. Programmed cell death and the control of cell survival: lessons from the nervous system. *Science* 1993; **262**: 695–700.
68. Burke RE. Programmed cell death and Parkinson's disease. *Movement Disord.* 1998; **13**: 17–23.
69. Hirsch E, Hunot S, Faucheux B, *et al.* Dopaminergic neurons degenerate by apoptosis in Parkinson's disease. *Movement Disord.* 1998; **2**: 383–4.
70. Banati RB, Blunt S, Graeber MB. What does apoptosis have to do with Parkinson's disease? *Movement Disord.* 1998; **2**: 384–5.
71. Jenner P. Oxidative mechanisms in nigral cell death in Parkinson's disease. *Movement Disord.* 1998; **13**: 24–34.
72. Dexter DT, Carter CJ, Wells FR, *et al.* Basal lipid peroxidation in substantia nigra is increased in Parkinson's disease. *J. Neurochem.* 1989; **52**: 381–9.
73. Sanchez-Ramos JR, Överick E, Ames BN. A marker of oxyradical-mediated DNA damage (8-hydroxy-2'-deoxyguanosine) is increased in nigro-striatum of Parkinson's disease brain. *Neurodegeneration* 1994; **3**: 197–204.
74. Schapira AHV. Evidence for mitochondrial dysfunction in Parkinson's disease: a critical appraisal. *Movement Disord.* 1994; **9**: 125–38.
75. Ahlskog JE. Neuroprotective strategies in the treatment of Parkinson's disease: clinical evidence. In: LeWitt PA, Oertel WH (eds). *Parkinson's Disease. The Treatment Options.* London: Martin Dunitz, 1999; 93–115.
76. Beal MF. Does impairment of energy metabolism result in excitotoxic neuronal death in neurodegenerative illness? *Ann. Neurol.* 1992; **31**: 119–30.

Epidemiology

W.J. Mutch and C. Lien

Study methods

Parkinson's disease (PD) is a common and disabling condition for which a considerable body of descriptive and analytical studies has been collected world-wide over many years. The variation in the reported prevalence of PD[1] may be due, at least in part, to the different methods used in studies, with diagnostic criteria and case-finding strategies being the most significant variables.

Diagnostic criteria

The diagnosis of PD is a matter of clinical judgement, and an incorrect diagnosis has been reported in almost 30 per cent of cases in two UK studies.[2,3] In older people, PD can be particularly problematic, and there are reports of many cases being missed in nursing homes,[4] as well as many older people being wrongly diagnosed, particularly in such institutions.[5] Extrapyramidal symptoms are not uncommon in 'successfully ageing' people,[6] and may also be present in older people in the community for reasons other than Parkinson's disease[7]. Hence, clearly defined criteria that may be applied consistently are essential for diagnosis to be successful.

When using commonly accepted criteria, the specificity of a diagnosis – irrespective of age – may be as low as 16 per cent,[8] and the actual set of criteria used clearly affects the prevalence rate.[9] Attempts have been made to produce criteria which are clearly defined and based on best evidence;[10,11] however, although variation remains it is focused (fortunately) on the classical features of resting tremor, rigidity and bradykinesia.

Case finding

Historically, studies have relied heavily on case records – a situation which can be particularly misleading when reports are confined to hospital or clinic records or to small groups of possibly atypical patients. Attempts have been made at a total census on a community-wide basis using cross-referencing from various sources of information and personal examination of all identified people.[2,3,5,12] This approach may work reasonably well in settings where access to, and quality of, medical care are good, but even then it will miss cases – particularly those in the first two to three years of overt disease who have not yet presented for clinical attention.

Door-to-door surveys are now considered to be the 'gold standard', and in the Euro-Parkinson study, 24 per cent of subjects were newly detected in this way.[13] These surveys can consist of a one-stage approach using a combined validated screening questionnaire and examination of all members of a household in a geographically defined area, or a two-stage approach where the screening and examination are carried out at separate times. However, it is possible that door-to-door studies using only questionnaires might miss some cases.[14] In general, non-response to surveys does not lead to bias except in the case of older women.[15] Surveys are extremely expensive to perform, but it may be possible to use anti-Parkinson drugs and death certificates as tracer or screening proxies; these may then be followed by more intensive descriptive or analytical studies.[16]

Comparing studies

The major difficulty in comparing studies on a world-wide basis and from different time periods has been the different age and sex structure of the respective populations. Conversion of data to a single standard population should overcome this,[1,13,17] but unfortunately not all investigators choose the same standard.[1,5,13]

To be of value, epidemiological studies must give (as a minimum) a full description of the methods used, the sample size, and the crude incidence or prevalence rates by age and sex.

INCIDENCE

There are remarkably few incidence studies of any value, the majority having unfortunately included post-encephalitic and vascular cases. What evidence there is suggests that the crude incidence of PD world-wide lies between 2 and 24 cases per 100 000 of the population per year,[1,18,19] and in Northern Europe these values are between 6 and 17 cases per 100 000 of the population per year.[1,2,5,20]

The incidence rises with patient age, and is greatest in the eighth decade of life.[1,21] Limited data indicate that the annual incidence is significantly higher in men than women in Rochester USA[22] and South-western Finland,[5] the trends also being in a similar direction in other studies.[1]

There is a significant lack of longitudinal data available, but isolated studies have suggested that in Japan the incidence may be falling in people aged under 50 years.[18] In Finland, during the past 20 years, the incidence may be falling in women yet rising in men (particularly those aged over 70 years) and in people living in rural areas.[5]

PREVALENCE

Much more data are available regarding the prevalence of PD. On a world-wide basis, the crude prevalence appears to vary from 10 to 657 cases per 100 000 of the population,[1,2,5,12,20,23–26] while in Europe it varies from 66 cases per 100 000 of the population in Sardinia[27] to 196 cases per 100 000 of the population in South-western Finland.[5] In the UK, the disease appears to affect at least 1 in 1000 of the population,[2,28] and possibly as many as 1 in 600.[3]

VARIATION IN PREVALENCE

Of major importance is whether the prevalence – and, by implication, the risk of the disease – truly varies world-wide. By using data adjusted against a standard population, it has been suggested[1] that world-wide prevalence could be divided into three groups: (i) a low-prevalence (<80 cases per 100 000 of the population); (ii) an intermediate prevalence (80–130 cases per 100 000); and (iii) high prevalence (>130 cases per 100 000) (Fig. 3.1).

Studies reflecting populations from different parts of the world were found in each of these groups. Subsequent studies from Wales,[2] Finland,[5] Faroe Islands,[12] Italy,[24] Australia,[26] England,[28] and Norway[29] have been found in the

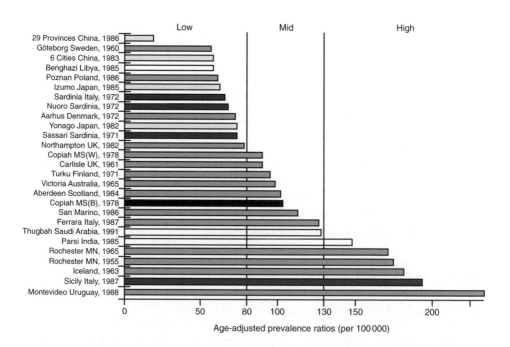

Fig. 3.1 World-wide comparison of age-adjusted prevalence ratios for Parkinson's disease by country for both sexes combined (adjusted to the 1970 US population). (Source: Zhang and Roman, 1993[1].)

mid- to high-prevalence groups, while one study from Sweden[20] has been found in the low group.

These data also inferred that studies conducted among oriental communities and black people living in Africa were only found in the low prevalence group, and this appeared to be confirmed by 'gold standard' door-to-door surveys. Subsequent studies, however, from Taiwan,[25] Japan[18] and Hawaii,[19] where only men of Japanese and Okinawan ancestry were examined, showed a prevalence that was mid-range.

Using a standardized population and similar case finding methods and diagnostic criteria, the Euro-Parkinson group suggested there was no convincing evidence for differences in prevalence across European countries.[13] Notably, the striking feature of studies performed during the 1990s has been the careful attention that has been paid to the methods applied.[2,5,12,13,18–20,24–26,28,29]

Many of the reported differences in PD prevalence – and, by implication, the risk world-wide – may well be due to artefacts, though further studies are required to clarify the situation in China and in black people living in Africa. A greater life expectancy in general, as well as longer survival after the onset of PD in more developed countries, may add to these differences in prevalence, though there is a lack of data to substantiate this.

If the prevalence of PD is truly different, then research on migrant populations (e.g. from Hawaii) might help to clarify the relationship between any genetic and environmental factors.

TEMPORAL CHANGES

It is possible that in some countries the prevalence of PD has changed with time. For example, an increased prevalence has been reported in Yonaga, Japan,[18] in Northampton, England[28] and in south-western Finland.[5] Whereas it might be possible to criticise the original study methods used in Japan and England, the data obtained in Finland were far more robust, there being a significantly increased prevalence in men and in all people (and especially those aged over 60 years) in rural settings. The occurrence in women appears to be relatively stable in Finland and Northampton, while in New Zealand the overall prevalence may have fallen.[30]

PARKINSON'S DISEASE IN THE VERY OLD

All studies agree that the prevalence of PD rises markedly with age,[1,13] but debate exists as to whether or not prevalence continues to rise in the very old. Zhang and Roman's review[1] indicated that five of 13 studies showed a continuing rise, while six subsequent studies[13,14,23,25,31,32] confirmed this and four did not.[12,24,28,29] There are particular diagnostic difficulties in older people. In addition, the absolute numbers in the very old is small, and therefore one patient might have an inordinate effect on the prevalence. It is possible that the only way to resolve this issue would be the careful follow up of a cohort of very old people.

GENDER-RELATED DIFFERENCES IN PD PREVALENCE

A further point for discussion is that of varying prevalence of PD between men and women. A detailed analysis performed in 1993 identified five studies in which the prevalence was significantly higher in men, while only one showed higher prevalence in women.[1] Subsequently, a male predominance was found in five further studies of which three were conducted in 'Nordic' countries.[5,12,20,23,28] Only the study from Finland[5] showed any significant inter-gender difference, but this was also marked by a change to male predominance over the past 20 years. Moreover, it is possible that these Finnish data were obtained from a cohort of susceptible men who were exposed to an environmental factor, while women did not receive such exposure. Other, more recent studies have demonstrated either a female predominance[30,33] or no difference.[13,14,25]

On balance, it is safe to say that on a world-wide basis PD is certainly as common in men as women, and indeed may be more common in men – particularly in 'Nordic' countries. Whether this is due to a differing susceptibility or to varying environmental exposure is not clear, though the more recently acquired Finnish data might be taken as evidence of the latter proposal.

AGE AT ONSET

Studies conducted during the past 30 years have suggested that the mean age at onset has remained within the seventh decade, with a remarkable focus on 64–66 years in 'Nordic' countries over the past 10 years.[5,12,20,29]

Mortality

Before the introduction of levodopa, people with PD were three times more likely to die compared with their peers.[34] Following the first use of levodopa however, mortality ratios (of 0.95 to 2.60)[7,19,35–38] have been reported in cohort studies, and ratios of 1.6[22] and 2.35[39] in the only case-controlled studies.

People aged over 70 years who have PD are significantly more likely to die than their peers.[7,19,39] Those whose disease has been present for more than 10 years,[19] and those with gait disturbance,[7,39] may also be more likely to die, though these findings were not confirmed in a cohort of American nursing home residents.[36]

In a detailed historical analysis, Clarke[40] has concluded that overall mortality fell in the 1970s and rose in the 1980s as the result of a cohort of frail older people whose death was delayed by levodopa. There is some evidence that, during the past two decades, mortality is decreasing world-wide in younger patients and increasing in those aged over 75 years,[41–45] though the reasons for this are unclear.[46] There are no data available regarding the effect of newer surgical interventions on mortality.

On balance, PD not only has significant functional import for older people but also probably hastens their death, even when levodopa is used.

Understanding aetiology

The cause of PD remains unknown. Epidemiology has contributed to our understanding of the condition by highlighting the potential role of environmental factors. Ben-Shlomo[46] has provided a thorough review of environmental risk factors, and has divided them into toxic, infections and miscellaneous (e.g. head injury, or drinking well water). Ben-Shlomo has highlighted the need for better measures of exposure, and to examine the circumstances and exposure in childhood. In addition, these studies highlighted that case-control studies are more liable to bias than cohort studies.

There is now a wealth of data on possible risk factors from around the world (Table 3.1). These data provide tantalising clues, but unfortunately lack consistency – in fact, growing old would appear to be the only unequivocal factor! With regard to occupational exposure, a recent Italian study could find no association, particularly for farmers[64] and, indeed, for Hispanics in America, farming as an occupation might actually be protective.[61] The role of diet remains an enigma.

A complex picture is emerging which, setting aside confounding factors, might suggest there are both common and different risk factors for different population groups. However, it should not be forgotten that no causal

Table 3.1 Possible environmental factors in Parkinson's disease

Study	Location	Factors
Godwin Austen et al. (1982)[47]	UK	Head injury, smoking
Barbeau et al. (1987)[48]	Quebec, Canada	Pesticides, paper mills, heavy metals
Aquilonius and Hartvig (1986)[49]	Sweden	Steel industry, metals
Rajput et al. (1987)[50]	Canada	Rural living
Golbe et al. (1988)[51]	USA	Dietary factors, nuts, salad oil, plums protect
Jimenez-Jimenez et al. (1988)[52]	Spain	Pesticides, metal industries, well water
Tanner et al. (1989)[53]	China	Industrial chemicals, printing, plants, quarries
Ho et al. (1989)[54]	Hong Kong	Rural life, farming, previous use of herbicides/pesticides, raw vegetables
Koller et al. (1990)[55]	USA	Rural life
Semchuck et al. (1992)[56]	Canada	Occupational herbicide use
Wang Wen-Zhi et al. (1993)[57]	China	Drinking river water, living near rubber plants
Hubble et al. (1993)[58]	USA	Pesticides, family history of neurological disease, depression
De Pedro Cuesta et al. (1996)[59]	Iceland	Pertussis
Liou et al. (1997)[60]	Taiwan	Paraquat, herbicides/pesticides in a dose–response
Marder et al. (1998)[61]	USA	Rural living, farming and well water in African Americans. Well water in Hispanics
Chan et al. (1998)[62]	Hong Kong	Family history, years exposed to pesticides
Smargiassi et al. (1998)[63]	Italy	Head injury, well water, occupational exposure industrial chemicals
McCann et al. (1998)[26]	Australia	Family history, rural living

relationship has yet been demonstrated for any of the putative factors. It is clear that further prospective cohort-based studies and studies comparing stable urban and rural populations in the same country would be of value.

Protection against PD

Whilst other factors relating to protection against PD may lack consistency, the inverse (protective) association with smoking seems clear.[65] A recent population-based case-control study has also demonstrated an inverse dose–response relationship between PD and smoking, and refutes bias or confounding factors.[66] In a prospective cohort study the age-adjusted incidence of PD was 50 per cent less in smokers of all ages above 50 years.[67]

Whilst confounding factors such as pre-morbid personality and certain genes which influence both the tendency to smoke and the risk of developing PD cannot be ruled out, it would appear likely that smoking is biologically protective. Accordingly, studies to show the biochemical mechanisms for such protection would be helpful.

It is interesting to note that in a study carried out in Hong Kong,[62] tea-drinking may be protective, and that anti-oxidants in the diet may also have some protective value.[46]

Family history

Many descriptive and case-control studies comment on the presence and significance of a family history.[68] The situation is complex, however, as there are recognized families with an autosomal dominant mode of inheritance of 'apparent' idiopathic PD.[69,70] The susceptibility gene for an Italian family[69] has been mapped to chromosome 4q21-q23,[71] while a further gene has been mapped to chromosome 2p13 in other families.[72] The former mutation appears to lead to an abnormal form of the presynaptic protein α-synuclein, which also appears to be a major constituent of Lewy bodies.[73] It is generally agreed that a single gene component may be important for a few younger patients with an 'apparent' idiopathic PD. Most patients, however, have no significant family history and, indeed, a recent large national twin study confirmed a lack of a classical genetic component in patients aged over 50 years.[74] Nonetheless, studies to elucidate these and any further genes, as well as α-synuclein, will also help our understanding of the more common idiopathic disease. In fact, most now agree that the aetiology of PD is complex and involves an increased susceptibility produced by functional polymorphisms in nuclear, and possibly also mitochondrial, genes.[75] These play a role in dopamine, drug and toxin metabolism,[76] and are triggered directly or indirectly by interactions with an appropriate environmental agent.

Parkinson's disease may well be truly heterogeneous in its causation and, if so, answers are likely to come from teams of epidemiologists, clinicians, geneticists and laboratory scientists working closely together. However, when issues appear very complex there is also sometimes value in standing back and asking if we are missing something.

References

1. Zhang Zhen-Xin, Roman GC. World wide occurrence of Parkinson's disease: an updated review. *Neuroepidemiology* 1993; **12**: 195–208.
2. Hobson JP, Meara RJ. A descriptive epidemiological study of Parkinson's disease in North Wales. *Age Ageing* 1999; **28** (suppl. 1): 63.
3. Mutch WJ, Dingwall-Fordyce I, Downie AW, Paterson JG, Roy SK. Parkinson's disease in a Scottish city. *Br. Med. J.* 1986; **292**: 534–6.
4. Larsen JP. Parkinson's disease as community health problem: study in Norwegian nursing homes. *Br. Med. J.* 1991; **303**: 741–3.
5. Kuopio A-M, Martilla RJ, Helenius H, Rinne UK. Changing epidemiology of Parkinson's disease in South Western Finland. *Neurology* 1999; **52**: 302–8.
6. Odenheimer G, Funkenstein HH, Beckett L, *et al.* Comparison of neurologic changes in 'successfully aging' persons v the total aging population. *Arch. Neurol.* 1994; **51**: 573–80.
7. Bennett DA, Beckett LA, Murray AM, *et al.* Prevalence of parkinsonian signs and associated mortality in a community population of older people. *N. Engl. J. Med.* 1996; **334**: 71–6.
8. Rajput AH, Rozkilsky B, Rajput A. Accuracy of a clinical diagnosis in parkinsonism: a prospective study. *Can. J. Neurol. Sci.* 1991; **18**: 275–8.
9. de-Ryk MC, Rocca WA, Anderson DW, Melcon MO, Breteler MMB, Maraganore DM. A population perspective on diagnostic criteria for Parkinson's disease. *Neurology* 1997; **48**: 1277–81.
10. Hughes AJ, Daniel SE, Kilford L, Lees AJ. Accuracy of clinical diagnosis of idiopathic Parkinson's disease: a clinico-pathological study of 100 cases. *J. Neurol. Neurosurg. Psychiatry* 1992; **55**: 181–4.
11. Koller WC, Montgomery EB. Issues in the early diagnosis of Parkinson's Disease. *Neurology* 1997; **49** (suppl. 1): S10–25.
12. Wermuth L, Joensen P, Bünger N, Jeune B. High prevalence of Parkinson's disease in the Faroe Islands. *Neurology* 1997; **49**: 426–32.
13. de-Rijk MC, Tzourio C, Breteler MMB, *et al.* Prevalence of parkinsonism and Parkinson's Disease in Europe: the Europarkinson collaborative study. *J. Neurol. Neurosurg. Psychiatry* 1997; **62**: 10–15.
14. Morgante L, Rocca WA, Di Rosa AE, *et al.* Prevalence of Parkinson's disease and other types of parkinsonism: a door-to-door survey in three Sicilian municipalities. *Neurology* 1992; **42**:1901–7.
15. Anderson DW, Rocca WA, de-Rijk MC, *et al.* Case ascertainment uncertainties in prevalence surveys of Parkinson's disease. *Movement Disord.* 1998; **13**: 626–32.
16. Strickland D, Bertoni JM, Pfeiffer RF. Descriptive epidemiology of Parkinson's disease through proxy measures. *Can. J. Neurol. Sci.* 1996; **23**: 279–84.
17. de Pedro Cuesta J. Parkinson's disease occurrence in Europe. *Acta Neurol. Scand.* 1991; **84**: 357–65.
18. Kusumi M, Nakashima K, Harada H, Nakayama H, Takahashi K. Epidemiology of Parkinson's disease in Yonaga City, Japan: comparison with a study carried out 12 years ago. *Neuroepidemiology* 1996; **15**: 201–7.
19. Morens DM, Davis JW, Grandinetti A, Ross GW, Popper JS, White LR. Incidence

and mortality in a prospective study of middle-aged men. *Neurology* 1996; **46**: 1044–50.

20. Fall PA, Axelson O, Fredriksson M, Hansson G, Lindvall B, Olsson JE, Granerus AK. Age-standardised incidence and prevalence of Parkinson's disease in a Swedish community. *J. Clin. Epidemiol.* 1996; **49**: 637–41.

21. Goldsmith JR, Herishanu YO, Podgaietski M, Kordysh E. Dynamics of Parkinsonism-Parkinson's disease in residents of adjacent kibbutzim in Israel's Negev. *Environ. Res.* 1997; **73**: 156–61.

22. Rajput AH, Offorf KP, Beard CM, Kurkland LT. Epidemiology of Parkinsonism: incidence, classification and mortality. *Ann. Neurol.* 1984; **16**: 278–82.

23. Melcon MO, Anderson DW, Vergara RH, Rocca WA. Prevalence of Parkinson's disease in Junin, Buenos Aires Province, Argentina. *Movement Disord.* 1997; **12**: 197–205.

24. Chio A, Magnani C, Schiffer D. Prevalence of Parkinson's disease in North Western Italy: comparison of tracer methodology and clinical ascertainment of cases. *Movement Disord.* 1998; **13**: 400–5.

25. Wang SJ, Fuh JL, Teng EL, *et al.* A door-to-door survey of Parkinson's disease in a Chinese population in Kinmen. *Arch. Neurol.* 1996; **53**: 66–71.

26. McCann SJ, LeCouteur DG, Green AC, *et al.* The epidemiology of Parkinson's disease in an Australian population. *Neuroepidemiology* 1998; **17**: 310–17.

27. Rosati G, Granieri E, Pinna L, *et al.* The risk of Parkinson's disease in Mediterranean people. *Neurology* 1980; **30**: 250–5.

28. Sutcliffe RLG, Meara JR. Parkinson's disease epidemiology in the Northampton district, England, 1992. *Acta Neurol. Scand.* 1995; **92**: 443–50.

29. Tandberg E, Larsen JP, Nessler EG, Riise T, Aarli JA. The epidemiology of Parkinson's disease in the county of Rogaland, Norway. *Movement Disord.* 1995; **10**: 541–9.

30. Caradoc-Davies TH, Weatherall M, Dixon GS, Carradoc- Davies G, Hantz P. Is the prevalence of Parkinson's disease in New Zealand really changing? *Acta Neurol. Scand.* 1992; **86**: 40–4.

31. de Rijk MC, Breteler MMB, Graveland GA, Ott A, Van Der Meche FGA, Hofman A. Prevalence of parkinsonism and of Parkinson's disease in elderly subjects: the 'Rotterdam Study'. *Ned. Tijdschr. Geneeskd.* 1996; **140**: 196–200.

32. Tison F, Dartigues JF, Dubes L, Zuber M, Alperovitch A, Henry P. Prevalence of Parkinson's disease in the elderly: a population study in Gironde, France. *Acta Neurol. Scand.* 1994; **90**: 111–15.

33. Mayeux R, Marder K, Cote LJ, *et al.* The frequency of idiopathic Parkinson's disease by age, ethnic group and sex in Northern Manhattan 1988–1993. *Am. J. Epidemiol.* 1995; **142**: 820–7.

34. Hoehn MM, Yahr MD. Parkinsonism: onset, progression and mortality. *Neurology* 1967; **17**: 427–42.

35. Diamond SG, Markham CH. Long-term experience with L-Dopa: efficacy, progression and mortality. In: Birkmeyer W, Hornykiewicz O (eds). *Advances in Parkinsonism.* Basel: Roche, 1976: 444.

36. Mitchell SL, Kiely DK, Kiel DP, Lipsitz LA. The epidemiology, clinical characteristics and natural history of older nursing home residents with a diagnosis of Parkinson's disease. *J. Am. Geriatr. Soc.* 1996; **44**: 394–9.

37. Curtis L, Lees AJ, Stern GM, Marmot MG. Effect of L-Dopa on the course of Parkinson's disease. *Lancet* 1984; **ii**: 211–12.

38. Ben-Shlomo Y, Marmot MG. Survival and cause of death in a cohort of patients with parkinsonism: possible clues to aetiology? *J. Neurol. Neurosurg. Psychiatry* 1995; **58**: 293–9.

39. Ebmeier KP, Calder SA, Crawford JR, Stewart L, Besson JAO, Mutch WJ. Mortality and causes of death in idiopathic Parkinson's disease: results from the Aberdeen Whole Population Study. *Scot. Med. J.* 1990; **35**: 173–5.

40. Clarke CE. Does Levodopa therapy delay death in Parkinson's disease? A review of the evidence. *Movement Disord.* 1995; **10**: 250–6.

41. Li TM, Swash M, Alberman E. Morbidity and mortality in motor neurone disease: comparison with multiple sclerosis and Parkinson's disease. *J. Neurol. Neurosurg. Psychiatry* 1985; **48**: 320–7.

42. Treves TA, de Pedro Cuesta J. Parkinsonism mortality: time and space patterns. *Acta Neurol. Scand.* 1991; **84**: 389–97.

43. Lilienfield DE, Chan A, Ehland J, *et al.* Two decades of increasing mortality from Parkinson's disease among the U.S. elderly. *Arch. Neurol.* 1990; **47**: 731–4.

44. Ben-Shlomo Y, Finnan F, Allwright S, Davey Smith G. The epidemiology of Parkinson's disease in Ireland: observations from routine data sources. *Ir. Med. J.* 1993; **86**: 190–4.

45. Imaizumi Y, Kaneko R. Rising mortality from Parkinson's disease in Japan, 1950-1992. *Acta Neurol. Scand.* 1995; **91**: 169–76.

46. Ben-Shlomo Y. How far are we in understanding the cause of Parkinson's disease? *J. Neurol. Neurosurg. Psychiatry* 1996; **61**: 4–16.

47. Godwin Austen RB, Lee PN, Marmot MG, Stern GM. Smoking and Parkinson's disease. *J. Neurol. Neurosurg. Psychiatry* 1982; **45**: 577–81.

48. Barbeau A, Roy M, Bernier G, Campanella G, Paris S. Ecogenetics of Parkinson's disease: prevalence and environmental aspects in rural areas. *Can. J. Neurol. Sci.* 1987; **14**: 36–41.

49. Aquilonius SM, Hartvig P. A Swedish county with unexpectedly high utilization of anti-parkinsonian drugs. *Acta Neurol. Scand.* 1986; **74**: 379–82.

50. Rajput AH, Uitti RJ, Stern W, *et al.* Geography, drinking water chemistry, pesticides and herbicides and the etiology of Parkinson's disease. *Can. J. Neurol. Sci.* 1987; **14**: 414–18.

51. Golbe LI, Farrell TM, Davis PH. Case-control study of early life dietary factors in Parkinson's disease. *Arch Neurol.* 1988; **45**: 1350–3.

52. Jimenez-Jimenez FJ, Mateo D, Gimenez-Roldan S. Exposure to well water and pesticides in Parkinson's disease: a case-control study in the Madrid area. *Movement Disord.* 1992; **7**: 149–52.

53. Tanner CM, Chen B, Wang W, *et al.* Environmental factors and Parkinson's disease: a case-control study in China. *Neurology* 1989; **39**: 660–4.

54. Ho SC, Woo J, Lee CM. Epidemiologic study of Parkinson's disease in Hong Kong. *Neurology* 1989; **39**: 1314–18.

55. Koller W, Vetere-Overfield B, Gray C, *et al.* Environmental risk factors in Parkinson's disease. *Neurology* 1990; **40**: 1218–21.

56. Semchuck KM, Love EJ, Lee RG. Parkinson's disease and exposure to agricultural work and pesticide chemicals. *Neurology* 1992; **42**: 1328–35.

57. Wang WZ, Fang XH, Cheng XM, Jiang DH, Lin ZJ. A case-control study on the environmental risk factors of Parkinson's disease in Tianjin, China. *Neuroepidemiology* 1993; **12**: 209–18.

58. Hubble JP, Cao T, Hassanein RE, Neuberger JS, Koller WC. Risk factors for Parkinson's disease. *Neurology* 1993; **43**: 1693–7.

59. de Pedro-Cuesta J, Gudmundsson G, Abraira V, *et al.* Whooping cough and Parkinson's disease. *Int. J. Epidemiol.* 1996; **25**: 1301–11.

60. Liou HH, Tsai MC, Chen CJ, *et al.* Environmental risk factors and Parkinson's disease: a case-control study in Taiwan. *Neurology* 1997; **48**: 1583–8.

61. Marder K, Logroscino G, Alfaro B, *et al.* Environmental risk factors for Parkinson's disease in an urban multi-ethnic community. *Neurology* 1998; **50**: 279–81.
62. Chan DK, Woo J, Ho SC, *et al.* Genetic and environmental risk factors for Parkinson's disease in a Chinese population. *J. Neurol. Neurosurg. Psychiatry* 1998; **65**: 781–4.
63. Smargiass A, Mutti A, De-Rosa A, De-Palma G, Negrotti A, Calzetti S. A case-control study of occupational and environmental risk factors for Parkinson's disease in the Emilia-Romagna region of Italy. *Neurotoxicology* 1998; **19**: 709–12.
64. Rocca WA, Anderson DW, Meneghini F, *et al.* Occupation, education, and Parkinson's disease: a case-control study in an Italian population. *Movement Disord.* 1996; **11**: 201–6.
65. Morens DM, Grandinetti A, Reed D, White LR, Ross GW. Cigarette smoking and protection from Parkinson's disease: false association or etiologic clue? *Neurology* 1995; **45**: 1041–51.
66. Gorell JM, Rybicki BA, Cole Johnson C, Peterson EL. Smoking and Parkinson's disease: a dose-response relationship. *Neurology* 1999; **52**: 115–19.
67. Morens DM, Grandinetti A, Davis JW, Ross GW, White LR, Reed D. Evidence against the operation of selective mortality in explaining the association between cigarette smoking and reduced occurrence of idiopathic Parkinson's disease. *Am. J. Epidemiol.* 1996; **144**: 400–4.
68. Wood N. Genes and Parkinsonism. *J. Neurol. Neurosurg. Psychiatry* 1997; **62**: 305–9.
69. Golbe LI, Iorio G, Bonavita V, *et al.* A large kindred with autosomal dominant Parkinson's disease. *Ann. Neurol.* 1990; **27**: 276–82.
70. Waters CH, Miller CA. Autosomal dominant Lewy body parkinsonism in a four generation family. *Ann. Neurol.* 1994; **35**: 59–64.
71. Polymeropolous MH, Higgins JJ, Golbe LI, *et al.* Mapping of a gene for Parkinson's disease to chromosome 4q21-q23. *Science* 1996; **274**: 1197–9.
72. Gasser T, Müller-Myhsok B, Wszolek ZK, *et al.* A susceptibility locus for Parkinson's disease maps to chromosome 2p13. *Nature Genet.* 1998; **18**: 262–5.
73. Spillantini MG, Schmidt ML, Lee VM, Trojanowski JQ, Jakes R, Goedert M. Alpha-synuclein in Lewy bodies. *Nature* 1997; **388**: 839–40.
74. Tanner CM, Ottman R, Goldman SM, *et al.* Parkinson's disease in twins: an etiologic study. *JAMA* 1999; **281**: 341–6.
75. Payami H, Zareparsi S. Genetic epidemiology of Parkinson's disease. *J. Geriatr. Psychiatry Neurol.* 1998; **11**: 98–106.
76. Bajaj NP, Shaw C, Warner T, Raychaudhuri K. The genetics of Parkinson's disease and Parkinsonian syndromes. *J. Neurol.* 1998; **245**: 625–33.

Part 2: Diagnosis and assessment of Parkinson's disease

Diagnosis and differential diagnosis

G.J.A. Macphee

Introduction

Parkinsonism is a clinical syndrome with three cardinal features: akinesia, rigidity and tremor. Akinesia is a requisite sign for diagnosis and is usually accompanied by rigidity; tremor is a variable finding.

It is now recognized that James Parkinson's essay of 1817 was a description of the syndrome of parkinsonism and that idiopathic Parkinson's disease (IPD) has many imitators. The causes of parkinsonism can be classified into three major groups: (i) IPD; (ii) atypical parkinsonian syndromes (parkinsonism plus) and other neurodegenerative disorders; and (iii) secondary or symptomatic causes (Table 4.1). Other aetiologies are increasingly reported for akinetic rigid syndromes,[1] and the table is not exhaustive.

The diagnosis of IPD presents a considerable challenge in older patients. Although IPD is the most common cause of parkinsonism at all ages, the prevalence of the atypical syndromes, drug-induced parkinsonism and tremor disorders (particularly non-specific 'shaking'[2]) also increases with advancing years. Age-associated changes in gait and station, often caused by cryptic neurodegenerative and cerebrovascular disease,[3] may cause diagnostic confusion with early parkinsonism.

Extrapyramidal signs (EPS) are common in elderly persons: EPS of variable severity were reported in 15 per cent of community-based subjects who were aged 65–74 years, and in 52 per cent of those aged over 85 years.[4] Clinically

Table 4.1   Differential diagnosis of parkinsonism

1. **Idiopathic Parkinson's disease

2.   Parkinsonism associated with neurodegenerative disorders

*Parkinsonism plus or atypical parkinsonian syndromes
- Progressive supranuclear palsy
- Multiple system atrophy
- Corticobasal degeneration

*Parkinsonism associated with other neurodegenerative disease
- *Dementia with Lewy bodies
- *Alzheimer's disease
- Pick's disease
- Amyotrophic lateral sclerosis
- Frontotemporal dementia

3. Secondary or symptomatic causes

*Drug-induced parkinsonism
- Neuroleptics
- Calcium channel blockers
- Other drugs

*Parkinsonism associated with cerebrovascular disease

Parkinsonism associated with hydrocephalus

Parkinsonism associated with infections
- Post encephalitic parkinsonism
- AIDS associated, e.g. HIV, cryptococcus, toxoplasmosis
- Viral encephalitides
- Neuroborreliosis
- Mycoplasma
- Prion diseases, e.g. Creutzfeld–Jacob disease
- Whipple's disease

Parkinsonism associated with toxic or metabolic disorders
- MPT (1-methyl-4-phenyl-1,2,3,6-tetrahydropyridine), carbon monoxide, carbon disulphide, methanol, manganese.
- Symptomatic massive basal ganglia calcification

Parkinsonism associated with head injury
- Dementia pugilistica (punch-drunk syndrome)

Parkinsonism associated with miscellaneous conditions
- Tumour, e.g. frontal meningioma
- Chronic subdural haematoma

Parkinsonism associated with inherited degenerative disease (usually young onset, but rare cases mid-life onset)
Wilson's disease, Huntington's disease, neuroacanthocytosis
Hallevorden–Spatz disease

Most common cause (**). Other main causes (*) in elderly

evident parkinsonism (two or more of the cardinal motor signs), in a similar population is lower at about 3 per cent.[5] This suggests a significant reservoir of subtle signs of parkinsonism in elderly subjects, who may or may not go on to develop IPD or another disorder. Parkinsonism occurring in the context of dementia becomes increasingly common in the ninth decade.[6]

Making a correct diagnosis of IPD is vital in establishing the prognosis for patient and family and initiating correct management. Equally important, IPD should be distinguished from imitators since outlook and management differ. Misdiagnosis may result in fruitless treatment with dopaminergic drugs, which may produce neuropsychiatric side effects in susceptible older subjects. Accurate diagnosis is also important for epidemiological and therapeutic research. For these reasons, all elderly persons with suspected parkinsonism should have specialist assessment.

This chapter will discuss the diagnosis of IPD and briefly review the conditions that most commonly mimic IPD, with particular emphasis on the atypical or 'parkinsonism plus' syndromes (progressive supranuclear palsy, multiple system atrophy and corticobasal degeneration).

Diagnostic problems

Clinicopathological studies confirm that the ante-mortem diagnosis of IPD, made by neurologists or geriatricians with a specific interest in parkinsonism is erroneous in 24 per cent of cases.[7,8] This is principally because the cardinal signs occur in conditions other than IPD. The main alternative diagnoses in the UK Brain Bank series of 100 cases were six cases of progressive supranuclear palsy (PSP), five of multiple system atrophy (MSA) and six of Alzheimer pathology.[7]

The diagnostic error rate is highest at disease onset and will fall over time, if the clinician is vigilant for the emergence of atypical features or 'red flags'[9] suggesting alternative diagnoses (Table 4.2). Only 65 per cent of patients with an initial diagnosis of IPD had confirmatory pathology at autopsy in one series,[8] but diagnostic accuracy had improved to 76 per cent at five years.

Nearly 25 per cent of subjects treated in general practice for Parkinson's disease have no evidence of true parkinsonism,[10] suggesting greater diagnostic error among non-specialists. Common misdiagnoses were essential tremor, ischaemic cerebrovascular disease, and extrapyramidal signs in Alzheimer's disease.

Clinical diagnosis

The diagnosis of IPD remains entirely clinical at present since there are no discrete biological markers. Some investigations are useful in recognising other causes of parkinsonism. Establishing a diagnosis of IPD (or other parkinsonian syndrome) is a two-step process:

Confirm the presence of true parkinsonism by clinical examination.

Table 4.2   Atypical features in idiopathic Parkinsons's disease

Early or prominent feature	Possible alternative diagnosis
Autonomic failure	MSA
Atypical levodopa dyskinesia	MSA
Atypical tremor	ET, DT, CBD, MSA
Minimal or absent tremor	MSA, PSP, VP, NPH
Early postural instability or falls	PSP > MSA, VP, NPH
Pyramidal signs	MSA, VP, PSP, NPH, CBD
Early dementia	DLB, AD, MID, PSP, CJD
Supranuclear gaze palsy	PSP > MSA, CBD
Marked asymmetry of motor signs	CBD
Myoclonus	CBD, MSA, DLB, CJD
Alien limb	CBD
Focal cortical signs	CBD
Pallilalia or pallilogia	PSP
Severe early dysarthria or dysphagia	PSP, MSA
Stridor, cold hands, marked antecollis	MSA
Wheelchair dependence	MSA

AD, Alzheimers disease; CBD, corticobasal degeneration; CJD, Creutzfeld–Jacob disease; DT, dystonic tremor; ET, essential tremor; MID, multi-infarct dementia; MSA, multiple system atrophy; NPH, normal pressure hydrocephalus; PSP, progressive supranuclear palsy; VP, vascular parkinsonism.

Consider the likely cause based on clinical features, progression of disease and response to treatment. This requires regular clinical review of the patient.

Cardinal features of parkinsonism

AKINESIA

Akinesia is the core feature of parkinsonism and must be present if the diagnosis is to be sustained. Akinesia is a symptom complex, comprising some or all of the following features: slowness (bradykinesia), poverty or lack of movement (hypokinesia), progressive early fatiguing and reduction in amplitude of repeated movements, impairment of sequencing or difficulty performing simultaneous motor actions. Fatiguing on repetitive motor tasks is a crucial finding since pyramidal tract lesions may also cause slowness of movement. Absence or poverty of movement is often best detected by casual observation including features such as decreased blink rate, paucity of facial expression, lack of fidgeting and reduced arm swing when walking. Confirmation of akinesia in the arms and face is important in supporting a diagnosis of IPD since 'lower-body parkinsonism' suggests cerebrovascular disease.

Formal tests for akinesia include asking the patient to tap the tip of the index finger regularly and rapidly on the distal thumb. In parkinsonism, the rhythm is ill-sustained and subject to periods of arrest followed by speeding up or complete breakdown of movement. Asking the patient rapidly to pronate and supinate the outstretched arms, or tapping the heel on the floor, may reveal similar motor timing difficulties. Watching the patient write may show disruption in a smooth flow of the pen, and the letters may progressively shrink in size. Handwriting may be small (micrographia) when compared with previous correspondence.

Some pitfalls exist in assessing akinesia in the elderly. Slowing of motor performance and reduction in diurnal activity are recognized with advancing age.[11,12] In contrast to the asymmetry which is characteristic of early IPD, age-related slowing is usually symmetrical and does not show the marked fatigability that defines true akinesia. Careful assessment of sensory function, tone, muscle power and reflexes should identify other diseases of both peripheral and central nervous systems, which slow motor performance. Focal pathology such as arthritis may also simulate bradykinesia. The psychomotor retardation of depression may be mistaken for bradykinesia, but depression itself is common in early IPD. Meticulous clinical assessment remains the principal tool in distinguishing imitators from early parkinsonism.

RIGIDITY

Rigidity is recognized as an increase in resistance to passive movements around a joint. It is described as plastic or 'lead pipe' when smooth, or 'cogwheel' when a ratchety feeling of fluctuating resistance occurs in the presence of a tremor which may or may not be clinically evident. Such resistance remains broadly constant throughout the range of excursion, independent of speed of movement. In contrast to rigidity, increased tone in *spasticity*, is velocity-dependent. During slow movements, little resistance may be felt; with swift movements a rapid rise in resistance is followed by resolution of resistance, the 'spastic catch'. *Gegenhalten* or paratonia is an uneven and often progressively increasing resistance to passive movement. Gegenhalten is associated with diffuse cerebral disease or cognitive dysfunction and may be mistaken for cogwheel rigidity.

Froment's manoeuvre may be useful in unmasking rigidity or cogwheeling, which is undetectable on routine testing. Increased tone may be found when the contralateral limb is activated (e.g. making a fist, drawing a circle in the air). Caution in interpretation is necessary since a mild increase in tone may be a non-specific response in healthy older persons. Asymmetrical augmentation of tone with cogwheeling is suggestive of IPD.

TREMOR

Tremor is an involuntary rhythmic oscillatory movement of a body part:

- *Action tremor* is any tremor that is present during voluntary contraction of muscle and includes postural and kinetic tremor.
- *Postural tremor* is seen with a sustained posture against gravity, for example with the arms outstretched.
- *Kinetic tremor* occurs during any movement.
- *Intention tremor* is a form of kinetic tremor and occurs when the amplitude of tremor increases during visually guided movements towards a target at the termination of the movement.
- *Resting tremor* emerges maximally when a body part is not voluntarily activated, and may be seen when a hand rests in the lap or dangles over an armrest. To be certain that a tremulous limb is completely supported against gravity, the examiner may need to rest the patient on a bed or couch.

POSTURAL INSTABILITY AND GAIT DISTURBANCE

Postural instability is often included as a fourth cardinal sign of parkinsonism, but has limited diagnostic specificity in the elderly. It may result from numerous other disorders affecting afferent and efferent neuronal pathways as well as central processing and musculoskeletal function.

Postural instability is usually the last cardinal feature to appear (by definition, stage 3 Hoehn and Yahr), but may occur prematurely in older patients.[13,14] The presence of falls early in the clinical course of parkinsonism usually suggests one of the atypical parkinsonian disorders (see Table 4.2).

The examiner tests postural stability by standing behind the patient, who should be asked to broaden their stance. Following explanation, the examiner should pull backwards on the patient's shoulders (the 'pull test') and be prepared to catch the patient if necessary. A normal response is resistance or recovery within one or two steps: the parkinsonian patient may take several steps to recover or begin to fall with retropulsion. Reduced arm swing is often the first sign of gait disturbance in IPD, followed by short-paced, shuffling steps. Breadth of base may be widened early in the disorder as a result of flexed posture but then narrows as a result of commanding rigidity.[15] Gait initiation may be troublesome, and turns may only be achieved *'en bloc'* with loss of truncal rotation. As disease progresses, impaired postural reflexes and flexed station may result in festination, where acceleration occurs in an attempt to retain balance. Falls may ensue if a wall or other object is not available for braking. Marked axial rigidity with modest distal parkinsonism and backward falls early in disease course suggests progressive supranuclear palsy.

Freezing may occur on starting to walk (start hesitation), while trying to turn or when approaching doorways. It is usually a feature of advanced IPD after significant duration of levodopa treatment. Freezing as an isolated or early feature may indicate subcortical cerebrovascular disease or normal pressure hydrocephalus.

Idiopathic Parkinson's disease

Definitions

Idiopathic Parkinson's disease is recognized as a levodopa-responsive parkinsonism with characteristic clinical features and natural history. At autopsy, the brain shows Lewy body degeneration of pigmented and other brainstem nuclei. A precise clinical definition of IPD is not established, but most experts consider the presence of two or more cardinal motor signs (one of which must include bradykinesia) and a consistent response to levodopa with the development of typical levodopa-induced dyskinesia indicative of IPD. Asymmetric onset[16] is a strong indicator of IPD.

Strict diagnostic criteria are discussed later, but most require pathological confirmation for definite IPD. Calne's clinical classification[17] is less rigid. It has the merit of defining clinically definite IPD, but the earlier caveats regarding postural instability as a cardinal feature in the elderly apply (Table 4.3).

Early features of IPD

Pathological changes and cell loss develop gradually in IPD during an unknown period of time. This preclinical period progresses until the symptomatic threshold of nigral cell loss is reached. A period of delay usually follows before diagnosis is suspected, with the onset of classical motor symptoms. Prodromal features include mood or personality changes, depression, impaired olfaction, limb pain and paraesthesiae, constipation and seborrhoeic dermatitis.[18] Unexplained fatigue may be prominent. Difficulty turning in bed is an early motor problem. Other common symptoms and signs of motor dysfunction in early parkinsonism are shown in Table 4.4.

Tremor in IPD

Tremor is present in 75 per cent of patients at presentation. Most patients with IPD develop tremor, but some may not.[19] Tremor usually begins unilaterally

Table 4.3 Calne classification (From Calne *et al.*, 1992)[17]

- CLINICALLY POSSIBLE IPD: one of the following; tremor (rest or postural), rigidity, or bradykinesia
- CLINICALLY PROBABLE IPD: two of the following cardinal features; resting tremor, rigidity, bradykinesia or postural instability *or* if resting tremor, rigidity, or bradykinesia are asymmetric
- CLINICALLY DEFINITE IPD: three of the cardinal features *or* two cardinal features with one of the first three presenting asymmetrically.

Table 4.4   Common symptoms and signs in early parkinsonism

Face	Reduced facial expression (hypomimia)
Speech	Softer, less distinct, 'boring' with lack of intonation
Postural	Difficulty turning in bed and getting out of chairs and cars
Fine motor tasks	Difficulties with handwriting, doing and undoing buttons, grooming and shaving, using kitchen utensils and tools
Gait	Slowing, dragging of one leg, lack of arm swing
Sensory	Stiffness, pain or discomfort in a limb. May present as 'frozen shoulder'

and distally in a limb, most commonly the arm but may commence in the leg or a single finger. Tremor often spreads proximally in the arm, before involving the ipsilateral leg and finally crossing to the contralateral limbs. Several types of tremor are recognized in IPD:[20]

- Classical 4–6 Hz resting tremor. (Higher-frequency tremor up to 9 Hz, may be found, particularly in the early stages).
- Postural/kinetic tremor may occur in addition to resting tremor; this may have a similar frequency to rest tremor, but can be faster (>1.5 Hz). The higher-frequency tremor may be disabling.
- Isolated postural/kinetic tremor with frequency between 4–9 Hz may occur in the absence of rest tremor.

The characteristic 'pill-rolling' rest tremor, often coupled with flexion extension movements of the fingers and arms is highly suggestive of IPD or drug-induced parkinsonism.[21] Such tremor will usually diminish on movement and during sleep but is enhanced by stress, anxiety and fatigue. As tremor decreases with voluntary movement it may increase asynchronously in the opposite hand. Asking the patient to count backwards will often reveal latent resting tremor. In some cases, the typical pill-rolling resting tremor of IPD is seen only during walking.

Rest tremor in IPD is usually accompanied by akinesia, but a monosymptomatic rest tremor may occur. There may be mild concurrent extra pyramidal signs such as reduced arm swing and facial expression, but other cardinal signs of PD are absent or uncertain. This variant has been labelled 'benign tremulous Parkinson's disease' since little or no progression may occur over a number of years. Functional neuroimaging demonstrates a dopaminergic deficit suggestive of IPD in the majority of such cases.[22]

DIFFERENTIAL DIAGNOSIS OF TREMOR

Essential tremor (ET) is frequently confused for IPD.[9,10] Like IPD, it becomes increasingly common in old age, with prevalence estimates ranging from 13 to 50 cases per 1000 persons over 60 years of age.[23]

ET is a 6–12 Hz bilateral generally symmetrical postural and kinetic tremor maximal in the hands and forearms. There is often a positive family history with autosomal dominant inheritance and a high rate of penetrance, usually before 65 years of age.[24] The severity may vary from a modest low-amplitude tremor with little disability that is partially responsive to alcohol, beta-blockers or primidone, to a severe high-amplitude tremor that causes significant handicap and is resistant to drug therapy. The tremor is generally greatest on sustained posture, but may increase at the termination of a movement. Spillage of cups of tea is a common complaint. Apparent rest tremor of the hands can occur in ET, causing confusion with IPD. ET is usually a vertical up-and-down tremor rather than pill-rolling. Other clues to the presence of ET include concurrent vocal, head (titubation) or neck tremor (no-no or yes-yes movements), all of which are uncommon in IPD. In contrast, jaw or leg tremor is highly suggestive of IPD. Cogwheeling may be found in ET, but not lead pipe rigidity or akinesia.

A postural or kinetic tremor may be seen in association with dystonia and may be misdiagnosed as ET.[25] This type of tremor is often asymmetric or unilateral, and may be task- or position-sensitive, affecting the forearms, hands, neck and voice.[20]

In elderly patients the distinction between ET, dystonic tremor and IPD can be very difficult. Some patients who meet the criteria of ET may manifest other mild extrapyramidal signs of uncertain significance such as modest reduction in facial expression or decreased arm swing. It is suggested that these patients are categorized as indeterminate tremor syndrome.[20] Ongoing clinical review and functional imaging studies may be necessary to clarify the diagnosis.

Other causes of tremor such as drugs (e.g. neuroleptics and anti-emetics), metabolic disorders (e.g. hyperthyroidism), various cerebral disorders including vascular disease, and peripheral neuropathies[20] should not be overlooked in differential diagnosis.

Other features of IPD

COGNITIVE DYSFUNCTION

Prodromal symptoms of IPD include changes in mood and behaviour, but mental status remains relatively normal in early IPD. Signs of significant cognitive impairment at disease onset should suggest other disorders (see Table 4.2). Cognitive problems in IPD are discussed in Chapter 8.

OCULAR DYSFUNCTION

Higher-order oculomotor functions are mildly perturbed in IPD,[26] but *clinically* most systems are preserved – in contrast to the atypical parkinsonian syndromes.[27] Some IPD patients do complain of blurred vision or difficulty reading caused by weak convergence or tracking problems. In a normal elderly population, broken pursuit movements and mild impairment of upward gaze and defective convergence are common.[27] Prominent visual symptoms or gaze paresis should suggest PSP.

Spontaneous eye blinking is reduced in IPD, but less severely than in PSP. Blepharospasm is usually a pointer to another disorder,[9] often PSP. Failure to habituate (continual blinking) when the forehead is tapped is a positive glabellar reflex, or Meyerson's sign. This primitive reflex is seen characteristically in IPD, with and without cognitive impairment, but is not specific for IPD.[3] Pertinent neuro-ophthamological examination in parkinsonism is well summarized by Hardie.[28]

SPEECH AND SWALLOWING, AND AUTONOMIC DYSFUNCTION

The speech of IPD is hypokinetic, typically monotonal, hypophonic and muffled. Early or prominent dysarthria or dysphagia suggest other forms of parkinsonism (see Table 4.2).

Orthostatic hypotension is common in IPD, particularly in the later stages.[29] Commanding or early autonomic dysfunction or bladder symptoms should bring to mind MSA. Concurrent morbidity or drug therapy (including antiparkinsonian drugs) may exacerbate or provoke postural hypotension or sphincter disturbance in IPD patients.

Clinical subtypes of IPD

The broad clinical expression of IPD has led to the concept of subtypes of IPD. Age has emerged as one potential determinant of disease course. More rapidly progressive disease is recognized in the elderly,[13,14] and may be associated with the early postural instability and gait difficulty (PIGD) subtype. Other levodopa-unresponsive features may coexist such as freezing, dysarthria and dementia.[18] Periventricular hyperintensities on magnetic resonance imaging (MRI), which increase with age are reported to be more widespread in patients with more rapid disease progression.[30] Atypical parkinsonian syndromes should be considered[31] in the differential diagnosis in these cases as well as overlap with common disorders such as stroke and Alzheimer's disease. In contrast to PIGD, tremor-dominant IPD is generally reported to be less aggressive and associated with preserved mental status and younger age at onset.[18,32] Other reports, however, suggest that severity of tremor is associated with older age, dementia and to a lesser extent rapid disease progression.[13,33] Variance exists in the literature on this topic and may reflect methodological differences in diagnostic criteria as well as bias in study populations. There is increasing awareness that the phenotype of IPD may have variable genetic causes (see Chapter 2).

Diagnostic criteria for IPD

A number of diagnostic criteria for IPD have been formulated[19,34,35] which usually require the presence of cardinal signs in association with exclusionary and supportive features. Because of the clinical variability in pathologically confirmed IPD, no criteria are ideal, i.e. 100 per cent sensitivity and 100 per cent specificity. Atypical features were present in 12 out of 100 pathologically confirmed cases of IPD.[36] Early autonomic failure occurred in 2 per cent of these cases, which would usually suggest an alternative diagnosis of MSA.

Levodopa responsiveness and dyskinesia are supportive features for IPD in most criteria, yet 2 per cent of autopsy-proven cases show a poor or absent response to levodopa.[36] Conversely, a positive response is not specific to IPD. Patients with both progressive supranuclear palsy and MSA may show an initial response to levodopa. Although this response is usually poorly sustained, some cases of MSA derive benefit from levodopa until death.[37]

Unilateral onset and persistent asymmetry of signs is considered characteristic of IPD, with symmetrical parkinsonism pointing to PSP or MSA. However, symmetrical disease may be more common in older patients with IPD (>70 years of age) compared with those of younger onset.[13] To add to the diagnostic difficulty, symptoms may begin asymmetrically in PSP[38] and may be unilateral in onset in MSA.[38]

Neuropathological brain examination in conjunction with the clinical history is the 'gold standard' for diagnosis of IPD. The United Kingdom Parkinson's Disease Society Brain Bank, clinical diagnostic criteria[34] were established on brain bank experience and are now widely accepted in the UK (Table 4.5). The retrospective application of these criteria in a pathological series[7] produced improvement in diagnostic accuracy from 76 per cent to 82 per cent, but clearly still left 18 per cent of cases misdiagnosed. Using a logistic regression model, selected criteria (asymmetrical onset, no atypical features and no alternative aetiology for parkinsonism) reduced the false positive rate to 7 per cent, but excluded 32 per cent of genuine cases.[16]

Different operational circumstances dictate the degree of stringency for diagnostic criteria. Therapeutic research demands high specificity, whereas epidemiological and clinical practice generally requires more sensitive criteria. This is recognized in using probable and possible categories in some recently developed criteria based on literature review.[19] These await prospective validation with neuropathology.

Pharmacological challenge tests

The response to an acute oral dose of levodopa or apomorphine injection is considered positive when there is an improvement of 20 per cent or better on the Unified Parkinson's Disease Rating Scale (UPDRS) (part 3, motor examination). These pharmacological challenge tests help to determine dopaminergic responsiveness in the short term with reasonable precision,[40] but their use as a diagnostic tool is not recommended by a recent UK guideline group,

Table 4.5 UK Parkinson's Disease Society Brain Bank clinical diagnostic criteria

STEP 1 *Diagnosis of parkinsonian syndrome*
Bradykinesia (slowness of initiation of voluntary movement with progressive reduction in speed and amplitude of repetitive actions) and at least one of the following:
(a) muscular rigidity
(b) 4–6 Hz rest tremor
(c) postural instability not caused by primary visual, vestibular, cerebellar or proprioceptive dysfunction

STEP 2 *Exclusion criteria for Parkinson's disease*
- History of repeated strokes with stepwise progression of parkinsonian features
- History of repeated head injury
- History of definite encephalitis
- Oculogyric crisis
- Neuroleptic treatment at onset of symptoms
- More than one affected relative
- Sustained remission
- Strictly unilateral features after 3 years
- Supranuclear gaze palsy
- Cerebellar signs
- Early severe autonomic involvement
- Early severe dementia with disturbances of memory, language and praxis
- Babinski sign
- Presence of cerebral tumour or communicating hydrocephalus on computed tomography scan
- Negative response to large doses of levodopa (if malabsorption excluded)
- MPTP exposure

STEP 3 *Supportive prospective positive criteria for Parkinson's disease; three or more required for diagnosis of definite Parkinson's disease*
- Unilateral onset
- Rest tremor present
- Progressive disorder
- Presistent asymmetry affecting the side of onset most
- Excellent response (70–100%) to levodopa
- Severe levodopa-induced chorea
- Levodopa response for 5 years or more
- Clinical course of 10 years or more

mainly because of low sensitivity in *de-novo* patients.[41] Other authorities support their utility.[29] One small study in an older parkinsonian group with a mean age of 85 years reported a low false negative rate using levodopa challenge testing.[42] Apomorphine testing avoids the theoretical risk of 'priming' for dyskinesia with levodopa in *de-novo* patients.

Challenge tests may be helpful in the later stages of disease if diagnostic and therapeutic uncertainties persist. A positive challenge test may be useful in demonstrating levodopa response objectively, if the therapeutic benefit is uncertain. A negative test should prompt re-evaluation of the benefit:risk ratio of continuing levodopa therapy, particularly if vascular parkinsonism is suspected. Older patients may be less tolerant of acute doses of levodopa/dopa de-carboxylase inhibitor (and apomorphine), despite domperidone cover.

Neuroimaging

Imaging of the brain is generally unnecessary in patients with features consistent with IPD and a good response to levodopa. However, in the presence of atypical features neuroimaging techniques may be helpful in supporting alternative diagnosis.

Computed tomography (CT) of the brain may identify patients with normal-pressure hydrocephalus, subcortical vascular disease and rarer causes of parkinsonism such as tumours.

MRI may demonstrate abnormalities on T2-weighted images consistent with MSA. Infratentorial abnormalities include atrophy and signal change in the pons and middle cerebellar peduncle. Striatal abnormalities include putaminal atrophy and a hyperintense putaminal rim. These findings have high specificity, but low sensitivity.[43] Atrophy of the mid brain and thinning of the quadrigeminal plate occurs in one-third of patients with PSP.[44] Asymmetrical atrophy of the parietal cortex on MRI is suggestive of corticobasal degeneration.[45] Unfortunately, these MRI changes in the atypical parkinsonian syndromes are usually absent in the early stages of disease when diagnosis is most difficult.

Functional imaging techniques such as single photon emission tomography (SPECT) and positron emission tomography (PET) provide data on dopaminergic system integrity *in vivo*.[46] In IPD, there is degeneration of the presynaptic dopaminergic neurones, but preservation of postsynaptic neurones.[47] Non-idiopathic parkinsonian syndromes such as PSP or MSA demonstrate both pre- and post-synaptic degeneration.[47]

PET scanning is a sensitive functional imaging technique but is expensive and is not widely available. SPECT is more accessible and less costly. SPECT permits the investigation of striatal post-synaptic D2 receptor status using tracers such as ^{123}I-iodobenzamide, a dopamine D2 receptor ligand.[47] This provides a semiquantitative evaluation of receptor status, which calculates the ratio of uptake in specific (striatal) to non-specific (e.g. occipital) areas. Assessment of pre-synaptic dopaminergic terminal function *in vivo* may also be performed using SPECT scanning. A number of SPECT tracers which monitor dopamine transporter function are now under active investigation. These include ^{123}I-beta-carbomethoxy-3-beta(4-iodophenyl)-tropane [beta CIT] and ^{123}I-FP-CIT.[47] Beta CIT requires 24 h of equilibration before scanning, which is inconvenient for both the patient and the laboratory; FP CIT scans can be achieved at 3–6 h after injection. These scans may become a useful diagnostic tool, since normal dopamine transporter status occurs in conditions such as essential tremor.

Present studies suggest that concomitant assessment of dopamine terminal and striatal function with PET or SPECT may help to discriminate atypical syndromes from IPD with up to 80 per cent specificity.[46] Such functional imaging is a burgeoning area of interest, but further studies – preferably with pathological correlation – are required to determine cost effectiveness in routine practice.

Magnetic resonance spectroscopy (MRS) is a non-invasive method of quantitating metabolite changes within the brain. This may be useful in distinguishing IPD from other disorders, but remains a research tool at present.[48]

Parkinsonism plus or atypical parkinsonian syndromes

Progressive supranuclear palsy

Progressive supranuclear palsy or Steele–Richardson–Olszewski syndrome is the most common atypical parkinsonian syndrome after IPD in old age.[49] It is characterized by a vertical supranuclear gaze palsy and early postural instability.

Subcortical-frontal pathways mediating volitional motor activity, saccadic eye movements, executive function, motivation and social behaviour are perturbed in PSP. Major neurotransmitter systems affected include dopaminergic striatonigral pathways, gaba-ergic and cholinoceptive striatal neurones, and the cholinergic brainstem and basal forebrain nuclei.[44]

The average incidence rate is estimated to be 5.3 new cases per 100 000 person-years for ages 50 to 99.[49] The prevalence rate for persons over 55 years is reported as 7 per 100 000.[50] These figures are conservative, since half the disease course usually elapses before diagnosis[45] and many cases are misdiagnosed.[51]

The incidence of PSP rises steeply with age, from 1.7 per 100 000 at 50–59 years to 14.7 per 100 000 at 80–99 years.[49] Median survival time from symptom onset is around 6 (range 2–16) years.[44] Men are more commonly affected than women (male:female ratio, 2:1).

The neuropathology of PSP demonstrates neurofibrillary tangles consisting of tau protein in the striatum, pallidum, subthalamic nucleus, substantia nigra, oculomotor complex, periaqueductal grey matter, superior colliculi, basis pontis and dentate nuclei and medulla with variable neuronal loss and gliosis.[45] Other neurodegenerative disorders such as corticobasal degeneration, post-encephalitic parkinsonism and the parkinsonism–dementia complex of Guam are also characterized by tau deposition in different forms. PSP and these disorders have been classified as 'tauopathies'.

The aetiology of PSP is unknown, but toxic and infectious aetiologies are postulated based on similarities to post-encephalitic parkinsonism and Guam complex. While usually considered a sporadic disease, familial cases are increasingly reported.[52] A recent study of 12 pedigrees suggested that hereditary PSP may be more common than previously thought,[53] probably due to variability in phenotype. Inheritance may be autosomal dominant with variable penetrance in these families.[53] There may also be a genetic predisposition to 'sporadic' PSP. There is an over-representation of the A0 allele of a polymorphic marker of the tau gene in patients with PSP,[54,55] but not corticobasal degeneration or Parkinson's disease.[55] Recent studies further suggest that PSP patients display several polymorphisms in tau, representing an extended tau haplotype (H1) which is more common than in the general population.[56] Interestingly, in Japan the tau A0 allele is as common in PSP patients as in a control population.[57] Non-genetic factors may trigger or accentuate neuronal degeneration in PSP.[44]

The clinical features of IPD, PSP, corticobasal degeneration (CBD) and MSA are shown in Table 4.6.

The onset of disease in PSP is insidious, with symptoms evolving in variable order. The initial features usually differ from those of IPD. Typically, patients present with early postural instability and falls. The gait is ataxic, usually wide-based and upright, and with more preservation of arm swing than IPD. Pseudobulbar palsy with dysphagia is often an early feature, unlike IPD, and may be misdiagnosed as motor neurone disease. Dysarthria is characterized by spasticity and ataxia rather than hypophonia as in IPD. The voice may have a growling quality with involuntary groaning. Perseveration, palilalia (repetition of words) and echolalia may intrude in speech.

Parkinsonism in PSP is characterized by symmetrical bradykinesia and axial more than limb rigidity. Distal limb rigidity and bradykinesia are milder than in IPD, while nuchal rigidity and dystonia are prominent. Levodopa treatment produces a poor or transient response. The rigid neck may become hyperextended and a hyperlordotic erect posture coupled with impairment of righting reflexes leads to *backward* falls. The facial appearance in PSP differs from the classic hypomimia of IPD, and is described as 'worried or astonished'. The eyebrows are often raised due to frontalis overactivity.

Neurobehavioural changes occur commonly in early disease, primarily apathy but also disinhibition, dysphoria, anxiety and emotional lability.[58] Patients may be misdiagnosed as having a dementia or psychosis. Mental and physical slowing and social withdrawal may be misinterpreted as normal ageing. Instability and disinhibition lead to impulsive, often dangerous behaviour at home and in traffic. Sitting is often achieved *'en bloc'* by toppling into a chair. Frontal lobe behaviours such as automatic imitation of gestures, motor perseveration, forced grasping and a tendency to grab objects placed nearby may be commanding as disease progresses.

Visual disturbances such as diplopia, blurred vision, burning eyes and light sensitivity may antedate the appearance of supranuclear gaze palsy.[59] Some patients complain bitterly of unsuitable spectacles, despite repeated attendance at opticians.

SUPRANUCLEAR GAZE PALSY

The hallmark of PSP is a paresis of downward vertical gaze, but this does not begin until a median of four years after disease onset.[50] Spillage of food may be a prominent symptom at this stage. Gaze restriction can be overcome by the oculocephalic or 'doll's head' manoeuvre, indicating a supranuclear origin. Assessment of reflex movements can be hampered by cervical rigidity. Limitation of upward gaze may antedate or exceed downward gaze problems, but this occurs in other neurodegenerative diseases and mild restriction is seen in normal ageing. Limitation of downward gaze is therefore more

Table 4.6 Clinical features of IPD (Idiopathic Parkinson's disease), PSP (progressive supranuclear palsy) CBD (corticobasal degeneration) and MSA (multiple system atrophy)

	IPD	PSP	CBD	MSA
Median age of onset	~ 60 years	~ 70 years	Not Known	~ 50 years
Median survival	~ Normal	~ 6 years	~ 6 years	~ 10 years
Pill rolling tremor	Common	Rare	Absent	Uncommon
Bradykinesia	Asymmetrical	Symmetrical	Strongly asymmetrical at onset	Symmetrical (but asymmetry well recognized)
Rigidity	Asymmetrical	Axial prominent May be extended neck	Strongly asymmetrical at onset	Symmetrical
Falls	Late	Early ~ 1st year Backwards	Late ~ 3+ years (unless leg affected early)	Early ~ 2–3rd year
Gait	Narrow base, stooped, flexed knees	Wide base, erect, extended knees	Variable base Apraxic Freezing	Narrow base, stooped, shuffling, may be ataxic
Autonomic dysfunction	Late, usually mild (may be drug induced)	Rare	Rare	Common, early and severe
Dysarthria and dysphagia	Late	Early	Early	Early
Facial expression	Hypomimia	Worried or astonished	Hypomimia	Hypomimia
Cognitive impairment	Late	Early	Usually later	Rare
Cortical signs	Absent	Absent	Present ± 'alien limb'	Absent
Supranuclear palsy	Absent	Vertical > horizontal	Horizontal = vertical	Horizontal > vertical
Blink rate	Low	Very low	Low	Low
Frontal behaviour	Absent or mild	Severe	Moderate	Absent or mild
Cerebellar signs	Absent	Rare	Rare	Common
Levodopa response	Good, sustained	Absent, poor or unsustained	No response	Absent, poor or unsustained (~30% may respond initially)

specific for PSP. Supranuclear gaze palsies are also reported in patients with dementia with Lewy bodies, MSA, cerebrovascular disease, Creutzfeld–Jacob disease and Huntington's disease.[45] Horizontal rather than vertical gaze is usually more affected in these disorders.

The earliest ocular sign of PSP is generally slowing of vertical saccades.[60] This is tested by asking the patient to make voluntary saccades on command to stationary targets directly ahead and down. Breakdown of optokinetic nystagmus in the vertical plane is also an early sensitive indicator of PSP.[61]

Vertical eye movements are characteristically more affected than horizontal movements in PSP, although in the later stages gaze may be affected in all directions. Pursuit movements are usually preserved initially but become saccadic as disease progresses. In the terminal stages the patient may lose all eye movements, including those to reflex manoeuvres.

Eyelid abnormalities are common in PSP. Blink rate is often reduced to less than 5 per minute, and artificial tears may be required to prevent exposure keratitis. Involuntary eye closure may be noted. Difficulty opening the eyes may be caused by true blepharospasm or levator inhibition due to apraxia. In late disease, the combination of eyelid abnormalities, facial dystonia and gaze abnormalities gives rise to a peculiar staring, non-blinking facies.[59]

COGNITIVE SYNDROME

The cognitive syndrome of PSP generally conforms to a specific pattern comprising cognitive slowing, impairment of executive function and forgetfulness.[62] The cognitive impairment may be severe enough to be considered dementia as disease progresses, although the deficits remain specific. PSP is considered the prototype of subcortical-frontal dementia. Cortical functions such as language, praxis and gnosis are generally unaffected, except for a reduction in spontaneous speech and mild word-finding difficulty.[45] Executive dysfunction and slow information processing is demonstrable with difficulties in initiation and fluency, concept formation and problem solving. Memory function improves in cued recall situations. Bedside and neuropsychological tests useful in defining cognitive abnormalities in PSP have been outlined.[60] In contrast to PSP, frontal lobe features in IPD and MSA are usually mild and often evident only on detailed neuropsychological testing[63] (see also Chapter 8).

Other clinical features of PSP include pyramidal tract signs, cerebellar ataxia, major depression, myoclonus,[59] focal dystonia,[64] sleep disturbances[65] and urinary frequency. Autonomic failure is not part of PSP, but urinary and faecal incontinence[66] as well as orthostatic hypotension can occur in advanced disease. Resting tremor is rare, and usually modest.[59]

CLINICAL VARIANTS

The full-blown picture of PSP is unmistakable, but the spectrum of clinical expression is extremely wide.[51] Lone parkinsonism may occur early in the disease course and be confused with IPD.[59] Some patients with an isolated cognitive syndrome without prominent motor signs may be misdiagnosed as dementia with Lewy bodies, Pick's disease, Creutzfeld–Jacob disease or even Alzheimer's disease, despite the lack of 'cortical' dementia.[51] Asymmetry of signs and limb apraxia, while uncommon and generally mild, may cause diagnostic confusion with corticobasal degeneration.[38]

Ophthalmoplegia never occurs in some cases.[67] These patients are often older with a trend to longer survival, and may represent a pathological subtype of PSP.[68]

Pure akinesia is a recently described syndrome first reported in Japan, characterized by progressive akinesia of gait, speech and handwriting without tremor, rigidity or dementia. It is suggested this is a clinical variant of PSP, and may occur before ocular abnormalities.[69]

Multiple lacunar infarcts in old age may mimic the clinical syndrome of PSP.[70]

DIAGNOSTIC CRITERIA

Different sets of criteria have been proposed for the diagnosis of PSP.[38,51,59] An international workshop[60] has published a set of diagnostic criteria based on literature review and expert consensus which aim to improve diagnostic accuracy specifying levels of diagnostic certainty. These criteria await external validation, but when tested in a detailed autopsy- confirmed set of cases, the criteria for probable PSP were highly specific (100 per cent) though not very sensitive (50 per cent). The possible criteria achieved 83 per cent sensitivity and 93 per cent specificity. The latter possible criteria are more suitable for clinical care, but show similar positive predictive value (~80 per cent) to Lees earlier criteria which are less rigid.[59]

Corticobasal degeneration

Corticobasal degeneration CBD (also known as corticobasal ganglionic degeneration) is a rare sporadic progressive neurodegenerative disorder with onset in the sixth decade or later. Recent evidence based on the neurochemistry of different tau isoforms suggests that PSP and CBD are closely related and comprise a distinct group of neurodegenerative disorders.[71] Neuropathological features in CBD may overlap not only with PSP, but also with Alzheimer's disease and focal or asymmetric cortical degenerations such as Pick's disease, frontotemporal dementia and amyotrophic lateral sclerosis with frontal dementia.[72] Immunohistochemistry[73] and molecular neuropathology[74] however will discriminate between these disorders, suggesting that CBD is a specific clinicopathological entity. Neuropathology shows neuronal loss and formation of ballooned achromatic neurones in the cortex and degeneration of substantia nigra. A tau immunoreactive neuronal inclusion body (corticobasal inclusion) found in the cortex and substantia nigra is characteristic.[73]

Other heterogeneous substrates including Pick's disease, Alzheimer's disease, PSP and cerebrovascular disease may produce a *clinical syndrome* of CBD if the lesions correspond to the classical topography of the disorder.[75] No data are available on prevalence or incidence, but CBD is probably underdiagnosed.[76] Median survival is 6–8 years.[77,78]

CLINICAL FEATURES[78]

The clinical features of CBD are listed in Table 4.6. CBD usually includes a combination of:

- movement disorders (asymmetric akinesia and rigidity not responsive to levodopa, limb dystonia, focal stimulus sensitive myoclonus, action tremor, postural instability);
- higher cortical dysfunction (ideomotor or ideational apraxia, alien limb, cortical sensory loss, dementia, aphasia, frontal release reflexes); and
- other manifestations (supranuclear gaze palsy, pyramidal tract signs, pseudobulbar palsy, cerebellar signs, pain).

The most common presenting complaint is clumsiness of one hand and arm.[79] Classically, patients develop a unilateral jerky, tremulous, akinetic rigid and apraxic extremity, usually the arm, with accompanying dystonia. The posture is often of a flexed hand and forearm with adduction of the arm. Cortical sensory signs develop concurrently in the form of agraphesthesia, astereognosis and tactile sensory extinction. Ideomotor apraxia[80] (difficulty initiating voluntary movements, making fine finger movements and copying hand postures) is a key finding[76] in CBD. Apraxia can be masked by concurrent rigidity and immobility as the limb progresses to functional uselessness. Examining the opposite limb may reveal an abnormality even if asymptomatic, indicating early involvement of the contralateral cortex.

The well-recognized 'alien limb phenomenon' (ALP) is very suggestive of CBD but is variably present[79] and not entirely specific.[81] Such an 'alien limb' has 'a mind of its own', drifting uncontrollably into space or crossing the midline and interfering with the contralateral limb or the examiner. Complex behaviour (groping and manipulation) should be present for true ALP rather than simple levitation with non-purposeful behaviour.

Symptoms and signs in CBD usually spread over a number of years to the ipsilateral or to the corresponding contralateral limb, but remain distinctly asymmetric. Rigid immobility ensues in the terminal phase with hypostatic complications.

DIAGNOSTIC PROBLEMS

The clinical features of CBD show considerable heterogeneity and may include dementia and altered behaviour with mild, delayed or absent motor symptoms in a minority of patients.[77,82] CBD can be confused with PSP, but cognitive problems and difficulty in walking usually occur rather later in CBD (unless the leg is affected first).[45] Limb dystonia may be an early feature in some cases of PSP which are misdiagnosed initially as CBD.[64]

In contrast to PSP, the supranuclear gaze palsy in CBD equally affects both horizontal and vertical gaze. The gaze abnormality in early disease is apraxic, with patients struggling to generate saccades to command.[26,45] Prominent eye blinks or head thrusts may be used to initiate saccade generation. Once achieved, gaze may be unrestricted. Such difficulties are most prominent in the direction of the more affected side of the body. These findings, combined with jerky pursuit movements maximal in the opposite direction, strongly suggest CBD as being the cause of the gaze palsy.[27]

In early disease an asymmetrical rigid syndrome may be mistaken for IPD. Helpful distinguishing features include lack of response to levodopa and cortical signs. The eye movement abnormalities exceed those of comparable IPD patients.[26] Myoclonus of the fingers and jerky action tremor are distinct from classical IPD rest tremor.[79]

Multiple system atrophy

Multiple system atrophy is a sporadic, progressive neurodegenerative disorder of unknown aetiology, characterized by any combination of parkinsonism and cerebellar, autonomic, urinary and pyramidal dysfunction. Neuropathology demonstrates neuronal loss and gliosis in some or all of the following: inferior olives, pons, cerebellum, substantia nigra, locus coeruleus, striatum and interomedial lateral columns of the spinal cord. Lewy bodies are usually absent.

MSA includes those disorders previously separated into three clinical syndromes referred to as: (i) striatonigral degeneration (SND), where parkinsonism predominates; (ii) sporadic olivopontocerebellar atrophy (OPCA), where cerebellar signs predominate; and (iii) Shy–Drager syndrome (SDS), where autonomic failure is commanding. It is now recognized that these divisions are rather artificial.[83] Although these subtypes express the predominant clinical presentation, as disease progresses a mixture of clinical features will emerge.[37,39] The discovery of abundant ubiquitin, tau and α-synuclein-positive glial cytoplasmic inclusion (GCI) bodies in the brains of patients with MSA has defined a characteristic pathological marker for the condition,[84] suggesting that SND, sporadic OPCA and SDS are different clinical phenotypes of the same disease.[85] The term MSA should not be used interchangeably for multisystem degeneration, being but one specific cause of neurodegeneration of multiple neuronal systems.

The epidemiology of MSA is poorly defined. Highly selective autopsy series suggest that MSA represents 3–22 per cent of incident cases of parkinsonism.[86] The only population study available reported an incidence rate of 3.0 per 100 000 for age 55–99 years for MSA, but age and sex subclasses were not stable.[49] Striatonigral degeneration (with postural hypotension in 50 per cent), accounted for 40 per cent of misdiagnosis of IPD at death in one autopsy series.[8]

MSA is reputed to occur most commonly in middle age,[87] but cases are seen until at least the ninth decade.[49] Median survival is around 8–10 years.[37,49] Older age at onset is associated with shorter survival.[37]

Clinical features

AUTONOMIC DYSFUNCTION

The clinical features of MSA (see Table 4.6) related to autonomic dysfunction, include orthostatic hypotension, urinary and male erectile dysfunction, constipation and decreased sweating.

Autonomic dysfunction (AuD) is invariable during the disease course,[37] but may be absent at disease onset. Orthostatic hypotension (OH) may be symptomatic or asymptomatic. Postural faintness is reported more commonly than recurrent syncope,[37] but this may represent selection bias of more prominent parkinsonism from movement disorder clinics. Since patients with IPD also develop AuD, distinction from MSA can be difficult. AuD in MSA tends to affect more than one autonomic domain, is generally more severe, and may antedate parkinsonism.[88] The older patient with parkinsonism may have other concurrent causes for OH such as drug treatment, diabetes mellitus and cerebrovascular disease. Neurovascular instability and OH may be prominent in dementia with Lewy bodies and Alzheimer's disease.[89] Diagnosis of MSA should be circumspect if AuD is limited to one domain.

Bladder dysfunction is an important indicator of possible MSA.[90] Atrophy of the brainstem leads to detrusor hyperreflexia, while loss of anterior horn cells in Onuf's nucleus produces sphincter weakness. Cell loss in the interomediolateral columns impairs parasympathetic innervation of the bladder and causes atonia with retention and overflow incontinence. Detrusor instability may be an early feature, with progression to failure of bladder emptying and high residual volume.[90] In the elderly, other potential causes of urinary dysfunction, such as abnormal detrusor behaviour, concomitant cerebral and urological pathology (including prostatic outflow obstruction in men) should be considered before attributing symptoms to MSA.

Impotence is the most common early sign of AuD in males with MSA, but is a non-specific feature in older men. Stridor is strongly suggestive of MSA.[87]

PARKINSONISM

Parkinsonism is the most common initial motor disorder in MSA, even allowing for ascertainment bias.[91] Severe and early dysphagia and dysarthria, as well as pseudobulbar crying or laughing, are characteristic of MSA. Speech is typically slurred with hypophonic monotony, sometimes with a scanning quality where cerebellar dysfunction is prominent, followed in later disease by a quivering strained quality of voice. Tremor in MSA tends to be jerky and irregular. Pill-rolling tremor is uncommon.

CEREBELLAR DYSFUNCTION

A pure cerebellar syndrome is uncommon in MSA,[85] but cerebellar features often coexist with parkinsonism.[39] Cerebellar signs seen in MSA include gait ataxia, finger nose or heel shin dysmetria, intention tremor and nystagmus. Various other eye signs are described with disproportionate impairment of slow phase eye movements.[27] Smooth pursuit movements commonly become saccadic. Mild supranuclear palsy may occur in any direction of gaze in MSA. Marked supranuclear downgaze palsy with significant slowing of saccades suggests PSP. Cerebellar signs may be difficult to discern in late disease, when parkinsonism is pronounced.

PYRAMIDAL DYSFUNCTION

Pyramidal tract signs (extensor plantar responses and hyperreflexia) are common in MSA, but weakness and spastic gait are not. Pyramidal tract signs in older patients with parkinsonism may be due to comorbid cerebrovascular disease or cervical myelopathy.

OTHER CLINICAL POINTERS TO MSA

Disproportionate antecollis, contracted or dusky violaceous extremities and wheelchair dependence are other pointers to MSA.[9] Rapid eye movement (REM) sleep behaviour disorder occurs in several neurodegenerative conditions including IPD, but is very common in MSA and may antedate other CNS symptoms by years.[92] Episodes of intense sleep-related vocalizations or extreme motor activity occur during REM sleep without loss of muscle tone and are accompanied by subsequent recall of vivid dreaming. Dementia is not part of MSA, but a dysexecutive syndrome similar to IPD may occur.[63] A mild peripheral neuropathy is reported in some cases.[87]

LEVODOPA RESPONSE

Absent, poor or waning response to levodopa is a hallmark of MSA; however, ~30 per cent of patients may have a good initial response to levodopa, falling to around 10 per cent in late disease.[37,87] Dyskinesia due to levodopa may be atypical and are often unilateral or dystonic, affecting the head, face and neck.[87]

DIAGNOSTIC PROBLEMS

There is a low clinical sensitivity for the diagnosis of MSA.[91] Neurologists with expertise in movement disorders correctly identified only 25 per cent and 50 per cent of patients with MSA at the first and last clinic visit, on average six years after symptom onset.[93] Early severe autonomic failure, absence of cognitive impairment, early cerebellar symptoms and early gait disturbance were identified as the best predictive features for MSA.[93] However, gait disturbance and instability within the first year of disease onset suggests PSP.[66] Gait abnormality in MSA usually emerges two to three years after symptom onset.

MSA presenting as pure parkinsonism causes most diagnostic confusion with IPD.[94] Rapid progression, symmetrical onset, absence of tremor at onset and no response to levodopa were reported to be more positively associated with MSA than IPD in 16 consecutive autopsy cases of MSA.[95] However, parkinsonism was asymmetric in 74 per cent of 100 patients in a clinical series,[37] and unilateral in onset in 49 per cent of 203 literature cases.[39]

DIAGNOSTIC CRITERIA

Diagnostic criteria for MSA have been formulated by Quinn and Wenning[87] and by a consensus committee of the American Autonomic Society and the American Academy of Neurology.[83,96]

Patients are classified as MSA-P if parkinsonian features predominate, or MSA-C if cerebellar features predominate.[83] These terms are intended to replace the SND and sporadic OPCA types of MSA.

Urogenital criteria which favour a diagnosis of MSA include urinary symptoms preceding or presenting with parkinsonism, urinary incontinence, post-micturition residual volume >100 ml, and worsening bladder control after urological surgery.[90]

In elderly patients, a high prevalence of concurrent pathology may simulate features of MSA and impair the specificity of diagnostic criteria. Characteristically, autonomic, urinary and corticospinal dysfunction should not be explained by drug therapy or other pathology.[96]

Laboratory tests including autonomic function tests, sphincter electromyography, neuroimaging and neuroendocrine testing[97] may support the diagnosis of MSA, but lack sensitivity in early disease.[83]

Other neurodegenerative disorders associated with parkinsonism

Dementia with Lewy bodies

Dementia with Lewy bodies (DLB) is characterized by a progressive dementia with a fluctuating course, extrapyramidal signs (EPS), visual hallucinations and increased sensitivity to neuroleptic drugs. Patients may present with cognitive impairment or with EPS. Whether DLB is a distinct nosological entity or represents one part of the spectrum of Lewy body diseases that includes IPD is uncertain. There is as yet, no clear agreement in the literature regarding a difference (if any) in the profile of the parkinsonian syndrome in DLB as compared with IPD; this may reflect bias in retrospective retrieval of data in autopsy studies as well as differing 'sampling' times during disease progression.

One autopsy-based study which examined early clinical features suggested that asymmetric parkinsonism, levodopa-induced dyskinesia and absence of cognitive impairment are likely indicators of IPD, while early hallucinations, absence of tremor, bradykinesia and dystonia point to DLB.[98] In contrast, another pathological study[99] reported that rest tremor was more common in IPD (85 per cent) than in DLB (55 per cent), and that myoclonus was more common in DLB (18.5 per cent) than in IPD (0 per cent), but found no other differences in EPS. A clinically based study[100] suggested that EPS in DLB were broadly similar to IPD, although symmetry of signs, absence of rest tremor and greater rigidity favoured a diagnosis of DLB.

Alzheimer's disease

Extrapyramidal signs are common in patients with Alzheimer's disease (AD).[101] Rigidity and bradykinesia are most prevalent, with resting tremor and abnormalities of gait less frequent.[101,102] EPS can be detected at any stage of the dementing process, but are more common in the later stages of illness.[102] AD patients with EPS have greater cognitive and functional impairment than those without EPS.[103]

AD and IPD are generally considered distinct nosological entities, but increasing evidence suggests that there are clinical and neuropathological overlaps,[101] with almost 30 per cent of the UK brain bank series having Alzheimer pathology.[7] Similarly, nigral Lewy bodies are commonly found in AD patients, suggesting an 'additional' diagnosis of IPD.[101]

Secondary causes of parkinsonism

Drug-induced parkinsonism

Drug-induced parkinsonism (DIP) is a common cause of parkinsonism in elderly patients,[6] and may affect up to 40 per cent of exposed individuals.[104] In a US Medicaid programme, elderly patients taking neuroleptics were 5.4 times more likely to begin anti-parkinsonian drugs than were non-users.[105]

Neuroleptic drugs (dopamine receptor-blocking compounds such as phenothiazines, butyrephenones, thioxanthenes and benzamides or dopamine-depleting drugs such as reserpine, tetrabenazine) are most often involved as precipitants. Substituted benzamides such as metoclopramide, or prochlorperazine (a phenothiazine derivative) are often prescribed for non-psychiatric conditions such as nausea or 'dizziness' in elderly patients, and these drugs are commonly implicated in DIP.

Apart from advancing age, reported risk factors for DIP include female gender[6] and high drug dosage,[105] but a clear dose–response curve has not been established.[104] Neuroleptic-induced parkinsonism generally starts within three months, usually 10–30 days after beginning treatment, but immediate onset within hours of exposure or more delayed emergence has been reported.[104]

Certain neuroleptic drugs such as thioridazine are considered to have less propensity to cause parkinsonism than haloperidol or chlorpromazine, but well-controlled studies are lacking. Newer 'atypical neuroleptics' such as clozapine, olanzapine or quetiapine may produce less extrapyramidal effects, but comparative dose–response studies in elderly subjects are required for confirmation.

Calcium channel-blocking drugs may possess anti-dopaminergic effects[104] and are recognized as a cause of DIP. Most substantiated are reports implicating the piperazine derivatives, flunarizine and cinnarizine.[106]

A number of other agents are reported to provoke DIP, but the putative mechanism and role of these agents in causation is unclear. Amiodarone and sodium valproate cause postural tremor,[20] and some cases of DIP have been described.[104,106] Isolated case reports of DIP exist for sundry drugs including lithium, sulindac, phenelzine, procaine, meperidine, amphotericin, captopril, cephaloridine and various cytotoxic agents.[104] Selective serotonin re-uptake inhibitor antidepressant drugs such as fluoxetine have been implicated in DIP, but a significant association appears unlikely.[1,106]

CLINICAL FEATURES

Drug-induced parkinsonism is classically a symmetrical akinetic rigid syndrome. Some cases may be indistinguishable from IPD, with asymmetric onset and resting tremor. Supporting features for the diagnosis of DIP include concurrent high-frequency (7–8 Hz) postural or action tremor, perioral tremor (rabbit syndrome), superimposed tardive dyskinesia and akathisia. Resolution of DIP usually occurs within three months following drug withdrawal, but some patients may have signs for up to one year before remission.[104] In a proportion of affected individuals, parkinsonism may persist or recur with progression to IPD. DIP appears to be a risk factor for subsequent development of IPD.[107] These patients may have a subclinical dopamine deficiency which has been unmasked by dopaminergic blockade or depletion. PET studies support this proposal. While reduced fluorodopa uptake on PET scanning does not invariably predict worsening parkinsonism in DIP, a normal PET scan correlates well with recovery.[108]

Normal-pressure hydrocephalus

At all ages, an akinetic rigid syndrome may complicate non-communicating hydrocephalus.[109] In older patients, normal-pressure hydrocephalus (NPH) has received most attention as a cause of parkinsonism.[110]

The clinical syndrome of NPH includes the gradual onset of gait disturbance, incontinence and dementia, but all three components may not always be present. The gait abnormalities may comprise elements of magnetic gait, start hesitation, apraxia and ataxia with a lurching quality. Characteristic features include a wide base, normal leg function when recumbent, poor tandem gait, brisk leg tendon jerks and spasticity. In addition to gait disturbance, other typical features of parkinsonism have been described in NPH, including rest tremor, hypomimia, hypophonia, decreased arm swing, akinesia and rigidity.[109] Parkinsonism may or may not improve with levodopa.[109]

Vascular parkinsonism

Macdonald Critchley introduced the term arteriosclerotic parkinsonism in 1929, reporting that a flexed posture, slowness of movement and a shuffling gait might be produced by 'cerebral arteriosclerosis'. Criticism of this concept followed, and Critchley redefined the syndrome in 1981 as arteriosclerotic pseudoparkinsonism,[111] as distinct from Parkinson's disease. He recognized that the disorder occurred mainly in elderly hypertensive patients, and was associated with a stepwise progression. Other clinical features included pyramidal and pseudobulbar signs, emotional lability, dementia, absence of tremor and a poor response to L-dopa (levodopa).

Since then, a number of different terms such as lower-body parkinsonism,[112] lower-half parkinsonism,[113] vascular pseudoparkinsonism[114] or simply vascular parkinsonism[115] have been employed in the literature to describe a similar syndrome occurring in association with neuroimaging evidence of subcortical ischaemia or lacunar infarcts. Although the relevance of these vascular lesions as a cause of the clinical features remains controversial,[116] increasing evidence supports a causal relationship. Intrinsic vascular lesions of the basal ganglia or disruption of frontostriatal pathways are suggested as plausible mechanisms.[115]

In MRI studies, subcortical white matter lesions appear more prevalent in patients with 'suspected vascular parkinsonism' (lower-half parkinsonism with frontal gait disorder) than in those with IPD or hypertension.[117] Two different types of vascular parkinsonism have been postulated.[117] First, an acute onset is reported with lesions predominantly affecting the subcortical grey nuclei (striatum, globus pallidus and thalamus); second, a more insidious onset is seen with diffuse subcortical white matter lesions. Territorial stroke is less commonly associated with parkinsonian signs than are lacunar events.[118]

Recent clinicopathological studies are of interest. Binswanger's disease (BD) or subcortical arteriosclerotic encephalopathy generally occurs in patients with vascular risk factors, and may present with a gait disorder with elements of parkinsonism and ataxia. Reports of levodopa-responsive parkinsonism (with no concurrent Lewy body pathology) and a progressive supranuclear palsy-like syndrome have recently extended the clinical spectrum of BD.[119]

Predominantly symmetrical axial parkinsonism occurring in two men in their ninth decade has been reported in association with dilatation of the perivascular spaces (*état criblé*) of the striatum confirmed with neuropathology.[120] One case also had typical pathology of IPD.

Because of the heterogeneity of clinical expression and course in previous studies, a precise definition of vascular parkinsonism is elusive. Typically, core features comprise predominant lower-body parkinsonism , pyramidal tract and pseudobulbar signs , associated risk factors for stroke, absence of tremor and poorer response to levodopa than in IPD.[112,121,122] Less commonly, basal ganglia lacunar states may produce a clinical syndrome that is indistinguishable from IPD, including levodopa responsiveness.[123,124] Resting tremor of non-pill-rolling type was reported in nearly 20 per cent of stroke patients with one or more parkinsonian signs.[118]

Most reports highlight the abnormality of gait[112,114,115,121] in VP, while noting a relative absence of parkinsonian features above the waist. A recent study of subcortical arteriosclerotic encephalopathy has emphasized the relationship to ataxia.[125]

The nosology of gait disorders associated with cerebral ischaemia remains confusing. Higher-level gait disorders as described by Nutt *et al.*[126] provide a useful operational classification, but overlap is common in practice. Variability in gait performance is often observed in these patients and may reflect the degree of emotional arousal or the presence or absence of internal or external cueing mechanisms.

The concept of vascular parkinsonism remains under debate but different phenotypes of parkinsonism, associated with cerebrovascular disease are recognized (Table 4.7). IPD and cerebrovascular disease are both common disorders of the elderly: coexistent pathology may produce an 'overlap syndrome' with some degree of slowing, rigidity or gait disturbance attributable to vascular disease. This should be considered as a cause of disproportionate motor disability and disappointing levodopa response in older patients with IPD.

Table 4.7 Cerebrovascular disease and associated parkinsonian syndromes

- Lower-body parkinsonism
  (prominent gait disturbance, absent or atypical resting tremor, poor levodopa response)
- Progressive supranuclear palsy-like syndrome
- Unilateral parkinsonism
- Parkinsonism indistinguishable from IPD
- Overlap syndromes associated with comorbid Lewy body and cerebrovascular pathology

Conclusions

Idiopathic Parkinson's disease and other parkinsonian syndromes are clinical diagnoses, and ongoing review of atypical features for IPD will increase the diagnostic accuracy. A summary of a practical clinical approach for diagnosis is shown in Fig. 4.1. Neuroimaging may be used as an adjunct to clinical diagnosis in the presence of atypical features or a poor or unsustained response to dopaminergic therapy.

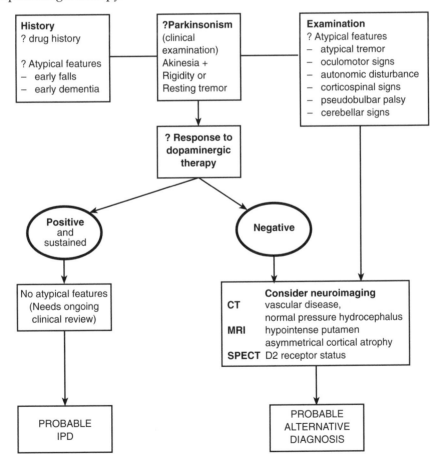

Fig. 4.1 Diagnostic approach for idiopathic Parkinson's disease (IPD).

References

1. Riley DE, Lang AE. Non Parkinson akinetic rigid syndromes. *Curr. Opin. Neurol.* 1996; **9**: 321–6.
2. Louis ED, Marder K, Cote L, *et al.* Prevalence of a history of shaking in persons 65 years of age and older: diagnostic and functional correlates. *Movement Disord* 1996; **11**: 63–9.
3. Waite LM, Broe GA, Creasey H, Grayson D, Edelbrock D, O'Toole B. Neurological signs, aging, and the neurodegenerative syndromes. *Arch. Neurol.* 1996; **53**: 498–502.
4. Bennet DA, Beckett LA, Murray AM, *et al.* Prevalence of parkinsonian signs and associated mortality in a community population of older people. *N. Engl. J. Med.* 1996; **334**: 71–6.
5. Moghal S, Rajput AH, D'Arcy C, Rajput R. Prevalence of movement disorders in elderly community residents. *Neuroepidemiology* 1994; **13**: 175–8.
6. Bower JH, Maraganore DM, McDonnell SK, *et al.* Incidence and distribution of parkinsonism in Olmstead County, Minnesota 1976–1990. *Neurology* 1999; **52**: 1214–20.
7. Hughes AJ, Daniel SE, Kilford L, Lees AJ. Accuracy of clinical diagnosis of idiopathic Parkinson's disease: a clinico-pathological study of 100 cases. *J. Neurol. Neurosurg. Psychiatry* 1992; **55**: 181–4.
8. Rajput AH, Rozdilsky R, Rajput A. Accuracy of clinical diagnosis in parkinsonism – a prospective study. *Can. J. Neurol. Sci.* 1991; **18**: 275–8.
9. Quinn N. Parkinsonism – recognition and differential diagnosis. *Br. Med. J.* 1995; **310**: 447–52.
10. Meara J, Bhowmick BK, Hobson P. Accuracy of diagnosis in patients with presumed Parkinson's disease. *Age Ageing* 1999; **28**: 99–103.
11. Rajput AH. Movement disorders and aging. In: Watts RL, Koller WC (eds). *Movement Disorders: Neurological Principles and Practice.* New York: McGraw Hill, 1997: 673–86.
12. van Hilten JJ, Braat AM, van der Velde EA, *et al.* Hypokinesia in Parkinson's disease: influence of age, disease severity, and disease duration. *Movement Disord.* 1995; **10**: 424–32.
13. Hely MA, Morris JGL, Reid WGJ, *et al.* Age at onset: the major determinant of outcome in Parkinson's disease. *Acta Neurol. Scand.* 1995; **92**: 455–63.
14. Diamond SG, Markham CH, Hoehn MM, McDowell FH, Muenter MD. Effect of age at onset on progression and mortality in Parkinson's disease. *Neurology* 1989; **39**: 1190.
15. Charlett A, Weller C, Purkiss AG, Dobbs SM, Dobbs RJ. Breadth of base whilst walking: effect of ageing and parkinsonism. *Age Ageing* 1998; **27**: 49–54.
16. Hughes AJ, Ben-Shlomo Y, Daniel SE, Lees AJ. What features improve the accuracy of clinical diagnosis in Parkinson's disease: a clinicopathologic study. *Neurology* 1992; **42**: 1142–6.
17. Calne D, Snow BJ, Lee C. Criteria for diagnosing Parkinson's disease. *Ann. Neurol.* 1992; **32**: 125–7.
18. Poewe WH, Wenning GK. The natural history of Parkinson's disease. *Ann. Neurol.* 1998; **44**: S1–9.
19. Gelb DJ, Oliver E, Gilman S. Diagnostic criteria for Parkinson disease. *Arch. Neurol.* 1999; **56**: 33–9.
20. Deuschl G, Bain P, Brin M, Ad Hoc Scientific Committee. Consensus Statement of the Movement Disorder Society on Tremor. *Movement Disord.* 1998; **13**: 2–23.

21. Quinn NP. Parkinson's disease: clinical features. In: Quinn NP (ed.). *Bailliere's Clinical Neurology: Parkinsonism*. London: Bailliere Tindall, 1997: 1–13.

22. Brooks DJ, Playford ED, Ibantz V, *et al.* Isolated tremor and disruption of the nigrostriatal pathway. *Neurology* 1992; **42**: 1554–60.

23. Louis ED, Ottman R, Hauser WA. How common is the most common adult movement disorder? Estimates of the prevalence of essential tremor throughout the world. *Movement Disord.* 1998; **13**: 5–10.

24. Bain P, Findley LJ, Thompson PD, *et al.* A study of hereditary essential tremor. *Brain* 1994; **117**: 805–24.

25. Schrag A, Muenchau A, Bhatia K, Quinn NP, Marsden CD. Overdiagnosis of essential tremor. *Lancet* 1999; **353**: 1498–9.

26. Vidailhet M, Rivaud S, Goulder-Khouja N, *et al.* Eye movements in parkinsonian syndromes. *Ann. Neurol.* 1994; **35**: 420–6.

27. Stell R, Bronstein AM. Eye movement abnormalities in extrapyramidal disease. In: Marsden CD, Fahn S (eds). *Movement Disorders 3*. Oxford: Butterworth Heinemann, 1994: 88–116.

28. Hardie R. The differential diagnosis of Parkinson's disease. *Rev. Clin. Gerontol.* 1995; **5**: 155–63.

29. Pogarell O, Oertel WH. Parkinsonian syndromes and Parkinson's disease. In: Le Witt P, Oertel WH (eds). *Parkinson's Disease: The Treatment Options*. London: Martin Dunitz, 1999: 1–10.

30. Piccini P, Pavese N, Canapicchi R, *et al.* White matter hyperintensities in Parkinson's disease. *Arch. Neurol.* 1995; **52**: 191–4.

31. Rajput AH, Pahwa R, Pahwa P, Rajput A. Prognostic significance of the onset mode in parkinsonism. *Neurology* 1993; **43**: 829–30.

32. Roos RAC, Jongen JCF, van der Velde EA. Clinical course of patients with idiopathic Parkinson's disease. *Movement Disord.* 1996; **11**: 236–42.

33. Friedman A. Old onset Parkinson's disease compared with young onset disease: clinical differences and similarities. *Acta Neurol. Scand.* 1994; **89**: 258–61.

34. Gibb WR, Lees AJ. The relevance of the Lewy body to the pathogenesis of idiopathic Parkinson's disease. *J. Neurol. Neurosurg. Psychiatry* 1988; **51**: 752.

35. Ward CD, Gibb WR. Research diagnostic criteria for Parkinson's disease. *Adv. Neurol.* 1990; **53**: 245–9.

36. Hughes AJ, Daniel SE, Blankson S, Lees AJ. A Clinicopathologic study of 100 cases of Parkinson's disease. *Arch. Neurol.* 1993; **50**: 140–8.

37. Wenning GK, Ben-Shlomo Y, Magalhaes M, Daniel SE, Quinn NP. Clinical features and natural history of multiple system atrophy: an analysis of 100 cases. *Brain* 1994; **117**: 835–45.

38. Collins SJ, Ahlskog JE, Parisi JE, Maraganore DM. Progressive supranuclear palsy: neuropathologically based diagnostic clinical criteria. *J. Neurol. Neurosurg. Psychiatry* 1995; **58**: 167–73.

39. Wenning GK, Tison F, Ben-Shlomo Y, Daniel SE, Quinn NP. Multiple system atrophy: a review of 203 pathologically proven cases. *Movement Disord.* 1997; **12**: 133–47.

40. Hughes AJ, Lees AJ, Stern GM. Apomorphine test to predict dopaminergic responsiveness in parkinsonian syndromes. *Lancet* 1990; **336**: 32–4.

41. Bhatia K, Brooks DJ, Burn DJ, *et al.* Guidelines for the management of Parkinson's disease. *Hospital Med.* 1998; **59**: 469–79.

42. D'Costa DF, Sheehan LJ, Phillips PA, Moore-Smith B. The levodopa test in Parkinson's disease. *Age Ageing* 1995; **24**: 210–12.

43. Schrag A, Kingsley D, Phatouros C, *et al.* Clinical usefulness of magnetic resonance imaging in multiple system atrophy. *J. Neurol. Neurosurg. Psychiatry* 1998; **65**: 65–71.

44. Litvan I. Progressive supranuclear palsy revisited. *Acta Neurol. Scand.* 1998; **98**: 73–84.
45. Litvan I. Progressive supranuclear palsy and corticobasal degeneration. In: Quinn NP (ed.). *Bailliere's Clinical Neurology: Parkinsonism.* London: Bailliere Tindall, 1997: 167–85.
46. Brooks DJ. The early diagnosis of Parkinson's disease. *Ann. Neurol.* 1998; **44**: S10–18.
47. Stoessl AJ, Ruth TJ. Neuroreceptor imaging: new developments in PET and SPECT imaging of neuroreceptor binding (including dopamine transporters, vesicle transporters and post synaptic receptor sites). *Curr. Opin. Neurol.* 1998; **11**: 327–33.
48. Davie C. The role of spectroscopy in parkinsonism. *Movement Disord.* 1998; **13**: 2–4.
49. Bower JH, Maraganore DM, McDonnell SK, Rocca MS, Rocca WA. Incidence of progressive supranuclear palsy and multiple system atrophy in Olmsted County, Minnesota, 1976 to 1990. *Neurology* 1997; **49**: 1284–8.
50. Golbe LI, David PH, Schoenberg BS, Duvoisin RC. Prevalence and natural history of progressive supranuclear palsy. *Neurology* 1988; **38**: 1031–4.
51. Valldeoriola F, Tolosa E, Valls-Sole J. Differential diagnosis and clinical diagnostic criteria of progressive supranuclear palsy. In: Battistin L, Scarlato G, Caraceni T, Ruggieri S (eds). *Advances in Neurology.* Philadelphia: Lippincott-Raven, 1996: 405–11.
52. Tetrud JW, Golbe LI, Forno LS, Farmer PM. Autopsy proven progressive supranuclear palsy in two siblings. *Neurology* 1996; **46**: 931–4.
53. Rojo A, Pernaute RS, Fontan A, *et al.* Clinical genetics of familial progressive supranuclear palsy. *Brain* 1999; **122**: 1233–45.
54. Higgins J, Litvan I, Pho L, Li W, Nee L. Progressive supranuclear palsy is in linkage dysequilibrium with the tau and not the alpha synuclein gene. *Neurology* 1998; **50**: 270–3.
55. Morris HM, Janssen JC, Bandemann O, *et al.* The tau gene A0 polymorphism in progressive supranuclear palsy and related neurodegenerative diseases. *J. Neurol. Neurosurg. Psychiatry* 1999; **66**: 663–7.
56. Baker M, Litvan I, Houlden H, Adamson J, Dickson D, Perez Tur J. Association of an extended haplotype in the tau gene with progressive supranuclear palsy. *Hum. Mol. Genet.* 1999; **8**: 711–15.
57. Conrad C, Amano N, Andreadis A, Xia Y, Namekataf K, Oyama F. Differences in a dinucleotide repeat polymorphism in the tau gene between Caucasian and Japanese populations: implication for progressive supranuclear palsy. *Neurosci. Lett.* 1998; **250**: 135–7.
58. Litvan I, Mega MS, Cummings JL, Fairbanks L. Neuropsychiatric aspects of progressive supranuclear palsy. *Neurology* 1996; **47**: 1184–9.
59. Lees AJ. The Steele–Richardson–Olszewski syndrome (progressive supranuclear palsy). In: Marsden CD, Fahn S (eds). *Movement Disorders 2.* Oxford: Butterworth Heinemann, 1987: 272–87.
60. Litvan I, Agid Y, Calne D, *et al.* Clinical research criteria for the diagnosis of progressive supranuclear palsy (Steel–Richardson–Olszewski syndrome): Report of the NINDS-SPSP International Workshop. *Neurology* 1996; **47**: 1–9.
61. Golbe LI. Progressive supranuclear palsy. In: Watts RL, Koller WC (eds). *Movement Disorders, Neurologic Principles and Practice.* New York: McGraw-Hill, 1997: 279–95.
62. Dubois B, Deweer B, Pillon B. The cognitive syndrome of progressive supranuclear palsy. In: Battistin L, Scarlato G, Caraceni T, Ruggieri S (eds). *Advances in Neurology.* Philadelphia: Lippincott-Raven, 1996: 399–403.
63. Pillon B, Goulder-Khouja N, Deweer B, *et al.* Neuropsychological pattern of stri-

atonigral degeneration: comparison with Parkinson's disease and progressive supranuclear palsy. *J. Neurol. Neurosurg. Psychiatry* 1995; **58**: 174–9.

64. Barclay CL, Lang AE. Dystonia in progressive supranuclear palsy. *J. Neurol. Neurosurg. Psychiatry* 1997; **62**: 352–6.

65. De Bruin VS, Machado C, Howard RS, Nirsch NP, Lees AJ. Nocturnal and respiratory disturbances in Steele–Richardson–Olszewski syndrome (progressive supranuclear palsy). *Postgrad. Med. J.* 1996; **72**: 293–6.

66. Litvan I, Campbell G, Mangone CA, *et al.* Which clinical features differentiate progressive supranuclear palsy (Steele–Richardson–Olszewski syndrome) from related disorders? A clinicopathological study. *Brain* 1997; **120**: 65–74.

67. Daniel SE, De Bruin VMS, Lees AJ. The clinical and pathological spectrum of Steele–Richardson–Olszewski syndrome (progressive supranuclear palsy): a reappraisal. *Brain* 1995; **118**: 759–70.

68. Daniel SE, Lees AJ, Anderton B, Revesz T. Neuropathological diagnosis of progressive supranuclear palsy. *Movement Disord.* 1997; **12**: 265.

69. Riley DE, Fogt N, Leigh RJ. The syndrome of 'pure akinesia' and its relationship to progressive supranuclear palsy. *Neurology* 1994; **44**: 1025–9.

70. Ghika J, Bougousslavsky J. Presymptomatic hypertension is a major feature in the diagnosis of progressive supranuclear palsy. *Arch. Neurol.* 1997; **54**: 1104–8.

71. Sergeant N, Wattez A, Delacourte A. Neurofibrillary degeneration in progressive supranuclear palsy and corticobasal degeneration: tau pathologies with exclusively 'exon 10' isoforms. *J. Neurochem.* 1999; **72**: 1243–9.

72. Schneider JA, Watts RL, Gearing M, Brewer RP, Mirra SS. Corticobasal degeneration: neuropathologic and clinical heterogeneity. *Neurology* 1997; **48**: 959–69.

73. Jackson M, Lowe J. The new neuropathology of degenerative frontotemporal dementias. *Acta Neuropathol.* 1996; **91**: 127–34.

74. Pollanen MS, Ksiezak-Reding H. The emerging molecular pathology of corticobasal ganglionic degeneration. *Movement Disord.* 1996; **11**: 350.

75. Maraganore DM, Boeve BF, Parisi JE. Disorders mimicking the 'classical' clinical syndrome of corticobasal degeneration. *Movement Disord.* 1996; **11**: 347.

76. Litvan I, Agid Y, Goetz CG, *et al.* Accuracy of the clinical diagnosis of corticobasal degeneration: a clinicopathologic study. *Neurology* 1997; **48**: 119–25.

77. Wenning GK, Litvan I, Jankovic J, *et al.* Natural history and survival of 14 patients with corticobasal degeneration confirmed at postmortem examination. *J. Neurol. Neurosurg. Psychiatry* 1998; **64**: 184–9.

78. Kompoliti K, Goetz CG, Boeve BF, *et al.* Clinical presentation and pharmacological therapy in corticobasal degeneration. *Arch. Neurol.* 1998; **55**: 957–61.

79. Rinne JO, Lee MS, Thompson PD, Marsden CD. Corticobasal degeneration: a clinical study of 36 cases. *Brain* 1994; **117**: 1183–96.

80. Leiguarda R, Lees AJ, Merello M, Marsden CD. The nature of apraxia in corticobasal degeneration. *J. Neurol. Neurosurg. Psychiatry* 1994; **57**: 455–9.

81. Ball JA, Lantos P, Jackson M, Marsden CD, Scadding JW, Rossor MN. Alien hand sign in association with Alzheimer's pathology. *J. Neurol. Neurosurg. Psychiatry* 1993; **56**: 1020–3.

82. Bergeron C, Pollanen MS, Weyer L, Black SE, Lang AE. Unusual clinical presentations of corticobasal ganglionic degeneration. *Ann. Neurol.* 1996; **40**: 893–900.

83. Gilman S, Low P, Quinn N, *et al.* Consensus statement on the diagnosis of multiple system atrophy. *Clin. Autonom. Res.* 1998; **8**: 359–62.

84. Lantos PL. The cellular and molecular pathology of multiple system atrophy. *Movement Disord.* 1997; **12**: 822.

85. Kaufmann H. Multiple system atrophy. *Curr. Opin. Neurol.* 1998; **11**: 351–5.

86. Jellinger KA. The neuropathologic diagnosis of secondary parkinsonian syndromes. In: Battistin L, Scarlato G, Caraceni T, Ruggieri S (eds). *Advances in Neurology*. Philadelphia: Lippincott-Raven, 1996: 293–303.

87. Quinn NP, Wenning GK. Multiple system atrophy. In: Battistin L, Scarlato G, Caraceni T, Ruggieri S (eds). *Advances in Neurology*. Philadelphia: Lippincott-Raven, 1996: 413–19.

88. Magalhaes M, Wenning GK, Daniel SE, Quinn NP. Autonomic dysfunction in pathologically confirmed multiple system atrophy and idiopathic Parkinson's disease – a retrospective comparison. *Acta Neurol. Scand.* 1995; **91**: 98–102.

89. Ballard C, Shaw F, McKeith I, Kenny R. High prevalence of neurovascular instability in neurodegenerative dementias. *Neurology* 1998; **51**: 1760–2.

90. Fowler C. Neurological disorders of micturition and their treatment. *Brain* 1999; **122**: 1213–31.

91. Wenning GK, Quinn NP. Multiple system atrophy. In: Quinn NP (ed.). *Bailliere's Clinical Neurology: Parkinsonism*. London: Bailliere Tindall, 1997: 187–204.

92. Plazzi G, Cortelli P, Montagna P, *et al.* REM sleep behaviour disorder differentiates pure autonomic failure from multiple system atrophy with autonomic failure. *J. Neurol. Neurosurg. Psychiatry* 1998; **64**: 683–5.

93. Litvan I, Goetz CG, Jankovic J, *et al.* What is the accuracy of the clinical diagnosis of multiple system atrophy? A clinicopathologic study. *Arch. Neurol.* 1997; **54**: 937–44.

94. Albanese A, Colosimo C, Lees AJ, Tonali P. The clinical diagnosis of multiple system atrophy presenting as pure parkinsonism. In: Battistin L, Scarlato G, Caraceni T, Ruggieri S (eds). *Advances in Neurology*. Philadelphia: Lippincott-Raven, 1996: 393–7.

95. Colosimo C, Albanese A, Hughes AJ, De Bruin VMS, Lees AJ. Some specific clinical features differentiate multiple system atrophy (striatonigral variety) from Parkinson's disease. *Arch. Neurol.* 1995; **52**: 294–8.

96. Consensus Committee of the American Autonomic Society and the American Academy of Neurology. Consensus statement on the definition of orthostatic hypotension, pure autonomic failure and multiple system atrophy. *Neurology* 1996; **46**: 1470.

97. Kimber JR, Watson L, Mathias C. Distinction of idiopathic Parkinson's disease from multiple system atrophy by stimulation of growth hormone release with clonidine. *Lancet* 1997; **349**: 1877–81.

98. Litvan I, MacIntyre A, Goetz CG, *et al.* Accuracy of the clinical diagnoses of Lewy body disease, Parkinson's disease, and dementia with Lewy bodies: a clinicopathological study. *Arch. Neurol.* 1999; **55**: 969–78.

99. Louis ED, Klatka LA, Liu Y, Fahn S. Comparison of extrapyramidal features in 31 pathologically confirmed cases of diffuse Lewy body disease and 34 pathologically confirmed cases of Parkinson's disease. *Neurology* 1997; **48**: 376–80.

100. Gnanalingham KK, Byrne E, Thornton A, Sambrook MA, Bannister P. Motor and cognitive function in Lewy body dementia: comparison with Alzheimer's and Parkinson's disease. *J. Neurol. Neurosurg. Psychiatry* 1997; **62**: 243–52.

101. Perl DP, Olanow CW, Calne D. Alzheimer's disease and Parkinson's disease: distinct entities or extremes of a spectrum of neurodegeneration? *Ann. Neurol.* 1998; **44**: S19–31.

102. Mitchell SL. Extrapyramidal features in Alzheimer's disease. *Age Ageing* 1999; **28**: 401–9.

103. Clark CM, Ewbank D, Lerner A, *et al.* The relationship between extrapyramidal

signs and cognitive performance in patients with Alzheimer's disease enrolled in the CERAD study. *Neurology* 1997; **49**: 70–5.

104. Montastruc JL, Llau ME, Rascol O, Senard JM. Drug-induced Parkinsonism. *Fundam. Clin. Pharmacol.* 1994; **8**: 293–306.

105. Avorn J, Bohn RL, Mogun H, *et al*. Neuroleptic drug exposure and treatment of parkinsonism in the elderly: a case-control study. *Am. J. Med.* 1995; **99**: 48–54.

106. Hubble JP. Drug-induced parkinsonism. In: Watts RL, Koller WC (eds). *Movement Disorders: Neurological Principles and Practice.* New York: McGraw-Hill, 1997: 325–30.

107. Chabolla DR, Maraganore DM, Ahlskog JE, O'Brien PC, Rocca WA. Drug induced parkinsonism as a risk factor for Parkinson's disease: a historical cohort study in Olmstead County, Minnesota. *Mayo Clin. Proc.* 1998; **73**: 724–7.

108. Burn DJ, Brooks DJ. Nigral dysfunction in drug-induced parkinsonism: an 18F-dopa PET study. *Neurology* 1993; **43**: 552–6.

109. Curran T, Lang AE. Parkinsonian syndromes associated with hydrocephalus: case reports, a review of the literature, and pathophysiological hypotheses. *Movement Disord.* 1994; **9**: 508–20.

110. Graff-Radford NR. Normal pressure hydrocephalus. *Neurologist* 1999; **5**: 194–204.

111. Critchley M. Arteriosclerotic pseudoparkinsonism. In: Rose FC, Capildeo R (eds). *Research Progress in Parkinson's Disease.* London: Pitman, 1981: 745–52.

112. Fitzgerald PM, Jankovic J. Lower body parkinsonism: evidence for vascular etiology. *Movement Disord.* 1989; **4**: 249–60.

113. Thompson PD, Marsden CD. Gait disorder of subcortical arteriosclerotic encephalopathy: Binswanger's disease. *Movement Disord.* 1987; **4**: 1–8.

114. Chang CM, Yu YL, Ng HK, Leung SY, Fong KY. Vascular pseudoparkinsonism. *Acta Neurol. Scand.* 1992; **86**: 588–92.

115. Winikates J, Jankovic J. Clinical correlates of vascular parkinsonism. *Arch. Neurol.* 1999; **56**: 98–102.

116. Fenelon G, Houeto JL. Vascular parkinsonism: a controversial concept. *Rev. Neurologique* 1998; **154**: 291–302.

117. Zijlmans JCM, Thijssen HOM, Vogels JM, *et al*. MRI in patients with suspected vascular parkinsonism. *Neurology* 1995; **45**: 2183–8.

118. van Zagten M, Lodder J, Kessels F. Gait disorder and parkinsonian signs in patients with stroke-related to small deep infarcts and white matter lesions. *Movement Disord.* 1998; **13**: 89–95.

119. Mark MH, Sage JI, Walters AS, Duvoisin RC, Miller DC. Binswanger's disease presenting as levodopa-responsive parkinsonism: clinicopathologic study of three cases. *Movement Disord.* 1995; **10**: 450–4.

120. Fenelon G, Gray F, Wallays C, Poirier J, Guillard A. Parkinsonism and dilatation of the perivascular spaces (etat crible) of the striatum: a clinical, magnetic resonance imaging, and pathological study. *Movement Disord.* 1995; **10**: 754–60.

121. Zijlmans JCM, Poels PJE, van der Straaten J, *et al*. Quantitative gait analysis in patients with vascular parkinsonism. *Movement Disord.* 1996; **11**: 501–8.

122. Yamanouchi H, Nagura H. Neurological signs and frontal white matter lesions in vascular parkinsonism: a clinicopathologic study. *Stroke* 1997; **28**: 965–9.

123. Murrow RW, Schweiger GD, Kepes JJ, Koller WC. Parkinsonism due to a basal ganglia lacunar state: clinicopathological correlation. *Neurology* 1990; **40**: 897–900.

124. Inzelberg R, Bornstein NM, Reider I, Korczyn AD. Basal ganglia lacunes and parkinsonism. *Neuroepidemiology* 1994; **13**: 108–12.
125. Ebersbach G, Sojer M, Valldeoriola F, *et al.* Comparative analysis of gait in Parkinson's disease, cerebellar ataxia and subcortical arteriosclerotic encephalopathy. *Brain* 1999; **122**: 1349–55.
126. Nutt JG, Marsden CD, Thompson PD. Human walking and higher-level gait disorders, particularly in the elderly. *Neurology* 1993; **43**: 268–79.

Assessment

5

R.J. Meara

Introduction

Assessment can be defined as the process of careful measurement and evaluation leading to an informed decision about possible interventions designed to improve functional ability and maximize independence.[1] In the broadest sense, assessment also includes re-evaluation to determine outcome. Assessment should be central to any purposeful health or welfare activity, and is particularly important in the rehabilitative approach to the long-term management of conditions such as Parkinson's disease (PD).[2] Without appropriate assessment, diagnoses can be missed and treatment opportunities overlooked. Remediable handicap can increase, and the effectiveness of interventions can never be established. Timely and appropriate assessment should lead to interventions that improve the quality of life for patients and carers.

Despite the importance attached to assessment several aspects of this process need to be examined. First, the need for assessment must be clear to both the subject of the assessment and the assessor – as must the goals of the assessment. The timing of the assessment in relation to drug therapy is also very important, since functional capacity can vary enormously in response to drug treatment. Who is most appropriate to undertake a given assessment and where this should take place must also be considered. Assessment can be purely 'clinical' based on history, examination and observation, or it may require the use of standardized and validated assessment tools. The results of the assessment should be discussed with the subject being assessed, as well as with other members of the multidisciplinary team. Assessment is a dynamic process that should involve the patient and carer as active partners in the assessment process. Lastly, assessment should lead to some form of health or welfare intervention that is known to be potentially effective in achieving a therapeutic goal.

Assessment is time-consuming, and every measurement undertaken leading to the recording of data can deflect time and resources from other important activities. Unfocussed assessment leading to mountains of data that are never reviewed and lead to no useful interventions is wasteful of time and effort and can be demoralising for all participants. Despite this, such aimless activity is an everyday occurrence in the NHS and in local authorities.

Comprehensive assessment in PD should cover physical, psychological, social and environmental domains,[3] and must also include the impact of PD on carers and families. Clearly, no health or social professional alone has the expertise to perform such an assessment in isolation, and PD needs to be managed by a multiprofessional health and welfare team. Not surprisingly, assessment in PD can present considerable challenges.

Challenges in the assessment of PD

Parkinson's disease is a progressive neurological disorder with a long clinical evolution. Although the primary lesion of PD involves the nigrostriatal tract, causing a disorder of motor control (akinesia, rigidity and tremor), primary and secondary changes resulting from PD can involve many areas of the nervous system, from the mesenteric plexus in the gut to the retina. This can result in a complex picture of neurological damage and diverse symptoms such as poor memory, anxiety, depression, apathy, constipation, urinary incontinence, dizziness, impotence and sleep disorder. As a result of this, assessment of motor function alone can rarely describe the full impact of PD on an individual's disadvantage and quality of life. For example, psychological dysfunction can occur directly as the result of the dopaminergic deficiency in PD and indirectly as a consequence of rapidly changing motor disability and physical handicap. The assessment process is also made more difficult by the fact that in older subjects PD commonly impairs language, communication and cognitive function.

Parkinson's disease shows a strong age-associated risk, and the large majority of people with PD are over the age of 70 years. This presents further difficulties in the assessment process as the effects of other disease states interact in complex ways with the impairments, disabilities and handicaps of PD. Often pre-existing cardiac, respiratory or joint disease can contribute more to frailty, handicap and disadvantage than PD. Recent clinicopathological studies have shown that several neuropathological processes coexist in older patients with PD[4,5], including vascular damage, Alzheimer's disease and Alzheimer-type pathology.

Why and when assessment is important in PD

To establish the presence and type of parkinsonism

Accurate diagnosis is essential for appropriate management and prognosis. The diagnosis of parkinsonism and what type of parkinsonism is present can present considerable difficulties in elderly subjects. Even in expert hands clinical diagnosis is far from secure[4,5], and this is even more evident in community studies of PD and parkinsonism.[6] Obtaining a good history, careful observation and neurological examination can often establish the diagnosis without much difficulty. However, the use of formal clinical diagnostic assessment criteria can improve the accuracy of diagnosis of PD[7] and similar use of criteria for essential tremor[8] and other disorders commonly mistaken for PD should also help to reduce diagnostic errors.

To monitor the response to treatment and early disease progression

Assessment of the response of the motor disorder to drug treatment in PD can help to confirm the diagnosis of PD and direct further treatment. Assessment of treatment response is a very important part of early management. In older people with suspected PD this usually means an evaluation of the response to levodopa. A good response can often be determined simply from the way the patient walks into the room and reports how they have been managing. However, the response to levodopa can be less clear-cut in elderly patients and may require formal assessment of the motor response using measures of akinesia, tremor and rigidity and comparing these with pre-treatment levels. This approach can also help to determine the best symptomatic individual response that can be achieved with drug treatment. Assessment of side effects from drug treatment is also important at this stage, particularly looking for postural hypotension, sleep disturbance, drowsiness, cognitive impairment and hallucinosis. The early development of such problems often indicates a poor prognosis and intolerance of maximally therapeutic levels of levodopa.

Formal brief challenge tests to indicate responsiveness to dopaminergic stimulation, using single large doses of levodopa or subcutaneous apomorphine, have been developed to predict the diagnosis and the likely response to longer-term treatment.[9,10] However, given the reported specificity and sensitivity of challenge tests, there is still no substitute for a therapeutic trial of levodopa treatment of several weeks' duration.[11]

Regular assessment of motor function, autonomic function and cognitive function can help to monitor disease progression and the continuing response of signs and symptoms to drug treatment. This approach will also demonstrate the development of disabling symptoms commonly seen in older patients with PD that do not appear to respond to dopaminergic drug treatment such as drooling, dysarthria, dysphagia, freezing and falls.

Similar regular assessment can help to establish the effectiveness of interventions designed to delay disease progression such as foetal transplantation, anti-oxidant therapy, selegeline and low-dose dopamine agonist therapy. Assessment for this indication will need to take place with the patient off all drug treatment in the maximally 'off' state. This can be extremely unpleasant and potentially dangerous for the patient concerned. Detailed assessment protocols (CAPIT) have been developed in surgical transplantation studies.[12]

To improve quality of life in advanced disease with complex problems

Comprehensive assessment becomes increasingly important with disease progression and often the development of other co-morbidities. The symptoms of late-stage disease often do not respond to dopaminergic drugs and increasing side effects limit treatment. Assessment can help to define the major problems and determine how these can be ameliorated. Very often, decisions need to be made about reducing dopaminergic drug treatment. Formal assessment of mood and anxiety with self-rating scales can help detect underlying depression and stress. This stage imperceptibly merges with the assessment needs of palliative care.

To meet the needs of family and carers

Caring in chronic disease is largely informal family care.[13] In response to this, the assessment of the needs of families and carers is being increasingly seen as an important part in the management of PD. Depression and anxiety are common in carers of people with PD, and risk factors for carer distress are becoming increasingly recognized.[14,15] Identification of such needs should lead to a reduction in carer distress by providing appropriate resources that support and do not undermine the carer's role. This may include the provision of physical care support, respite care, social support and financial aid. On occasions, the perceived needs of carers may be in conflict with the needs of the person for whom they are caring.

Specific assessment tools such as the Geriatric Depression Scale[16] can be useful in detecting depressive illness in carers. Standardized assessments of health-related quality of life, cognitive function and anxiety might also prove to be useful in carers.

To support research in PD

Basic medical research, pharmaceutical company-sponsored drug research and health service research into PD can all require specialized assessment techniques. The level and intensity of assessment in research is necessarily greater than that normally possible in everyday clinical practice. The observation that patients in clinical trials do better than those given normal clinical care may partly reflect this fact.

Assessment domains in PD

Disease-specific clinical rating scales

The need for more formal assessment of impairments in PD was developed from the discovery of drug treatment for the condition[17]. The assessment of the motor impairments of rigidity, tremor and akinesia is usually carried out as part of the bedside neurological examination, and mentally assigned a subjective value. The sensitivity of this approach is likely to be fairly crude and the discriminative power very limited. In an attempt to formalize the bedside approach many clinical rating scales have been developed based on sign-and-symptom test items and/or the effect of PD on activities of daily living (ADL). Examples of the first include items such as walking pattern, finger movements, standing up from a chair, or amplitude of resting tremor. Examples of the second include the effect of PD on washing, dressing, feeding and household chores. Well recognized clinical rating scales include the Hoehn and Yahr scale[18], the Columbian Rating Scale[19], the Northwestern University Disability Scale[20], the Webster Scale[21] and the Unified Parkinson's Disease Rating Scale[22] (UPDRS). Existing clinical rating scales cover many domains of assessment in PD and also tend to blur the distinction between impairments, disabilities and handicaps or disadvantages. Sections of clinical rating scales can either be scored independently or can be summated to reach a grand total. The validity and reliability of these scales have not generally been established, and this is discussed critically in a recent review.[23] The lack of any weighting of scores on test items makes the clinical interpretation of overall global scores and changes in scores difficult. Clinical rating scales are often used as outcome measures in drug studies in PD, though the manipulation of such numerical 'results' are difficult to interpret given the subjective nature of the rating scales.[24]

As the most popular clinical rating scale in present use, the US-derived UPDRS deserves further comment.[22] This is a very large scale, largely derived from several other scales. The UPDRS has been the subject of a recent reliability and validity studies.[25-27] The scale takes around 20–40 min to administer, and as a result is rarely used in clinical practice in its entirety outside of research studies. Although an attempt at a comprehensive assessment of PD, the UPDRS fails to cover adequately the important features of PD in elderly subjects such as cognitive function, bladder and bowel symptoms and axial and balance problems. However, despite its limitations it has become the new 'gold standard' clinical rating scale, supplanting the hopelessly inadequate and flawed Hoehn and Yahr scale.

The reliability of sign-and-symptom tests has been investigated by showing video recordings of patient performances to a group of neurologists and non-medical undergraduates. This study demonstrated that reliability was unsatisfactory in both groups, and that this was largely due to the inherent peculiarities and ambiguities of particular patient performances and contextual factors.[28] This same study also investigated the convergent validity of five clinical rating scales, both ADL and sign-and-symptom based, in 49 patients with PD.[28] There was good evidence of convergent validity between the scales studied, but considerable redundancy in the number of test items was apparent. The investigators concluded that the sensitivity of rating scales to clinical interventions was limited by the raters' capacity for absolute categorical judgement and that valid objective measures needed to be developed.

Physical domain

Motor

As discussed above, bedside examination is usually the most detailed assessment of the impairment of motor function in PD that is carried out in normal clinical practice. However, a more formal assessment is probably required to establish the magnitude of response to drug therapy and the progression of motor symptoms. One approach that can be used is to employ the motor subsection of the UPDRS. This takes around 10 min to complete. Motor impairment can be further assessed in the clinic by simple and practical objective tests of motor function. These could include a timed 10-m walk and a simple measure of hand akinesia such as finger tapping on a counter device or touching each armrest of a chair with each hand in turn over a period of 1 min (two-touch test). To date, normative values in elderly subjects for these tests do not exist. More detailed tests of motor function involving reaction and movement times and mechanically estimated measures of limb rigidity have been described, but are still largely confined to use in movement disorder laboratories.[29,30]

Sensory

Painful symptoms are common in PD, and either result from the primary disease process or arise secondarily from rigidity. Painful symptoms often occur as part of sleep disturbance at night or as part of an acute 'off' response when drug treatment temporarily fails to work. No specialized assessment scales have been developed for this symptom, though painful symptoms are represented, albeit poorly, in one item of the UPDRS.

Autonomic function

Autonomic dysfunction is common in PD due to direct involvement of the autonomic system and as a result of the drug treatment of PD. Severe autonomic dysfunction raises the possibility of diagnoses other than PD. Impairment of autonomic function may also arise from co-morbidity as well as from concurrent drug therapy, such a thiazide diuretics to treat hypertension. Postural hypotension can be extremely disabling and potentially very hazardous, leading to falls and injury. Assessment of PD must include lying and standing blood pressure and pulse. The blood pressure should be taken under standardized conditions.[31] This assessment should be undertaken at frequent intervals, particularly if medication is changed. Other symptoms of autonomic impairment such as frequency of micturition, constipation, impotence and abnormal sweating also need to be recorded. An autonomic symptom checklist has been developed for use in PD.[33] Symptoms of autonomic dysfunction correlate poorly with objective tests of autonomic function. Older patients with PD in a movement disorder clinic rarely complete details of any sexual problem on the checklist (personal observations).

Activities of daily living

The impact of PD on functional capacity is easily captured by the use of existing generic ADL scales. An instrumental ADL scale such as the Nottingham Extended ADL Index[31] can be used in this situation, combined with the Barthel ADL scale.[34] The UPDRS contains a subsection of ADL elements that could also be used.

Self-reported disability has also been investigated in PD, and patients' perceptions have been shown to be accurate compared with assessments made by relatives and observers.[35] A brief self-report ADL scale has been found to correlate well with measures of disease severity and quality of life in PD.[36]

Mental domain

Mood

Depression is common in PD, and once detected can respond well to antidepressant medication. Discussion of mood with the patient and recognition of the part that mood disorders play in the clinical expression of PD can in itself be a therapeutic exercise.

Several self-rated mood questionnaires exist to detect depression and anxiety, such as the Geriatric Depression Scale,[37] the Beck Depression Inventory[38] and the Hospital Anxiety and Depression Scale.[39] At appropriate cut-off scores these scales show acceptable sensitivity and specificity for syndromic depression when compared with formal psychiatric diagnosis.[40] Depression can predate the motor onset of PD, and the risk of depression seems particularly high around the time of diagnosis and when major changes in disability occur. These findings reflect both the biological and reactive elements of depression in PD.

A busy outpatient clinic is not an ideal place to administer such instruments unless a quiet room that affords privacy can be provided. Although designed as self-rated instruments, in reality the nurse or relative often helps to fill in the responses. This can directly affect the results – as can the sight of the scoring sheet or any suggestion that the questionnaire is designed to detect 'depression'.

Cognitive function

Cognitive impairment is also common in PD, ranging from mild evidence of frontal lobe dysfunction to frank dementia. Many elderly patients and their carers complain of problems with apathy, passivity, poor concentration and impaired short-term memory. A considerable proportion of elderly patients with late-onset PD will progress to dementia. Screening tests of cognitive function are important to define groups of patients at risk of dementia and to identify patients who will be poorly tolerant of certain treatment such as dopamine agonist drug therapy. The rate of cognitive decline in the individual patient can help in determining future treatment strategy and in providing a prognosis for the patient and carer. Better knowledge of the risk factors for dementia in PD may in the future permit early interventions that are designed to slow the development of dementia in at risk groups.

Two useful tests of cognitive function are the Mini Mental State Examination (MMSE)[41] and the CAMCOG assessment.[42] The CAMCOG test has recently been revised with the addition of more specific tests of executive function (CAMCOG-R).[43] The MMSE is a brief global test of cognitive function, but suffers from lack of specificity and ceiling effects. Age and past educational achievement influence performance on the MMSE. The sensitivity and specificity of the CAMCOG and the MMSE in detecting dementia has been reported in patients with clinically probable PD recruited from a community-based disease register.[44] This study found that in PD the CAMCOG assessment is more sensitive to early cognitive decline than the MMSE. Since the CAMCOG takes 30 min to administer, a useful strategy would be to use the MMSE as a screening tool and to reserve the CAMCOG assessment for patients with borderline scores on the MMSE and for patients with evident cognitive impairment that requires further definition.

Social environmental domain

Assessment of social support and leisure activities is an important aspect of comprehensive assessment in PD. Housing, driving ability and the availability of public transport or access to shopping are likely to be major determinants of quality of life in PD. Driving assessments are considered in Chapter 12. The social support of patients and carers may be an important determinant of access to, and utilization of, health and social services.[45]

Health-related quality of life measures can be used in PD to measure the complex interaction of PD and quality of life. Generic measures such as the Short Form-36 have largely been found to be unsuited to elderly people. Disease-specific measures such as the PD-39 and the PDQL have recently been developed and validated in PD.[46-48] More detailed discussion of quality of life in PD can be found in Chapter 6.

Table 5.1 Suggested minimum assessment guideline for older patients with Parkinson's disease (PD)

Body weight
Supine and standing blood pressure and pulse
Clinical diagnostic criteria for PD
Motor subsection of UPDRS
Mini Mental State Examination (MMSE)
Geriatric Depression Scale (GDS)
Barthel ADL/Nottingham Extended ADL Index
Timed 10-m walk
Two-touch test of upper-limb akinesia
PDQL

A practical approach to assessment in PD

Detailed assessments take time, and outside of research programmes are not feasible – particularly for the practitioner working without the support of a large team. Several of the suggested assessments are self-rated, though often elderly patients will require some help with completion of these or missing data will make such assessments invalid. Non-medical personnel given adequate training can administer the UPDRS, MMSE and CAMCOG assessments. Nursing staff can often fulfil this role, and assessment is seen as an important function of Parkinson Disease Specialist Nurse (see Chapter 16).

A suggested minimum assessment guideline in PD on first referral is shown in Table 5.1. How often such assessments need to be repeated probably reflects the rate of disease progression and how frequently treatment is changed. Assessment of motor function needs to be taken at a standardized time for each patient in relation to drug treatment if significant dose response fluctuations occur. In most cases, this means assessing motor function when the patient is reasonably 'on' in terms of response to drug treatment. In many older patients response fluctuations are not evident, and motor evaluation can be carried out at any time.

Specialist assessment in PD

Initial assessment will often indicate the need for more specialist assessments by a wide range of health and welfare professions, including the physiotherapist, occupational therapist, speech and language therapist, dietician, dentist, chiropodist, orthoptist, clinical psychologist, neurosurgeon, ophthalmologist, old age psychiatrist and urologist.

References

1. Barer D. Assessment in rehabilitation. *Rev. Clin. Gerontol.* 1993; **3**: 169–86.
2. Ward CD. Rehabilitation in Parkinson's disease. *Rev. Clin. Gerontol.* 1992; **2**: 254–68.

3. Struck AE, Siu AL, Wieland GD, Adams J, Rubenstein LZ. Comprehensive geriatric assessment: a meta-analysis of controlled trials. *Lancet* 1993; **342**: 1032–6.

4. Hughes AJ, Daniel SE, Kilford L, Lees AJ. The accuracy of clinical diagnosis of idiopathic Parkinson's disease: a clinicopathological study. *J. Neurol. Neurosurg. Psychiatry* 1992; **55**: 181–4.

5. Rajput AH, Rozdilsky B, Rajput A. Accuracy of diagnosis in Parkinsonism – a prospective study. *Can. J. Neurol. Sci.* 1991; **18**: 275–8.

6. Meara RJ, Bhowmick BK, Hobson JP. Accuracy of diagnosis in patients with presumed Parkinson's disease in a community based register. *Age Ageing* 1999; **28**: 99–102.

7. Gibb WRG, Lees AJ. The relevance of the Lewy body to the pathogenesis of idiopathic Parkinson's disease. *J. Neurol. Neurosurg. Psychiatry* 1988; **51**: 745–52.

8. Findley LJ, Koller WC. Definitions and behavioural classifications. In: Findley LJ., Koller WC (eds). *Handbook of Tremor Disorders. Neurological Disease and Therapy, Vol. 30.* New York: Marcel-Dekker Inc., 1995: 1–5.

9. D'Costa DF, Sheehan LJ, Phillips PA, Moore-Smith B. The levodopa test in Parkinson's disease. *Age Ageing* 1995; **24**: 210–12.

10. Hughes AJ, Lees AJ, Stern GM. Apomorphine test to predict dopaminergic responsiveness in parkinsonian patients. *Lancet* 1990; **336**: 32–4.

11. Hughes AJ, Lees AJ, Stern GM. Challenge tests to predict the dopaminergic response in untreated Parkinson's disease. *Neurology* 1991; **41**: 1723–5.

12. Langston JW, Widner H, Goetz CG. Core assessment programme for intracerebral transplantation (CAPIT). *Movement Disord.* 1992; **7**: 2–13.

13. Nolan M, Grant G, Keady J. (eds). *Understanding Family Care.* Buckingham: Open University Press, 1996.

14. Miller E, Berrios GE, Politynska BE. Caring for someone with Parkinson's disease: factors that contribute to distress. *Int. J. Geriatr. Psychiatry* 1996; **11**: 263–8.

15. Meara RJ, Mitchelmore E, Hobson JP. Use of the GDS-15 as a screening instrument for depressive symptomatology in patients with Parkinson's disease and their carers in the community. *Age Ageing* 1999; **28**: 35–8.

16. Yesavage JA, Brink TL. Development and validation of a geriatric depression screening scale: a preliminary report. *J. Psychiatr. Res.* 1983; **17**: 37–49.

17. Marsden CD, Schachter M. Assessment of extrapyramidal disorders. *Br. J. Clin. Pharmacol.* 1981; **11**: 129–51.

18. Hoehn MM, Yahr MD. Parkinsonism: onset, progression and mortality. *Neurology* 1967; **17**: 427–42.

19. Lang AET, Fahn S. Assessment of Parkinson's disease. In: Munsat TL (ed.). *Quantification of Neurologic Deficit.* Stoneham MA: Butterworths, 1989: 285–309.

20. Canter CD, de la Torre A, Mier M. A method for evaluating disability in patients with Parkinson's disease. *J. Nerv. Ment. Dis.* 1961; **133**: 143–7.

21. Webster DD. Clinical analysis of the disability in Parkinson's disease. *Mod. Treat.* 1968; **5**: 257–82.

22. Fahn S, Elton RL. Members of the UPDRS Committee. Unified Parkinson's Disease Rating Scale. In: Fahn S, Marsden CD, Calne DB, Goldstein M (eds). *Recent Developments in Parkinson's Disease.* Florham Park NJ: Macmillan Health Care Information, 1987: 153–64.

23. Wade DT (ed.). *Measurement in Neurological Rehabilitation.* Oxford: Oxford University Press, 1992.

24. Martinez-Martin P. Rating scales in Parkinson's disease. In: Jankovic J, Tolosa E. (eds). *Parkinson's Disease and Movement Disorders.* Baltimore: Williams and Wilkins, 1993: 281–92.

25. Martinez-Martin P, Gil-Nagel A, Morlan Gracia L, Balseiro Gomez J, Martinez-Sarries J, Bermejo F, and The Co-operative Multicentric Group. Unified Parkinson's Disease Rating Scale Characteristics and Structure. *Movement Disord.* 1994; **9**: 76-83.
26. van Hiltern JJ, van der Zwan AD, Zwinderman AH, Roos RAC. Rating impairment and disability in Parkinson's disease: evaluation of the Unified Parkinson's Disease Rating Scale. *Movement Disord.* 1994; **9**: 84–8.
27. Stebbins GT, Goetz CG, Lang AE, Cubo E. Factor analysis of the motor section of the Unified Parkinson's Disease Rating Scale during the off-state. *Movement Disord.* 1999; **14**: 585–9.
28. Henderson L, Kennard C, Crawford TJ, Day S, Everitt BS, Goodrich S, Jones F, Park DM. Scales for rating motor impairment in Parkinson's disease: studies of reliability and convergent validity. *J. Neurol. Neurosurg. Psychiatry* 1991; **54**: 18–24.
29. Teravainen H, Calne D. Quantitative assessment of Parkinsonian deficits. In: Rinne UK, Klinger M, Stamm G. (eds). *Parkinson's Disease – Current Progress, Problems and Management.* Holland: Elsevier/North Holland Biomedical Press, 1980: 145–64.
30. Ward CD, Sanes JN, Dambrosia JM, Calne DB. Methods for evaluating treatment in Parkinson's Disease. In: Fahn S, Calne DB, Shoulson I. (eds). *Advances in Neurology, vol. 37: Experimental Therapeutics of Movement Disorders.* New York: Raven Press, 1983: 1–7.
31. Mathias CJ, Bannister R. Investigation of autonomic disorders. In: Bannister R., Mathias CJ. (eds). *Autonomic Failure.* Oxford: Oxford University Press, 1992: 255–90.
32. Berrios GE, Campbell C, Politynska BE. Autonomic failure, depression and anxiety in Parkinson's disease. *Br. J. Psychiatry* 1995; **166**: 789–92.
33. Nouri FM, Lincoln NB. An extended activities of daily living scale for stroke patients. *Clin. Rehab.* 1987; **1**: 301–5.
34. Collin C, Wade DT, Davis S, Horne V. The Barthel ADL index: a reliability study. *Int. Disability Stud.* 1988; **10**: 61–3.
35. Brown RG, MacCarthy B, Jahanshahi M, Marsden CD. Accuracy of self-reported disability in patients with parkinsonism. *Arch. Neurol.* 1989; **46**: 955–9.
36. Edwards NI, Meara RJ, Hobson JP. The Parkinson's disease Activities of Daily Living scale: a new simple and brief subjective measure of disability in Parkinson's disease. *Age Ageing* 1999; **28** (suppl. 2): 107.
37. D'Ath P, Katona P, Mullan E, Evans S, Katona C. Screening, detection and management of depression in elderly primary care attenders. I: The acceptability and performance of the 15 item Geriatric Depression Scale (GDS15) and the development of short versions. *Family Practice* 1994; **11**: 260–6.
38. Beck AT, Ward CH, Mendelson M, Mock J, Erbaugh J. An inventory for measuring depression. *Arch. Gen. Psychiatry* 1961; **4**: 53–63.
39. Zigmond AS, Snaith RP. The Hospital Anxiety and Depression Scale. *Acta Psychiatr. Scand.* 1983; **17**: 361–70.
40. Jackson R, Baldwin B. Detecting depression in elderly medically ill patients: the use of the Geriatric Depression Scale compared with medical and nursing observations. *Age Ageing* 1993; **22**: 349–43.
41. Folstein MF, Folstein SE, McHugh PR. 'Mini-Mental State'. A practical method for grading the cognitive state of patients for the clinician. *J. Psychiatr. Res.* 1975; **12**: 189-98.
42. Huppert FA, Brayne C, Gill C. CAMCOG – A concise neuropsychological test to assist dementia diagnosis: socio-demographic determinants in an elderly population sample. *Br. J. Clin. Psychol.* 1995; **34**: 529–41.
43. Leeds L, Meara RJ, Woods RT, Hobson JP. A validation of the new executive

functioning sub-tests of the revised CAMCOG with the Ravens Coloured Progressive Matrices and the Weigl-Grewel Neuropsychological tests in elderly stroke survivors. *Age Ageing* 1999; **28** (suppl. 2): 62.

44. Hobson JP, Meara RJ. The detection of dementia and cognitive impairment in a community population of elderly Parkinson's disease subjects by use of the CAMCOG neuropsychological test. *Age Ageing* 1999; **28**; 39-43.

45. Hobson JP, Meara RJ. Coping and support networks for people with Parkinson's disease. In: Percival R, Hobson JP (eds). *Parkinson's Disease – Studies in Psychological and Social Care*. Leicester: BPS Books (The British Psychological Society), 1999: 217–28.

46. Jenkinson C, Peto V, Fitzpatrick R, Greenhall R, Hyman N. Self-reported functioning and well-being in patients with Parkinson's disease: comparison of the Short-form Health Survey (SF-36) and the Parkinson's Disease Questionnaire (PDQ-39). *Age Ageing* 1995; **24**: 505–9.

47. de Boer AGEM, Wijker W, Speelman JD, de Haes JCJM. Quality of life in patients with Parkinson's disease: development of a questionnaire. *J. Neurol. Neurosurg. Psychiatry* 1996; **61**: 70–4.

48. Hobson JP, Holden A, Meara RJ. Measuring the impact of Parkinson's disease with the Parkinson's Disease Quality of Life questionnaire (PDQL). *Age Ageing* 1999; **28**: 341–6.

Quality of life

6

D.R. Forsyth

Introduction

Parkinson's disease (PD) has a major adverse impact on the lives of both sufferer and carer(s). Patients not only suffer functional impairment, but the disease may also affect their emotional and social life. Given the pervasive nature of PD, there is without doubt a need for self-rated quality of life assessment scales in the assessment of any new treatments. This is especially so, as there appears to be poor correlation between the physician's perception of their patient's quality of life and the patient's own perception. Neurological assessment scales, for example the Unified Parkinson's Disease Rating Scale (UPDRS) simply describe the signs and symptoms of PD without attending to the many dimensions of the disease, including its emotional and social impact on sufferer and carer.

Concern over other people's perception of the PD sufferer, or the carer, reduce the opportunities to socialize (Table 6.1). Anxiety exacerbates tremor and dysphonia, heightening self-awareness, embarrassment and risk of depression; this frequently results in further social isolation for both sufferer and carer. Mobility problems make travelling difficult, and nocturnal symptoms disturb both partners! Carers are also restricted by their anxieties over leaving the PD sufferer unattended, for example, the fear of their falling. Patient well-being has been shown to be proportional to their perception of control over their symptoms. The extent to which the individual feels in control of their disease/life also influences their level of dependency upon others; with more optimistic individuals requiring less assistance.[1] It is therefore not surprising that caregiver strain has also been shown to be inversely proportional to the sufferer's perception of control over their symptoms.[2]

Table 6.1 Social impact of Parkinson's disease

Stigma	% suffering
Complain of poor social functioning	29
No longer participate in social activities	40
Feel rejected by family (sometime/all the time)	38/14
Feel miserable and depressed	78
Plan life around medication	75
Experience side effects of medication	64
Experience 'wearing-off'	45
Sleep disturbance	75
Balance problems	72
Difficulties with walking	75
Complain of poor memory	75

Quality of life assessment

In the absence of a cure for PD, therapies are directed at maintenance of function and limitation of symptoms. It is clearly important (whether in the context of clinical trials or routine clinics) that, when assessing the impact of any therapy (pharmacological or physical), we consider the whole patient and not just the motor components. For quality of life (QOL) must be a better indicator of successful management, than say the degree of reduction in 'off' time. What matters is how the patient feels, rather than how the doctors think they ought to feel on the basis of clinical measurement.

Generic scales

Generic scales, such as the Sickness Impact Scale (SIP), which contains 153 questions, and the Nottingham Health Profile (NHP), which contains 38 questions, assess the impact of disease on quality of life but do not focus on the specific problems of PD. The NHP was developed to measure effects on QOL at the severe end of ill health and thus may not detect small improvements in QOL.[3] The Short Form 36 (SF36) consists of 19 items relating to physical, psychological and social function; 11 to well-being; and five to general health perception. The items relating to vigorous activities/work in the SF36 are not pertinent to those aged over 65 years, and lead to an age-related increase in omissions. The SF36 has also been criticised for its possible floor effects. Although the items relating to physical and social function in the SF36 appear to correlate with Hoehn and Yahr scores, the SF36 is unlikely to be a sensitive measure of change in disease after any intervention.[4,5]

Disease-specific scales

Disease-specific scales, such as the PDQL and PDQ-39, can be self-rated and measure the impact of PD upon QOL. The PDQL has 37 items: 14 relate to

Parkinsonian symptoms; nine to emotional functioning; seven to systemic symptoms; and seven to social functioning. In 136 PD sufferers assessed using the PDQL, older age, depression, cognitive impairment and disease severity were all associated with lower health-related QOL.[6] The PDQL requires longitudinal validation, and thus cannot yet be recommended for assessing the impact of any therapeutic interventions.[7]

The PDQ-39 has 10 items relating to mobility; six to activities of daily living; six to emotional well-being; four to stigma; three to social support; four to cognition; three to communication; and three to bodily discomfort. The mobility and the activities of daily living (ADL) domains of the PDQ39 do show a correlation with the severity of the disease, as assessed by the Hoehn and Yahr scale. These domains also appear to be responsive to disease progression. This longitudinal validity means that the profile response to the PDQ39 may be useful in studying the impact of a therapeutic intervention upon different aspects of function and well-being in PD. A summary index (PDSI) can also be used from the responses to the PDQ39 to summarize the impact of disease and overall effect of therapeutic interventions upon function and well-being. The PDSI has also been shown to correlate with disease severity assessed by both Hoehn and Yahr, or the Columbia rating scale.[8,9]

Impact of PD on the patient's family

Parkinson's disease does not just affect the sufferer, it also impacts upon their family and friends. O'Reilly et al.[10] compared 154 carer spouses of PD sufferers with 124 non-carer controls from the perspective of social functioning, psychological well-being and physical health. Carer spouses faired worse in all three domains. They were less likely to get out of the house at least once per week, or to have had a holiday in the last year. There was an almost five-fold increase in psychiatric morbidity in the carers, and they were more likely to suffer chronic illness. The physical, social and psychological strain on carers increases in proportion to the level of care they are having to provide. Thus, the needs of these 'informal' carers must not be forgotten and should be assessed.

Carer's needs fall broadly into the following areas: information; reduction in physical and psychological burden; a good night's sleep; knowledge of and access to benefits, e.g. Attendance Allowance; and respite care. The impact of the disease upon the carer can be assessed using the Caregiver Strain Index (CSI). This is a 13-item (brief), easily administered questionnaire that assesses the physical, social and emotional impact of dependency and caring upon the carer. The CSI has been shown to be valid across generations.[11] Carter et al.[12] examined the experience of 380 spouse caregivers at 23 different sites across the USA. As the disease progresses, so caregiver strain accumulates: a tripling of caregiver tasks by Stage 4/5; depression in the carer is more common by Stage 4/5; caregivers' lives are less predictable as the disease progresses; and the positive quality of the relationship declines from Stage 2 onwards. Carer stress has also been shown to correlate strongly with levels of depression in the PD sufferer.[13]

Impact of PD on the patient

Whilst there is no doubt that physician and patient alike seek to optimize the control of the disease, we cannot hope to improve the quality of our patients' lives if we do not understand how the disease affects them as individuals. Nocturnal problems are common in PD, including early and frequent wakening, cramps, pains and nightmares.[14] These have an important impact upon the QOL of both sufferer and spouse. Just as PD is protean in its manifestations, so we must be diverse in our efforts to improve the QOL of the PD sufferer and their carers. A functional-status approach alone is not appreciated; this only leads to dissatisfaction among sufferers and carers and comments such as: '. . . they just seem to keep changing the tablets or the dose and that's all we get from them . . .'; '. . . they don't seem to consider the things that are important to us'. For example, a reduction in 'off-time' attests to the physical impact of a treatment, but tells us nothing about the quality of the 'on-time' gained, or any effect of the treatment on the quality of the remaining 'off-time'. What patients and carers also want is: information; to be listened to; support – both practical and emotional; and access to other professionals as required. This was summarized by one patient: '. . . if someone takes an interest that is more important to me than all the tablets I've been given'.

Specialist services

The provision of specialist PD services, with the specialist nurse as the prime coordinator, addresses much of this dissatisfaction. The Parkinson's disease nurse specialist (PD nurse) has a pivotal role in the coordination and delivery of high-quality care to the PD sufferer and their carer(s). The PD nurse will provide advice and support both to the PD patient, their family and all other professional groups with which they may be involved. S/he is also an educational resource to all involved in the management of PD. This requires a high level of skill in liaison, supervising, and coordinating services to ensure that multidisciplinary teams are utilized effectively. At local, national and individual levels, the PD nurse specialists have initiated improvements to the overall standard of care by raising awareness of the problems associated with living with PD. The QOL of PD sufferers who have contact with a PD nurse is enhanced because they are less likely to fall, suffer fractures, or be institutionalized.[15] These practical benefits of PD nurses are probably attributable to their effects on monitoring and giving advice on drug therapy within primary care.

Team working is essential in providing a quality service to the PD sufferer and their carers.[16] Multidisciplinary clinics, with ready access to physiotherapist, occupational therapist, speech and language therapist, and availability of other disciplines as needed, for example dietician and clinical psychologist, help to improve the quality of care provided. Consideration must also be given as to how one meets the needs of PD sufferers in nursing homes, who may not be able physically to attend these clinics.

At some time in their life, the PD sufferer may require some form of surgery, not necessarily as a direct consequence of their disease. A recent survey of PD sufferers in Scotland has shown that this can be a traumatic experience, with many experiencing postoperative confusion, loss of symptom control, or other complications of the disease, due to failure to receive their medication on time.[17] Such experiences lead to PD sufferers wanting to avoid hospital admission.

The Global Parkinson's Disease Survey (GPDS) (Table 6.2), inspired by the European Parkinson's Disease Association (EPDA), is the first in-depth international survey of QOL in PD.[18] We already know that therapies focus on controlling symptoms and that control of motor symptoms contributes to a better QOL. The GPDS demonstrated that QOL in PD is affected by factors other than disease severity and medication usage. Only 17.3 per cent of the variation in QOL was explained by the disease stage (Hoehn and Yahr) and medication usage. Almost 60 per cent of the variation in QOL can be explained by knowing the disease stage, medication usage, presence of depressive symptoms (measured by Becks Depression Inventory), the patient's level of satisfaction with the explanation of the diagnosis and their current level of optimism. Thus, the GPDS has helped to identify those factors which might be important in improving the QOL of PD sufferers.

Depressive symptoms may be present in around two-thirds of PD sufferers and one-third of carers.[19] Carers are more likely to suffer depression when the PD sufferer is depressed. In a community-based study of 233 PD sufferers, depressive symptoms, presence of sleep disturbance, and low degree of independence were associated with higher stress levels and reduced QOL.[20] Thus, it is important to screen for depression, for it is common, potentially treatable, significantly affects the QOL of PD sufferers, and adds to the distress of caregivers. The Geriatric Depression Scale (GDS-15) is a self-reported screening

Table 6.2   Profile of Parkinson's patients and carers from six countries participating in the Global Parkinson's Disease Survey

	Patient profile	Carer profile
Males (%)	60	23
Age 60–74 years (%)	52	43
Access to carer (%)	74	–
Retired (%)	–	45
Median caregiving (h/day)	–	17
Median time as carer (years)	–	6.5
Levodopa treatment (%)	88	–
Dopamine agonist treatment (%)	60	–

Source: Findley (1999)[18].

instrument, which has been validated in elderly community-dwelling Parkinson's sufferers and their carers.

A better understanding of those features of PD that have the greatest impact on patient and carer well-being, will be important in the development of new and improved management strategies. Current treatment algorithms focus on drug therapy and pay little attention to other aspects of the disease or non-drug therapies. Whilst control of symptoms is important, the PD team must also recognize the strong relationship between depression and QOL in PD, and consider measures to manage this. Attention must also be given to the explanation of the diagnosis and maintaining patient optimism. The importance of the first consultation cannot be overemphasized as providing the foundation upon which to build a supportive, patient-focused, disease management strategy.

Future research might wish to explore three particular questions: (i) What is the impact on QOL of treating depression in PD? (ii) What coping strategies are effective? (iii) How do we best measure the impact of the PD team in the giving of the diagnosis, support and provision of information?

References

1. Shifren K. Individual differences in the perception of optimism and disease severity: a study among individuals with Parkinson's disease. *J. Behav. Med.* 1996; **19**: 241–71.
2. Wallhagen MI, Brod M. Perceived control and well-being in Parkinson's disease. *West. J. Nurs. Res.* 1997; **19**: 11–31.
3. Jenkinson C, Fitzpatrick R, Argyle M. The Nottingham Health Profile: an analysis of its sensitivity in differentiating illness groups. *Soc. Sci. Med.* 1988; **27**: 1411–14.
4. Hayes V, Morris J, Wolfe C, *et al.* The SF-36 health survey questionnaire: is it suitable for use in older adults? *Age Ageing* 1995; **24**: 120–5.
5. Jenkinson C, Peto V, Fitzpatrick R, *et al.* Self-reported functioning and well-being in patients with Parkinson's disease: comparison of the short-form health survey (SF-36) and the Parkinson's Disease Questionnaire (PDQ-39). *Age Ageing* 1996; **24**: 505–9.
6. Hobson P, Holden A, Meara J. Measuring the impact of Parkinson's disease with the Parkinson's Disease Quality of Life Questionnaire. *Age Ageing* 1999; **28**: 341–6.
7. de Boer AG, Wijker W, Speelman JD, *et al.* Quality of life in patients with Parkinson's disease: development of a questionnaire. *J. Neurol. Neurosurg. Psychiatry* 1996; **61**: 70–4.
8. Fitzpatrick R, Peto V, Jenkinson C, *et al.* Health-related quality of life in Parkinson's disease: a study of outpatient clinic attenders. *Movement Disord.* 1997; **12**: 916–22.
9. Jenkinson C, Fitzpatrick R, Peto V, *et al.* The Parkinson's Disease Questionnaire (PDQ-39): development and validation of a Parkinson's disease summary index score. *Age Ageing* 1997; **26**: 353–7.
10. O'Reilly F, Finnan F, Allwright S, *et al.* The effects of caring for a spouse with Parkinson's disease on social, psychological and physical well-being. *Br. J. Gen. Pract.* 1996; **46**: 507–12.
11. Robinson BC. Validation of a Caregiver Strain Index. *J. Gerontol.* 1983; **38**: 344–8.
12. Carter JH, Stewart BJ, Archbold PG, *et al.* (Parkinson's Study Group). Living with

a person who has Parkinson's disease: the spouse's perspective by stage of disease. *Movement Disord.* 1998; **13**: 20–8.

13. Miller E, Berrios GE, Politynska BE. Caring for someone with Parkinson's disease: factors that contribute to distress. *Int. J. Geriatr. Psychiatry* 1996; **11**: 263–8.

14. Lees AJ, Blackburn NA, Campell VL. The night time problems of Parkinson's disease. *Clin. Neuropharmacol.* 1988; **6**: 512–19.

15. Jarman B. The Imperial College School of Medicine Parkinson's disease nurse specialist project. Presented at: *'The science and practice of multidisciplinary care in Parkinson's disease'.* The Royal College of Physicians, London. 12 June, 1998.

16. Firth-Cozens J. Celebrating teamwork. *Qual. Healthcare* 1998; **7** (suppl. I): S3–7.

17. Barber M, Stewart D, Scott S, *et al.* Patient and carer perception of the management of Parkinson's disease in the peri-operative period. *Age Ageing* 1999; **28** (suppl. 2): 99 (Abstract 149).

18. Findley L. Investigating factors which may influence quality of life in Parkinson's disease. *Proceedings of 13th International Congress on Parkinson's disease,* Vancouver, 24–28 July 1999 (Abstract).

19. Meara J, Mitchelmore E, Hobson P. Use of the GDS-15 geriatric depression scale as a screening instrument for depressive symptomatology in patients with Parkinson's disease and their carers in the community. *Age Ageing* 1999; **28**: 35–8.

20. Karlsen KH, Larsen JP, Tandberg E, *et al.* Influence of clinical and demographic variables on quality of life in patients with Parkinson's disease. *J. Neurol. Neurosurg. Psychiatry* 1999; **66**: 431–5.

Part 3: Specific problems in Parkinson's disease

Caring for carers

7

R. Cousins, A.D.M. Davies, J.R. Playfer and
C.J. Turnbull

Introduction

Most research on Parkinson's disease (PD) has focused on the person with the diagnosis. In recent years, however, there has been a move towards recognizing that PD has a major impact upon the spouse and other family members who assume the responsibility for giving care to the person with the diagnosis. As Parkinson's disease is both a movement disorder and a neuropsychological disorder, carers of people with Parkinson's disease are faced with a variety of challenges from physical and psychological symptoms of the illness. Addressing the needs of the PD patient in the community places demands on carers that warrant them being described as 'the hidden patients',[1] for '... caregiving is potentially a fertile ground for persistent stress'.[2] In this chapter, the argument will be made that interventions to improve the quality of life for people with PD must include in their focus the welfare of the caregiver.

Background

Developments in medicine and technology during the past century have led to a dramatic change in lifespan. Coupled with increases in the number of older adults are increases in the number of older adults with functional disabilities, chronic impairments and progressive diseases (such as PD) where age is a proven risk factor. To remain in the community, the frail elderly need support in activities of daily living which, for the large part, is provided by the family. The family provides nursing care, task-related assistance and also moral support, though at a cost. Study after study indicates that unpaid, unanticipated care of the elderly is a stressful life event.

The focus of recent research of caring has been to provide predictors of distress, depression and burden. The underlying aim is to provide recommendations for effective interventions to relieve carer distress, and as a consequence, keep the care-receiver in the family home. The potentials of providing informal care are related to the possibility of institutionalization.[3-7] It was reported as early as 1972 that, when institutionalization does occur, it is usually because of a breakdown in caregivers' health.[8]

Interest in the plight of carers, and their recent rise in status to a group that requires public recognition and support, has not emerged without a challenge. Criticism has come from the disability movement for what it views as a disproportionate emphasis on the needs of carers at the expense of those for whom they care.[9,10] The assertion is that the goal of public policy should be to enable disabled people to live independently, and therefore do away with the need for caring relationships. The thrust of the argument being that to focus on the carer's needs distracts attention from the (by implication) greater needs of the disabled person. However, the social base of the disability movement is among younger people with physical disability, and therefore reflects its ideals and aspirations.[11] The energy of this movement may serve to direct attention away from the needs of carers of the elderly, and especially people with neuropsychological illness who are not in the position to strike for independence. Pertinent to this discussion, the progressive nature of Parkinson's disease means that people with PD have to expect to get to a stage where they can only remain at home with the support of a 'full-time' carer.

Family obligations and love are the driving force of informal care of people with PD.[12,13] Acting in love does not negate the actuality that complying with the demands of PD will have consequences on the carers' own lives. While this remains the case, there is a necessity to address carer distress alongside the needs of the person with PD. Ultimately carer well-being has as much an effect on patient well-being as the other way round. That is, PD provides a family illness situation in which both the patient and their carer have legitimate requirements for quality of life, and the needs of both individuals need to be finely balanced for mutual benefit.

Model of the illness situation

The notion that PD is a family illness can be illustrated by an adaptation of Young's model of illness in later life (Fig. 7.1). Young[14] argues that the consequences of illness in the family should be conceptualized as a mutual encounter, as both the patient's response and the carer's response to the illness situation in turn affect the situation. The patient–caregiver interaction model

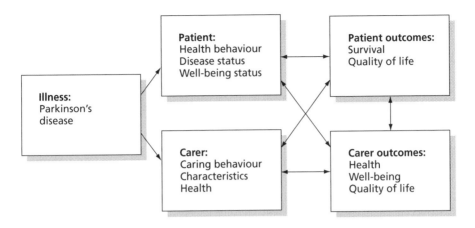

Fig. 7.1   Patient–caregiver interaction model. (Adapted from Young.[14])

shows the way that quality of life in PD is dictated by the complex dynamic interplay of patient and caregiver responses to the illness situation.

The illness

Parkinson's disease is characterized by an insidious onset, and even when the first symptom is the typical finger tremor, it is frequently not recognized as PD. In general, patients and their carers have very little prior knowledge of PD: they learn about it through experience.[15,16] When we looked at the experience of onset and diagnosis of 83 PD patients and caregiver dyads,[12,13] it was found that ignorance of the cause of the first symptoms was the rule rather than the exception. Moreover, carers reported that the uncertainty of not knowing the prognosis of the manifest changes in behaviour was a source of stress. That is, the family can be faced with the stress of uncertainty from an undefined illness situation for a significant period of time. Even when dyads sought medical advice, over 25 per cent of our sample of elderly people with PD initially came away without a diagnosis of the condition.[12] Thus, PD can have a negative impact on the incapacitated person and their carer, even before diagnosis.

Patient behaviour

A diagnosis of PD constitutes a fundamental threat to quality of life and emotional well-being for the patient. The need for care increases alongside this physical deterioration. PD is also associated with a variety of subtle cognitive impairments and an increased risk of dementia.[17] About one-third of PD patients will experience hallucinations in the advanced stages.[12] Depression is a serious and frequent problem for Parkinson's patients,[18] and there are also changes in personality.[12,13] About one-half of our sample of carers perceived personality change and hence changes in behaviour in the people with PD. There were common themes in the changes reported: apathy, withdrawal and deterioration in communication; also a reduction in confidence, and an increase in worrying and agitation. Moreover, patients note such changes themselves.[19]

Carer behaviour and outcomes

Care for people with PD is provided first by the family. In general, there is substantial evidence that indicates that if a spouse is alive and well, then they will assume the responsibility for the welfare of an incapacitated elder. Where there is no spouse, close relatives are preferred to distant ones, any relative is preferred to no relative, and female relatives are preferred to male relatives.[20]

A decline in health is the starting point of the complex interactions between patient and carer, as in any illness situation. The carer addresses both physical and psychological needs, taking on a job with ever-increasing hours as demand grows alongside progression of illness. The input of dopaminergic medication initially brings some relief, but then sooner or later the 'honeymoon' is over and the medication may even bring additional problems to deal with. The best predictor of carer depression is patient depression.[21] The decrease in communication from the patient is a notable challenge for many carers.

From our study we found that there were specific patient variables that affected carer outcomes:

1. The time demands of PD caregiving have consequences on carers' social life, and are associated with burden, depression, and poor psychological health.

2. Physical demands are strongly associated with all aspects of carer distress.

3. Demands from psychological change in PPD (personality, depression, mental status, hallucinations) are associated with an impact on the dyadic relationship, emotional burden and lowered life satisfaction in carers.[12]

Carers bring their own characteristics into the caring situation. As indicated in the model (see Fig. 7.1), carer characteristics have an affect on outcomes, as well as their response to the demands of the people with PD. We found that carers' emotionality and coping style were major predictors of caregiver outcomes.[12,13] Coping style is amenable to change. As mentioned above, we also found that carers were not well informed about PD, particularly the psychological aspects of the disease. Objective tests of physical demand and psychological demand indicated that it was those carers that were looking after more advanced PD patients who knew more; hence we gave the tentative conclusion that they were learning 'on the job'.[16] Following from this, and interviews with carers, we support the view that 'forewarned is forearmed'. A judicious explanation of likely prognosis based on current symptoms should be available, perhaps by through PD nurse specialists.

Patient outcomes

Patient survival and quality of life is determined by the interaction of their own disease status and behaviour, carer characteristics and behaviour, and carer outcomes. Non-compliance to medication is a negligible problem in PD in so far as patient delivery is concerned, the equation being no medication equals poor movement. Where the carer has taken on the responsibility for medication delivery however, we found a minority of carers who were prepared to withhold medication for a short periods, to keep the person with PD immobile, enabling them to complete other tasks (e.g. basic housework).

This particular example demonstrates how outcomes for patients are bound up with ethical issues that arise in caring. If one considers that there are three broad goals of caring activity:

1. to carry on living as before;

2. to achieve well-being for the care-receiver; and

3. to achieve well-being for the carer (self),

then dilemmas can arise when actions are perceived to serve one goal, but not another. Therefore carers are called on to prioritise and make choices that are not mutually beneficial.
For example:

- 'It is easier for me to do things, than to let someone with PD struggle'
- 'I sometimes feel "on edge" when I let the PD patient do things himself/herself'
- 'Sometimes I have to override the PD patient's wishes to get things done'
- 'I am afraid to leave the PD patient alone while I go out'
- 'I dress the PD patient and choose his/her clothes every day'
- 'The constant demands of caring for a PD patient limits the needs of someone else'.

Each of these examples demonstrates ethical conflicts that arise constantly in caring. A problem first occurs when welfare outcomes for the person with PD and their carer differ. A perceptive carer reported, 'Sometimes I do want to do things for Colin, just to help him because he might be struggling a bit. But then I think no, it helps him if he can do it himself. We found that there were frequent situations where slowness caused great frustration and irritation. The dilemma centres on when to help – and when to stand back.

Because in PD, caring is typically a family affair that is not overseen by others, there is the potential for conflicts in determining personal autonomy: the freedom to determine one's own actions. In family caregiving, intrusion upon autonomy can go unchecked and unseen. Care can slip into control, not from malevolence, but in the guise of good intentions. The carer takes over, and this can ultimately induce a dependency situation. Alternatively, the situation can arise where the carer is totally at the PD patient's beck and call – 'From the moment he opens his eyes in the morning to the time he shuts them at night, I am on call. He will not do anything for himself, and he will not be left. The position is that carers constantly have to make judgements about the value of the consequences of their actions. Carer's judgements will adjust as information and experience is accumulated, but ultimately their actions result from the application of their own code of ethics. The handling of ethical dilemmas and issues surrounding personal autonomy is a neglected area in caregiving.

Conclusions

It is recognized that carers are important in PD: a breakdown in caregiving leading to institutionalization is as likely to be the result of a breakdown in the caregiver's health, as to be caused by the person with PD being too ill to be cared for. The model presented in this chapter illustrates that PD in the community is a family illness. Patient symptoms and behaviour have an effect on the carer, and the characteristics and behaviour of both patient and carer predict carer distress levels. Patient outcomes are influenced naturally not only by the illness itself, but also by the care they receive. Therefore, it is imperative that carers are recognized as being part of the illness process, and do not remain 'hidden patients'.

References

1. Fengler AP, Goodrich N. Wives of elderly disabled men: the hidden patients. *Gerontologist* 1979; **19**: 175–83.
2. Pearlin LI, Mullan JT, Semple SJ, Skaff MM. Caregiving and the stress process: an overview of concepts and their measures. *Gerontologist* 1990; **30**: 583–94.
3. Aneshensel CS, Pearlin LI, Schuler R. Stress, role captivity and the cessation of caregiving. *J. Health Soc. Behav.* 1993; **34**: 54–70.
4. Cohen CA, Gold DP, Shulman KI, et al. Factors determining the decision to institutionalize dementing individuals: a prospective study. *Gerontologist* 1993; **33**: 714–20.
5. Colerick EJ, George LK. Predictors of institutionalization among caregivers of Alzheimer's patients. *J. Am. Geriatr. Soc.* 1986; **34**: 493–8.
6. Gerritsen JC, van der Ende PC. The development of a care-giving burden scale. *Age Ageing* 1994; **23**: 483–91.
7. Moritz D, Kasl S, Berkman L. The health impact of living with a cognitively impaired elderly spouse: depressive symptoms and social functioning. *J. Gerontol.* 1989; **44**: S17–27.
8. Isaacs B, Livingstone M, Neville Y. *Survival of the Unfittest: A Study of Geriatric Patients in Glasgow*. London: Routledge & Kegan Paul, 1972.
9. Oliver M. The Politics of Disablement. London: Macmillan, 1990.
10. Morris J. *Pride Against Prejudice: Transforming Attitudes to Disability*. London: Women's Press, 1991.

11. Twigg T. Carers, families, relatives: socio-legal conceptions of caregiving relationships. *J. Soc. Welfare Family Law* 1994; **3**: 279–98.
12. Cousins R. *A Study of Psychological Distress in Caregivers of Parkinson's Patients.* University of Liverpool: Unpublished PhD Thesis, 1997.
13. Davies ADM, Cousins R, Turnbull CJ, Playfer JR, Bromley DB. The experience of caring for people with Parkinson's disease. In: Percival R, Hobbs P (eds). *Parkinson's Disease: Studies in Psychological and Social Care.* London: BPS Books, 1999: 154–98.
14. Young RF. Elders, families, and illness. *J. Aging Stud.* 1994; **8**: 1–15.
15. Cousins R, Davies ADM, Stirling W, Playfer JR, Turnbull CJ. Knowledge of Parkinson's disease. *Proc. Br. Psychol. Soc.* 1995; **3**: 2.
16. Davies ADM, Cousins R, Bromley DB, Playfer JR, Turnbull CJ. Wiser but sadder? The role of knowledge of Parkinson's disease on care-giver distress. *Welfare Research Conference of the Parkinson's Disease Society of the United Kingdom.* London, 1997.
17. Dubois B, Boller F, Pillon B, Agid Y. Cognitive deficits in Parkinson's disease. In: Boller F, Grafman J (eds). *Handbook of Neuropsychology, Vol. 5.* Amsterdam: Elsevier, 1991: 195–240.
18. Sano M, Mayeux R. Biochemistry of depression in Parkinson's disease. In: Huber SJ, Cummings JL (eds). *Parkinson's Disease: Neurobehavioural Aspects.* Oxford: Oxford University Press, 1992: 229–39.
19. Chesson R, Cockhead D, Romney-Alexander D. Quality of life with Parkinson's disease: views of Scottish consumers and providers. In: Percival R, Hobbs P (eds). *Parkinson's Disease: Studies in Psychological and Social Care.* London: BPS Books, 1999: 93–130.
20. Qureshi H, Walker A. *The Caring Relationship: Elderly People and their Families.* London: Macmillan, 1989.
21. Meara J, Michelmore E, Hobson P. Use of the GDS-15 geriatric depression scale as a screening instrument for depressive symptomatology in patients with Parkinson's disease and their carers in the community. *Age Ageing* 1999; **28**: 35–8.

8 Neuropsychiatry

J.V. Hindle

Introduction

Parkinson's disease (PD) is a complex disorder with neurological and psychiatric components. The older term for the condition was paralysis agitans, with paralysis at that time meaning abolition of movement and sensation. Dr. James Parkinson, in his essay on the *Shaking Palsy*, famously described the senses and intellect as being uninjured.[1] Parkinson was open to the possibility of psychiatric disturbance in the condition, and quoted one case of a patient who became melancholy and dejected, mute, then spitting.[1] An historical re-reading of the 'senses and intellect uninjured' suggests the true interpretation to be that sensory modalities remain uninjured (distinguishing it from other causes of paralysis) and that intelligence is normal.[2] Although psychiatric abnormalities were recognized in the nineteenth century by Charcot in Paris and Gowers in London, they were only judged to be an intrinsic part of the condition in the early twentieth century. Benjamin Ball, the first professor of psychiatry in Paris, was an exception and, in 1881, quite correctly stated that 'a large number of parkinsonian patients present psychological disorders extending from simple irritability to psychosis; I would say that a slight degree of cognitive impairment is the rule'.[2] We now recognize that psychiatric problems in PD can include cognitive impairment, dementia, depression, psychosis, anxiety, and more rarely drug-induced mania and hypersexuality.

There are complex interactions between motor function, emotions, the effects of treatment, the effects of chronic disability and cognition. Today, the most problematic psychiatric disorders are often secondary to the combined effects of the disease and treatment.

The importance of mental state

The maintenance of mental health in PD may be more important than the physical state. Depression and cognition may affect the quality of life of patients and stress their carers more than physical disability.[3,4] Psychosis is disruptive to normal life, and often involves a substantial increase in demands on the primary healthcare team. The development of psychosis may even predict institutionalization and early death.[5] Cognitive impairment may limit performance of complex psychomotor tasks such as driving.[6] Mild cognitive impairment can be detected even early in the disease. An understanding of the psychiatry of PD is therefore important.

Heterogeneity in the psychiatry of PD

The complexity of the psychiatry of PD is a manifestation of the heterogeneity of the condition itself. This heterogeneity has no simple explanation. The psychiatric symptoms are a manifestation of the system failure brought about by the underlying disease processes. In older patients, the variation in psychiatric manifestations may be greater due the effects of ageing and the effects of co-morbid conditions such as cerebrovascular disease. An interaction between genes, the environment, the biology of the brain and ageing may bring an increased liability to develop neurodegeneration. The hallmark of this neurodegenerative process in PD is the intracellular inclusion body known as the Lewy body. Variations in the distribution of this pathology may lead to a spectrum of conditions with varying motor and psychiatric features, including idiopathic PD and dementia with Lewy bodies (DLB).[7]

It is useful to attempt to distinguish primary psychiatric phenomena, which are due to the disease itself, from secondary phenomena which may be due to the effects of treatment, other superimposed conditions or the effects of the psychosocial stress of chronic disability. The primary psychiatric abnormalities were well described prior to the use of levodopa and surgery by Mjones in 1949, who summarized these as abnormalities of personality, memory, depression and anxiety.[8] In considering these, it is important not to include those patients suffering from parkinsonism secondary to the encephalitis lethargica pandemic in 1917–21, which caused more florid psychiatric phenomena including severe personality change and psychosis.

Parkinsonian 'personality'

Early in the twentieth century there was increasing interest in descriptive psychopathology. The influence of Freud and his pupils produced a fascination with the power of the mind and personality. Theories of the effects of suppressed emotion and psychogenesis of disease increased interest in the effects of personality as a cause of PD. Preceding the motor syndrome, patients were said to be industrious, introverted, punctual, inflexible, reliable, exacting, morally rigid and exhibited reduced novelty-seeking behaviour.[9] It now seems most likely that these traits are in fact a manifestation of mild affective and cognitive changes very early in the disease.[9] Abnormalities of neurotransmitters, which precede the motor symptoms, may manifest in psychological changes. For example, it is possible that deficiency of serotonin may contribute to pre-morbid shyness. A recent study of personality, depression and pre-morbid lifestyle in twin pairs discordant for PD gives some support for the existence of a genetically determined non-motor syndrome of PD prior to the onset of motor symptoms.[10]

Psychogenic parkinsonism has been described in patients with normal positron emission tomography (PET) scans, some of whom had spontaneous remission. This condition is extremely rare and is a diagnosis of exclusion.[11] More commonly, psychogenic symptoms can complicate the presentation of PD.

Measurement in neuropsychiatry

Psychometric testing, electrical measurement and imaging techniques can be used in the assessment of cognitive and psychiatric processes in PD. A battery of psychometric tests and rating scales is required to examine the spectrum of cognitive and psychological abnormalities in PD (Table 8.1). Clinical assessment of the mental state is also covered in Chapter 5, on the assessment of PD.

The standard electroencephalogram (EEG) is not very helpful in PD and should be normal. Specific EEG responses to a single stimulus, known as event related potentials (ERP), have been extensively studied. The time to a positive deflection on the ERP is called the latency. The peak at 200 millisecond (P_{200}) is due to activation of association areas, and the peak at 300 milliseconds (P_{300}) is due to thinking time and reflects uncertainty. The latency of

Table 8.1   Neuropsychological tests in Parkinson's disease

Function	Examples of tests
Global cognition	Mini mental state examination (MMSE) Cambridge cognitive examination (CAMCOG) Rivermead behavioural memory test (RBMT)
Executive function and set shifting	CAMCOG-R (extra subsection for executive function) Wisconsin card sorting test STROOP test
Frontal lobe	Verbal fluency 'F,A,S' test Proverbs/Similarities Go-no-go tests Cognitive estimates
Working memory	Digit span
Visuospatial	Picture completion -Weschler adult intelligence scale (WAIS) Clock drawing

these peak responses is delayed in PD, and also in Alzheimer's and Huntington's diseases, reflecting abnormal central processing.[12] In addition, the EEG can be studied in relation to preparation for movement – the movement-related potential (MRP). A negative deflection (bereitschaftspotential) prior to a movement reflects the ability to anticipate and prepare for an action. This is also impaired in PD.[13] Brain electrical activity mapping (BEAM), which gives a contoured map of the intensity of electrical activity in response to a stimulus, has also been studied.[12] Equipment using 24 and 32 leads gives poor resolution, but the recent availability of 120-lead machines has vastly improved resolution for more detailed studies. Structural imaging using computed tomography (CT) and magnetic resonance imaging (MRI) has been used to measure the size of subcortical areas. However, functional imaging is much more useful in the study of cognition since areas of increased cerebral blood flow and metabolism can be demonstrated during the performance of specific tasks. Scans are performed at rest and during activation, then subtracted to demonstrate specific areas of activation. PET is performed in specialist centres using a cyclotron to manufacture the short-lived isotopes. Single photon emission tomography (SPECT) utilizes CT techniques to enhance isotope brain scans produced from improved radiotracer biochemicals that emit gamma rays. The technique is not as quantifiable as PET, and the resolution is poorer, but it is more accessible and has been used in the differential diagnosis of PD.[13] A more rapid change in cerebral blood flow can be detected using functional magnetic resonance scanning (FMRI). This technique uses MRI technology to monitor the change in resonance, which occurs when oxyhaemoglobin changes to deoxyhaemoglobin, thus measuring blood flow and metabolism. FMRI has only recently been utilized in PD, but promises to be the most sensitive technique in functional studies of cognition in this condition. Proton magnetic resonance spectroscopy, which measures metabolite signals from neurones, has been used to study small changes in cortical metabolism in early non-demented PD patients.[15]

Cognitive functions of the basal ganglia

In order to understand the effects of PD on cognition it is important to have a basic understanding of the functional anatomy of the basal ganglia. In a very simplified model it is useful to consider the basal ganglia connections as a series of parallel circuits (Fig. 8.1). The motor loop, which is involved in automatic motor function and automatic (implicit) learning, is under-active in PD. Implicit processes include conditioning, priming and automatic motor skills, which are not available to conscious thought. The complex loop, which is involved in explicit learning, problem solving and attention, is also under-active in PD.[16] Explicit processes are available to conscious thought, and include short- and long-term memory. Short-term or working memory can either be verbal or visuo-spatial, long-term memory can be either be episodic (recalled in a specific time frame) or semantic (recalled outside a time frame, e.g. grass is green).[17] The number of neurones in the lateral part of the substantia nigra compacta correlates with the motor severity of PD, whereas the number of neurones in the medial substantia nigra compacta correlates with abnormalities of cognition.[18] Compensatory over-activity of the cerebella motor pathways occurs in PD,[20] and these pathways involve more conscious processes such as attention and cueing.

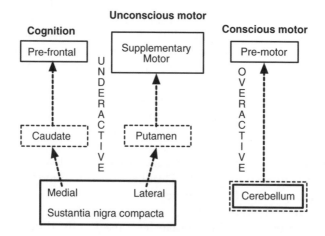

Fig. 8.1 Basal ganglia pathways in Parkinson's disease.

Cognitive and behavioural changes in PD

Cognition is the process by which knowledge is acquired, and this includes perception, intuition and reasoning.[17] Modern studies of cognition in PD began with Aubrin, who in 1937, supervised by Guillaine-Barré, performed one of the earliest experiments to use psychometric instruments for the measurement of cognition in PD.[2]

Patients with PD demonstrate slowing of movement (bradykinesia), and in addition show variable degrees of slowing of thought and speech. This was thought to be similar to the psychomotor retardation seen in depression by the French psychiatrist Ball in 1881.[2] This slowing of thought processes was defined as bradyphrenia by Naville in 1922.[2] Bradyphrenia is most severe in progressive supranuclear palsy (PSP), in which patients may take minutes to respond. Although bradyphrenia represents some slowing of central processing it is important to distinguish this from other forms of cognitive deterioration seen in PD.

Cognitive processes can be distributed or localized in the brain (Table 8.2),[17] and the fact that many of these functions are impaired in PD reflects the extensive connections of the basal ganglia with other brain areas. Higher animals are able to produce adaptive behaviour through connections between the basal ganglia and the prefrontal cortex (Fig. 8.2). The basal ganglia tend to select routine over-learned or safe behaviours. In normal circumstances these behaviours are suppressed through connections with the prefrontal cortex,

Table 8.2   Structure of cognition and memory

Cognition – Distributed	Cognition – Localized
• Attention – Reticular activating system and association areas • Memory – Limbic, hippocampus, diencephalon • Higher functions – Frontal	• Dominant hemisphere – Language, calculation, praxis • Non-dominant – Spatial attention, visuoperceptual skills, construction, language prosody, vigilance
Memory – Explicit	**Memory – Implicit**
• Short term (working memory) – verbal, spatial • Long term – Episodic, semantic	• Conditioning • Priming • Motor skills

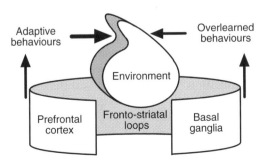

Fig. 8.2   Behaviour and basal ganglia.

which interacts more with the environment to produce adaptive behaviour appropriate to the situation. Interruption of this system in the prefrontal cortex tends to produce perseveration and disinhibition, whereas a basal ganglia lesion tends to produce a difficulty in acquiring new behaviours and a predominance of over-learned behaviour.[21]

The basal ganglia are involved in the generation, maintenance, switching and blending of motor, cognitive and behavioural patterns or sets. A basal ganglia lesion leads to difficulties with procedural mobilization, that is problems selecting, activating and maintaining behaviours, difficulty formulating strategies and preparing for action.[16,21] In the non-demented PD patient, the core deficit is of planning abilities sometimes called the dysexecutive syndrome.[22] This produces abnormalities of the executive functions of abstract reasoning, planning, set shifting, working memory, semantic memory, temporal sequencing, and abnormal procedural learning evidenced by slowing of serial reaction times.[22] These abnormalities of frontal lobe function may be associated with apathy. There is also evidence of visuospatial dysfunction with reduction in central processing speed and reduced useful visual field.[23] These visual abnormalities may predict poor performance in complex psychomotor tasks such as driving a car. Recent studies have shown that slowing of the processing of visual information is the best predictor of poor driving ability in PD[6] and of accident risk in older adults.[24]

Underactivation of the prefrontal and supplementary motor areas with compensatory increased activation of lateral prefrontal, cerebellar and hippocampal areas have been shown on PET scans.[25] These abnormalities occur not only when a task is actually performed but also when subjects imagine performing the task. This evidence supports the use of compensatory strategies, which utilize the activated brain areas in therapy.

Age of disease onset is a critical determinant of cognitive deterioration in PD. Regression analyses have demonstrated that older age of disease onset consistently predicts cognitive decline above and beyond normative ageing and disease duration, with specific deterioration in visuospatial ability, immediate and delayed verbal memory and executive functions.[26]

The effects of treatment on cognition are confusing. Levodopa would be expected to improve function mediated by dopaminergic pathways, but the effects are difficult to separate from the effects of disease severity and motor performance. This may explain why some studies have suggested that levodopa contributes to frontal dysfunction. There is conflicting evidence regarding any specific cognitive deficit associated with modern stereotactic surgery in PD. Subgroup analysis shows that postoperative cognitive decline may be more common in older patients and patients taking higher doses of levodopa undergoing pallidal stimulation.[27] The effects of subthalamic stimulation on cognition are yet to be studied.

In summary, the deficits in PD tend to lead patients to be rather more reactive rather than predictive in relation to the environment in cognitive, behavioural and motor activities, and this deficit increases with older age of disease onset.

Dementia in PD

The term 'dementia' has been used for centuries, but it first acquired a medical connotation in the eighteenth century. In the *Encyclopedie* of 1765, Diderot and D'Alembert described people with dementia as having weakening of understanding and memory, cannot remember anything, have no judgement and are sluggish and retarded.[2] This may have been the first description of dementia with parkinsonism. The syndrome of dementia is a more global decline of intellect, memory and personality than the cognitive deficits of PD described above, and interferes with everyday activities through changes in emotional control, motivation or social behaviour. Dementia is more common with an age of onset of PD >60 years and in late-stage disease with more severe extrapyramidal syndrome, particularly in patients who develop psychosis and confusion on levodopa.[28] Early abnormalities on tests of verbal fluency, the picture completion section of the Wechsler Adult Intelligence Scale, and the interference section of the STROOP test (a test of divided attention), may also predict the development of dementia.[28]

The age-specific prevalence of dementia (from all causes) in the normal population increases with increasing age. The relative risk of developing dementia in PD at all ages is higher than that of age-matched controls, but also increases with increasing age. In clinical practice, therefore, dementia is common in the older PD patient but relatively less common in the young. The most accurate prevalence figures for dementia in PD are derived from community studies. A recent community study using the CAMCOG (cognitive section of the Cambridge Examination for mental disorders) as a screening tool showed a total of 44 per cent to meet DSM-IV criteria for dementia. The demented subjects were significantly older, demonstrated more depression, and tended to have more severe motor problems. This study also confirmed the high false-positive rate of the commonly used mini mental state examination (MMSE) for detecting dementia in PD.[29]

It is clear that the dementia in PD is not one condition but is heterogeneous and contributed to by a spectrum of pathologies. Patients may develop a severe disturbance of planning (dysexecutive syndrome), slowing of thought (bradyphrenia) and a memory deficit which responds to external cues or reminders which is described as subcortical dementia. This deficit of recall is not primarily due to memory disruption, and there is debate about the use of the term dementia in these patients. The term 'subcortical dementia' was first used in 1974, and although there is still some debate, recent papers have supported the clinical usefulness of distinguishing subcortical from cortical dementia.[18] Since patients demonstrate frontal lobe dysfunction, including impaired verbal fluency, the condition is more correctly termed a subcorticofrontal dementia. This may be due to PD itself, but severe dysexecutive syndromes are more of a feature of PSP and this condition must be excluded.

Aetiology: pathology

In post-mortem studies dementia may be associated with increasing density of cortical intracellular inclusion bodies (Lewy bodies) which, in its most advanced form, is called dementia with Lewy bodies (DLB). In a recent study there was a direct correlation between the density of α-synuclein cortical Lewy bodies and the severity of dementia, with a high sensitivity (91 per cent) and high specificity (90 per cent) of these markers for dementia in PD.[30] In other studies there is no clear relationship in PD between the density of cortical Lewy bodies and dementia. DLB may however represent 15–20 per cent of all causes of dementia in general, and is the most important differential diagnosis in PD with dementia. These patients have early onset of cognitive deficit with fluctuation, early hallucinosis, more severe visuospatial dysfunction, disturbances of consciousness and severe motor problems.[31] The consensus criteria for the clinical diagnosis of DLB (Table 8.3) have been validated prospectively over a one-year follow-up.[32] In this study, comparing DLB with Alzheimer's disease (AD), the DLB patients suffered more visual hallucinations, disturbances of consciousness and parkinsonism than the AD patients. A small proportion of patients with AD (6.7 per cent) may develop parkinsonism, but this is usually late in the disease.[32].

When comparing DLB with PD, the DLB patients tended to have more rigidity and more visuospatial disturbances, as evidenced by difficulty on the draw and copy stages of the clock-drawing test. Patients with AD had difficulty drawing clocks but responded better to copying clocks.[33] PD dementia can also be due to concurrent AD or cerebrovascular disease, or to a mixture of causes. In a recent pathological study of dementia with no PD, 85 per cent had Alzheimer pathology, 29 per cent infarcts and 15 per cent Lewy bodies.

Table 8.3 A summary of international consensus criteria for the diagnosis of dementia with Lewy bodies

1. **Progressive cognitive decline interfering with normal social and occupational function.** Evident with progression. Prominent subcorticofrontal, attentional and visuospatial deficits
2. **Core features**
  - Fluctuating cognition
  - Recurrent visual hallucinations
  - Spontaneous motor features of Parkinsonism
3. **Supportive features**
  - Falls
  - Syncope/transient loss of consciousness
  - Neuroleptic sensitivity
  - Systematized delusions
  - Other hallucinations
4. **Diagnosis less likely in the presence of:**
  - Stroke on clinical examination or imaging
  - Any other disorder sufficient to account for the condition

The most significant finding was the high prevalence of mixed pathology (38.8 per cent).[34] Although this study was not specifically concerned with PD, it does confirm the heterogeneity of dementia and the fact that clinical diagnostic criteria may not be good at picking up this mixed pathology. In a postmortem pathological study of hospitalized PD, patients with dementia have a higher degree of cortical Alzheimer pathology, but the correlation of neurofibrillary changes, cortical Lewy bodies and dementia was poor.[35] Despite this, some workers have hypothesized that PD-specific lesions when combined with Alzheimer pathology increases the likelihood that a patient will dement. There are common biochemical abnormalities in both conditions. The Lewy body neurofilaments and Alzheimer tangles share common characteristics, and these two pathologies appear more together than expected by chance, suggesting some relationship between them. Although pathological abnormalities of subcortical structures (nucleus basalis of meynert, locus ceruleus and limbic structures) occur in PD, it seems to be the development of cortical Lewy bodies and/or Alzheimer pathology which is most associated with the onset of dementia.[35]

The role of white matter vascular lesions in the dementia of PD is unclear. Vascular mixed pathology in dementia without PD is more common than pure vascular dementia, and it may be the case in PD that vascular lesions add to the burden of pathology causing dementia.

The pathological causes of dementia and cognitive impairment in PD are likely to be heterogeneous, and there may be a spectrum of pathological changes, which increases the probability of dementia. These changes can be summarized as follows:

- Atrophy of the substantia nigra.
- Atrophy of the substantia nigra and nucleus basalis (cholinergic).
- Atrophy of the substantia nigra and nucleus basalis with cortical Lewy bodies.
- Atrophy of the substantia nigra and nucleus basalis with cortical Lewy bodies and plaques (DLB).
- Atrophy of the substantia nigra and nucleus basalis with cortical Lewy bodies, plaques and tangles (AD).

Aetiology: neurochemistry

Dopaminergic, cholinergic and noradrenergic mechanisms have been postulated for the cognitive changes in PD. Methyl-phenyl-tetrahydropyridine (MPTP) selectively destroys nigrostriatal neurones, and people exposed to this develop parkinsonism, with deficits in planning and internal control. Dopaminergic stimulation has only a weak positive effect on cognition in off-periods in PD. This dopamine deficiency is compounded by loss of inputs from the cholinergic and noradrenergic systems. Atrophy of the nucleus basalis in PD produces a marked cholinergic underactivity. Cognitive deficits increase with reduced cortical cholinergic and particularly nicotinic receptor binding.[36] Nicotine increases the availability of dopamine, improving motor function and some aspects of cognition in normals, AD and possibly PD.[36] Smoking reduces the incidence of AD and PD, and a neuroprotective role has been postulated. The effects of acetylcholinesterase inhibitor drugs may be partly mediated through nicotinic receptors and these drugs, which are being tested in DLB, may be useful in PD. Noradrenergic deficiency may produce attention deficits, which may be potentially correctable with noradrenaline precursors or re-uptake inhibitors.[37]

Management of dementia

The difficulty of diagnosis of dementia in PD is compounded by fluctuation in the condition, the presence of the motor deficit, depression and the effects of treatment. Since the dementia of PD is due to a spectrum of disorders, including AD, the principles of clinical management of patients with dementia in PD are no different to other forms of dementia. These principles of management of dementia, which focus on carers, cognition, assessment, liaison and medical treatment can be summarized using the mnemonic, 'CALM' (Table 8.4). Patients may benefit more from external cues for memory and movement . Sedation, especially neuroleptics, should be avoided if possible, but where agitation and restlessness is a problem small doses of benzodiazepines can be tried. Once anti-parkinsonian medication is optimized, acetylcholinesterase inhibitors should be considered. This should be done with careful titration of small increments of treatment, while monitoring the patient's mental, physical and cognitive state, as in AD. Management of hallucinations is of major importance, particularly for the relatives (see below). It is easy for these patients to 'fall between two stools' because of the combination of major physical and cognitive symptoms. Therefore, early liaison with psychogeriatric services is important in order to develop a joint management plan, which must involve liaison with social services and provision of appropriate social and respite care. Access to detailed and repeated neu-

Table 8.4 The management of dementia in Parkinson's disease: 'CALM'

- **Carer support** – Appropriate and timely social and respite care, support groups
- **Cognitive strategies** – Use of cueing and attentional strategies for movement and memory
- **Assessment** – Full and regular interdisciplinary assessment – cognition, capacity, mood, psychosis, motor, ADL and social function
- **Liaison** – Early psychogeriatric referral. Close liaison between specialist and primary healthcare teams. Key role of PD nurse specialist
- **Medical care** – Avoid neuroleptics, consider acetylcholinesterase inhibitors, manage sleep disturbance, manage hallucinosis, avoid hospitalization and anaesthesia where possible

ropsychological assessment by a clinical psychologist integrated with the interdisciplinary team is helpful in the assessment and management of cognitive changes and dementia in PD. These patients may worsen in hospital because of the change in environment and accidental alteration of drug timing. In some areas there is provision of respite care for the patient and carer together. Anaesthesia often produces deterioration in cognitive and physical function. Support for carers is vital, since the 24- h burden of care is stressful and demanding. Many cases will ultimately not be manageable in the home environment. Assessment of the capacity of patients to make decisions can be difficult due to speech problems and the fluctuation of cognition. It is important to understand that patients must be assumed to have capacity unless specific criteria are met, since there is a tendency to try to make decisions for patients without their full participation. Loss of capacity may occur when abilities to understand, retain and manipulate information are lost, or when/if the patient is unable to communicate choice. Decisions must be free from coercion, and this includes internal coercion from delusions and psychosis. Loss of capacity is not assumed because a diagnosis of PD dementia has been made. Often capacity may vary and may need to be assessed in relation to a specific decision at a specific point in time. An independent assessment from a psychogeriatrician can be helpful in these circumstances. It is useful for patients and relatives to complete an enduring power of attorney at an early stage. This process allows an appointed attorney to continue to look after the affairs and interest of the patient if they lose capacity. Where loss of capacity is demonstrated, it is important for the carers to be fully involved in decisions on respite and long-term residential or nursing home care, since they possess vital knowledge of those for whom they care.

Depression in PD

Depressive symptoms are common in PD, especially in elderly patients,[4] but there are problems defining depressive illness since many standardized tests are affected by the physical symptoms of PD. Autonomic symptoms are more common in elderly PD patients and can be associated with depression and anxiety. The psychomotor retardation of PD can be confused with depression. Diagnostic criteria for depression in medical conditions are confusing and difficult to apply in practice.

The prevalence of depression in PD depends upon the definition used. The use of a simple rating scale such as the Geriatric Depression Scale may aid assessment of patients, but may reflect the presence of depressive symptomatology rather than depressive illness. In a recent community study using the GDS as a screening tool the prevalence of depression was 64 per cent in patients and 34 per cent in carers.[4] Other community studies using DSM-IV criteria for medical mood disorder reported much lower frequencies of 3–8 per cent.[38] In a meta-analysis of 52 studies containing 5000 subjects, the prevalence of minor depression was 44 per cent, major depression 11.8 per cent and anxiety 25.3 per cent.[39] Apathy, with or without depression, is common in PD and seems to be associated more with cognitive impairment than with depression, with patients demonstrating abnormalities particularly on frontal lobe function.[40]

Aetiology

Many possible associations of depression in PD have been studied (Table 8.5). There is some evidence for a laterality of mood with studies showing more depression in right hemi-PD.[41] Transcranial magnetic stimulation of the dominant hemisphere may improve mood.[42] More severe akinesia and motor fluctuation may increase depression. There is conflicting evidence as to whether psychosis or cognitive impairment are associated with depression. Studies comparing depression in PD and depression without PD have shown similar cognitive deficits in both conditions, with reduced verbal fluency and attention deficits in depression and problems of abstract reasoning and set shifting in PD depression.[43] Patients with depressive pseudodementia respond to cueing in a similar manner to PD patients with subcortical dementia, which suggests that similar neural pathways are involved.[44] Some studies have shown that increasing age is a risk factor for PD depression. Other studies suggest that the increased handicap of having PD at a young age increases the risk of depression. Women are proportionately more likely to suffer depression in PD. Marked sleep disturbance is associated with PD depression, with findings of abnormalities of melatonin and circadian rhythm in fluctuating PD being similar to those in non-PD depression.[45]

It is still unclear how much the depression of PD is due to the biology of the disease or is the result of psychosocial effects of chronic disease. An organic basis for depression is supported by some studies showing a possible familial aggregation of unipolar depression and PD.[46] Depression is more pronounced in off-periods, possibly due to the deregulation of the locus ceruleus similar to that found in rapid cycling bipolar affective disorder.[41] Noradrenergic deficiency and cell loss in the locus ceruleus may be associated with the bradyphrenia and attention deficits of PD. Dopamine deficiency in basal ganglia, orbitofrontal and limbic circuits is associated in animal studies with dysfunction of the reward system. This can lead to anhedonia or the reduced

Table 8.5 Depression in Parkinson's disease: associations and aetiology

Associated conditions	Organic features	Psychosocial features
• Anxiety	• Biochemical changes	• Similar prevalence in other
• Psychosis	• Familial aggregation	chronic diseases
• Cognitive impairment	• Mesencephalic changes	• No relation to PD severity
• Sleep disturbance	on sonography and MRI	• No relation to PD
• Female	• ERP changes	progression
• ? Younger	• Produced by deep brain	• Related to handicap
• Akinesia	stimulation	• Multifactorial
• Motor fluctuation	• Motor fluctuation	
• Right hemi-PD	• Response to rTMS, ECT and	
	drugs	

experience of reward seen in PD. Serotonergic abnormalities in the medial raphé projection to the diencephalon and limbic areas may produce the psychomotor retardation of PD and depression. In addition to these neurochemical disturbances, abnormalities of the mesencephalon on MRI and transcranial ultrasound, frontal cortical under-activity on PET scans and reduced caudate metabolism all suggest an organic basis for depression in PD.[41] Cerebrovascular disease is an important determinant in the aetiology of depression,[47] especially in the elderly, and may also be an important contributory factor to the development of depression in the elderly PD patient. The possible neuroanatomical relationship between depression and the basal ganglia was emphasized by a recent description of acute severe depression brought on by deep brain stimulation. In this case, stimulation of the left subthalamic nucleus improved symptoms of PD, but additional stimulation of the left substantia nigra evoked unequivocal depressive symptoms.[48] This case raises the possibility of specific neural pathways in the brain for mood, in addition to motor functions.[49]

There is, however, considerable disadvantage and handicap associated with a chronic neurological disorder. There is no good evidence for a direct correlation between disease severity and depression. Some workers have gone so far as to suggest a mainly psychosocial model for depression in PD.[50] It is difficult to attribute functions of the human mind to purely neurochemical and structural changes, and intuitively it seems most likely that PD depression has a major organic predisposition interacting with psychosocial factors influencing its presentation.

Management of depression

The treatment of depression in PD has not been well studied but, as in the case of dementia, the principles can be summarized using the mnemonic, 'CALM' (Table 8.6). Provision of support, advice and counselling to both patients and carers may be combined with antidepressant therapy. A clear explanation that depression is a common intrinsic part of PD is needed in order for patients and carers to accept appropriate help and treatment. Cognitive therapy can

Table 8.6 The management of depression in Parkinson's disease: 'CALM'

- **Carer** – Support and counselling for patient and carer. Assessment of carer stress and depression
- **Cognition** – Possible role for cognitive therapy
- **Assessment** – Regular interdisciplinary assessment including diagnosis and severity of depression, associated cognitive impairment, exclude pseudodementia, psychosis, motor and mood fluctuation, ADL and social function
- **Liaison** – Psychogeriatric referral if resistant or severe. Close liaison between primary healthcare team and specialist
- **Medical** – Optimize dopaminergic therapy. Appropriate antidepressant. Avoid TCA. Careful use of SSRI monitoring motor function. Combined re-uptake inhibitors SNRI and especially NaSSA may prove beneficial. Possible role for moclobamide. ECT effective in severe depression

benefit depression in the elderly and may have a role in PD. Support groups held through PD clinics or the Parkinson's Disease Society, can provide an informal form of group therapy. Counselling and support can be provided for patients and carers by social workers and counsellors with a special interest in PD, or through the welfare officer of the local Parkinson's Disease Society. The PD nurse specialists have a key role in the provision and coordination of these support services in the management of depression.

The first option in the drug treatment of PD depression is to ensure optimal dopaminergic treatment. Mood elevation and anxiety reduction can be demonstrated using levodopa infusions, and therefore smoothing out fluctuations may be important in the control of depression in PD.[51] There is currently no real evidence that any antidepressant has greater safety or efficacy than any other in PD. The presence of anxiety may influence the choice of antidepressant to a more sedative one or a selective serotonin re-uptake inhibitor (SSRI) antidepressant. In a recent review of all adequate trials of drug treatment of PD depression, five out of 12 trials were using the monoamine oxidase inhibitor selegeline.[41] Despite this, the consensus is that selegeline is not a very effective antidepressant. There is a very slight risk of producing a serotonin syndrome (hyperpyrexia, agitation, confusion) when selegeline is combined with tricyclics or long-acting SSRI antidepressants such as fluoxetine. There is a theoretical risk of increased parkinsonism with SSRI antidepressants, and some case reports exist of akathisia, tardive dyskinesia and dystonia,[52] but there is no clinical evidence that these effects are significant. The favourable side-effect profile means many clinicians use SSRI antidepressants as the first-line treatment in PD, although trial evidence for efficacy these drugs in PD is based mainly on open studies.[53] There is not yet any trial evidence that the SSRI antidepressants help depressive symptoms outside a depressive illness. Studies are being conducted using SSRI antidepressants in mood fluctuations in PD. Tricyclic antidepressants (TCA) were prescribed widely in PD because of the belief that the anticholinergic effect may also help the motor symptoms. Desimipramine can increase tremor in PD, but other studies show that imipramine is most effective in patients with rigidity.[54] In elderly patients the anticholinergic side effects of these drugs, including urinary retention, blurred vision, faecal impaction and dry mouth interfering with dentures, reduce their tolerability. Since anticholinergic drugs are now avoided by most experts in the treatment of PD, tricyclic antidepressants are now second-line drugs in the treatment of PD depression.

The newer noradrenaline and serotonin combined re-uptake inhibitors may have an increasing role in PD depression. Their relative lack of side effects such as nausea, sleep disturbance, agitation and sexual dysfunction provide a useful alternative to the TCA and SSRI drugs. They have yet to show advantages over SSRI drugs, and there is limited experience in PD. Venlafaxine, a serotonin and noradrenaline re-uptake inhibitor (SNRI), has an anxiolytic effect with a rapid onset of action in the elderly at 1–2 weeks.[55] These effects have not been demonstrated in PD, but may be due to combined actions on serotonin and noradrenaline (which occurs at higher doses) and an ability to titrate the dose rapidly. Mirtazepine, a derivative of mianserin, is a noradrenaline and specific serotonin antidepressant (NaSSA) and may also have a more rapid onset of action.[55] Antidepressant actions of NaSSA are produced through increasing noradrenaline by antagonism of pre-synaptic α_2 autoreceptors and indirect enhancement of serotonin neurotransmission by 5-HT_1 receptors. This profile of neurotransmitter action may be theoretically useful in PD, reducing both depression and motor symptoms.[56] It is possible that serotonergic manipulation could lead to hallucinosis in PD, and there is an early case report of psychosis possibly induced by mirtazapine.[57] Other drugs include Reboxitine, which is a selective noradrenaline re-uptake inhibitor and may cause insomnia, increased sweating and dry mouth, and Nefazodone, which has SSRI actions with additional 5-HT_2 action and reduced side effects.

Moclobamide, a reversible monoamine oxidase A (MAOA) inhibitor, may be considered as an option in resistant depression in PD. It has a combined effect on serotonin and noradrenaline and possibly other transmitters. In clinical practice in patients without PD, moclobamide is only a weak antidepressant. An ideal antidepressant in PD would combine inhibition of re-uptake of dopamine, serotonin and noradrenaline with no hypertensive effect. To this end, some workers have combined MAOA inhibition with MAOB inhibition, showing enhanced antidepressant activity with no cheese (hypertensive) effect.[58]

The best approach to PD depression is to optimize dopaminergic therapy, followed by a trial of at least 6 weeks of adequate doses of antidepressant with careful monitoring of the patient's mood and motor function. The choice of which antidepressant to use comes down to personal experience and preference. Many workers use the SSRI group as first-line therapy with a combined re-uptake inhibitor (SNRI or NaSSA) as second choice. More studies are needed of the possible extrapyramidal side effects of the SSRI group and the motor effects of the combined re-uptake inhibitors. The pattern of liver enzyme induction varies from one SSRI to another, and this may influence the choice of drug. The response to an antidepressant is best reviewed after 6 weeks of a therapeutic dose. If, after this period, there is no response, a change of antidepressant can be considered. Some workers have suggested a cascade of antidepressant treatment, utilizing a different group every 6 weeks, until there is a response. Future clarification of the efficacy of different antidepressant groups in PD may allow the clinician to choose the most effective drug at the outset, avoiding the need for frequent change in therapy. Treatment should be continued for six months following response before gradually tailing off. Two or more episodes of depression may be an indication for long-term treatment.

Direct-acting dopamine agonists (e.g. pergolide, pramipexole) may have an antidepressant effect, and this may be partly due to an effect on psychomotor retardation. Catechol-O-methyl transferase (COMT) inhibitors may have a similar effect through enhancement of dopaminergic transmission and reduction in motor fluctuation.

Medication failure, the development of suicidal ideas or life-threatening complications at any stage, should be taken seriously, and electroconvulsive therapy (ECT) considered. ECT has been shown to be effective in the treatment of depression, motor fluctuations and drug-induced mania. Motor symptoms, especially rigidity, have been shown to respond and relapse more quickly than depression, the response being greater in the elderly.[41,59]

Repetitive transcranial magnetic stimulation (rTMS) has been used experimentally to treat depression. This technique produces induced electrical activity in the brain by repetitive activation of a surface electromagnet. The effects on depression may only last 2 weeks, and concurrent antidepressants are needed. rTMS may, in future, be a useful alternative to ECT, since it has a more focal effect, reducing adverse cognitive symptoms and avoiding the need for a general anaesthetic. Stimulation over the motor cortex can reduce motor slowing and improve cognition in elderly PD patients. rTMS requires further evaluation, but has a promising future role in the treatment of depression in PD.[41,42]

Drug-induced phenomena in PD

Anxiety

Symptoms of anxiety are common in PD, occurring in at least 25 per cent of patients.[39] Anxiety can be a part of a depressive illness and can be helped by appropriate sedative antidepressant therapy. Increasing anxiety may be a manifestation of cognitive changes in PD, with new situations or changes from regular routine feeling threatening to patients who are cognitively less flexible. Anxiety can also be a drug-induced side effect, occurring at peak dose or in an off-period.[60] It is important therefore to take a good history from patients and carers in order to ascertain the cause of anxiety in PD.

Restlessness at peak dose can be severe, with mental over-activity and rarely the development of mania. This may be a dopaminergic phenomenon, since dopamine agonists have been reported to produce mania in the absence of PD.[60]

Explanation, support, advice and relaxation exercises, combined with appropriate pharmacotherapy are the mainstays of treatment of anxiety in PD. SSRI antidepressants, sedative tricyclic antidepressants, small doses of benzodiazepines and only rarely low-dose atypical neuroleptics could be used in severe anxiety.

Sexual dysfunction

Sexual dysfunction is common in PD. Impotence may be due to side effects of drugs such as antidepressants, or part of the disease. Hypersexualism is usually a peak-dose phenomenon,[60] and can lead to complaints from the partner of unreasonable sexual demands. Sometimes unwelcome thoughts or behaviours are intrusive and similar in nature to obsessive compulsive disorder. Hypersexualism is not associated with cognitive changes at peak dose, and the cause in not well understood.[61] Priapism due to levodopa has been reported and was noticed more in the days of high-dose treatment.[60] Loss of libido is common but less well recognized, and has been reported to be a problem in women.[62] Issues of sexuality are overlooked or avoided in elderly people, who may be less willing to respond to direct questions on sexual matters in quality of life assessment tools. The PD nurse specialist may be able to provide counselling and advice to patients and partners. This may be best done in the patient's own home rather than in clinic.

Psychosis

Aetiology

During the first five years following diagnosis, 30 per cent of patients will develop hallucinosis. There may be a kindling effect, with patients progressing down a 'neuropsychiatric slippery slope', one type of symptom increasing the likelihood of the next (Fig. 8.3). Although this effect is debatable, once elderly patients start to hallucinate, the hallucinations can be very difficult to eliminate, and become permanent in 80 per cent of patients.[63] These hallucinations are thought to be due to excessive dopaminergic and serotonergic activity.[60] Dopaminergic treatment may only precipitate psychosis in predisposed individuals who have a limbic predominance of Lewy bodies.

The first sign of problems may be vivid dreams, illusions of shapes in shadows or patterns, or a peculiar sense of presence in the room. This may progress to stereotyped non-threatening visual hallucinosis in a clear sensorium. Hallucinations are visual, vivid and vital, or living, including images of people who may be small (Lilliputian syndrome). They may occur in the evening and at night, in the shadows, in patterns on the furniture and carpets, and are often seen through windows or in mirrors. They become intrusive

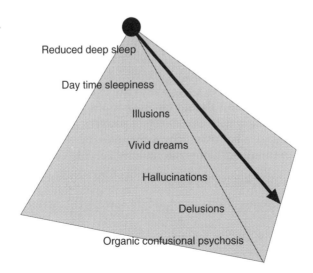

Reduced deep sleep

Day time sleepiness

Illusions

Vivid dreams

Hallucinations

Delusions

Organic confusional psychosis

Fig. 8.3   The neuropsychiatric 'slippery slope'.

when patients start to act upon hallucinations, by laying extra places at table or beating off non-existent intruders. Patients may then develop systematic delusions surrounding the hallucinations, losing their ability to distinguish reality. There are some rare reports in PD of delusional misidentification, in which the misidentification of a near relative is associated with secondary delusions. This may be due to the coexistence of psychosis and frontal lobe impairment.[64] A more serious form of hallucinosis is evidenced by the development of mixed visual, auditory and tactile hallucinations. These may frightening, with visions of animals and insects, and occur throughout the day and night. This is an organic confusional psychosis and is similar to delirium tremens. Improvement using physostigmine suggests a cholinergic deficit as the basis for these hallucinations.[60] Auditory hallucinations only occur in patients who are also experiencing visual hallucinations. The voices are external, talking in the first or second person, are separate from the usually silent visual hallucinations, and do not usually have any affective component.[65] Patients can also experience tactile hallucinations, either in association with or separate from the visual hallucinosis.

There may be a bimodal onset of hallucinosis, with early onset (<5.5 years) associated with motor fluctuations and large doses of medication, and late onset >5.5 years) associated with cognitive impairment.[63] Hallucinations and delusions are more common in patients with a low mental test score. Pre-existing cognitive impairment and hallucinosis may be made worse by the use of direct-acting dopamine agonists, and elderly patients should be assessed carefully before commencing these drugs.[63]

Management of psychosis

Intercurrent illness as a cause for delirium should be ruled out. The severity of the psychosis and the degree of disruption to normal life are assessed. Many rating scales are used in psychiatry to assess psychosis, but are not specifically designed for PD and are research tools. A simple severity scale can be used in clinic (Table 8.7), together with measures of cognition (MMSE) and motor function, to assess severity and to monitor the effectiveness of intervention. Carers often experience more distress than patients, particularly because the hallucinations tend to be worse in the evening or at night, giving poor sleep. Careful explanation should be given to the patient and carer. Sensory regulation is important, with avoidance of patterns and provision of adequate lighting to reduce shadows. The principles of the management of psychosis can be summarized using the mnemonic, 'ERA' (Table 8.8). Drug

Table 8.7 Parkinson's disease hallucinosis score

Symptom	Score
• None	0
• Vivid dreams, illusions, sense of presence	1
• Dreams encroaching on waking hours, occasional tolerable visual hallucinations	2
• Regular evening and night-time intrusive visual hallucinations	3
• Disturbing visual, auditory or tactile hallucinations, occur day and night, delusions	4

therapy must be reduced in a stepwise manner, removing the most hallucinogenic drugs first, down to the minimum L-dopa (levodopa) dose required for motor function (Fig. 8.4).[66] It is not yet clear whether the new COMT inhibitor, entacapone, causes a similar frequency of hallucinosis as the direct-acting dopamine agonists, but many clinicians would opt for COMT inhibitors as adjunctive therapy for patients with previous hallucinosis or cognitive impairment. Subcutaneous apomorphine may allow reduction of other drugs, with a consequent reduction in hallucinosis. Occasionally, where these strategies have been ineffective, specific antipsychotics may be needed. Hallucinosis may be associated with 5-HT over-activity and cholinergic deficit

Table 8.8   The management of Parkinson's disease psychosis: 'ERA'

- **Exclude delirium** – Screen for intercurrent physical illness
- **Explain to carer** – Worries the carer more than the patient!
- **Reduce sensory deprivation and sensory overload** – adequate lighting, avoid excessive patterned furniture and fittings
- **Reduce drugs in stepwise fashion**
- **Anti-psychotics** – Careful use of atypical drugs. Monitor ECG, cognitive and motor function. Do not use traditional antipsychotics
- **acetylcholinesterase inhibitors** – Careful use monitoring cognition and motor function

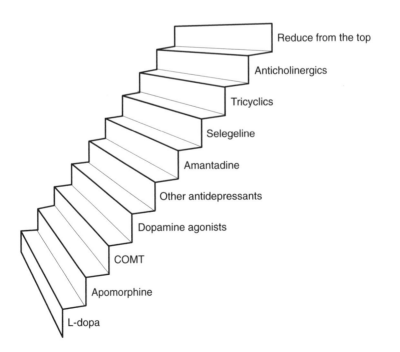

Fig. 8.4   Psychosis: stepwise reduction in drug treatment.

centrally. Small open-label studies have shown efficacy of the anti-emetic ondansetron (5-HT$_3$ antagonist) and some atypical neuroleptics in the treatment of PD psychosis. Atypical neuroleptics must be used in the smallest possible doses, such as olanzapine (2.5 mg), quetiapine (25 mg) and risperidone (1 mg). In practice, risperidone and olanzapine[67] can cause sedation and worsen motor function; olanzapine may worsen cognition and appears to offer no advantage over other antipsychotics in DLB. Quetiapine may be better tolerated, but is a weaker antipsychotic agent.[68] Clozapine is the most studied antipsychotic in PD and is effective in reducing psychosis, anxiety and hypersexuality,[69] but a licensing restriction limits its use in the UK. Zotepine has a similar antipsychotic efficacy to clozapine, and has an antidepressant effect by blocking noradrenaline re-uptake. This profile of action is potentially beneficial in PD but requires further study.

All of the atypical neuroleptics cause prolongation of the QT interval on ECG, especially in elderly patients. An ECG must be performed prior to therapy, and it is advisable to re-check the ECG at regular intervals. Atypical neuroleptics tend to accumulate in the elderly and therefore the doses used must be as small as possible with careful observation of the effects on motor and cognitive symptoms. Traditional antipsychotics (e.g. thioridazine) should be avoided because of their marked extrapyramidal side effects. A trial of acetylcholinesterase inhibitors may be warranted in dementia with psychosis, since enhancement of cholinergic activity may improve cognition and psychosis.[70] In an open study, rivastigmine reduced neuropsychiatric symptoms, and improved reaction times and cognitive performance, without worsening motor function.[70] These drugs must be given under the supervision of a specialist who can monitor cognition, motor function and the severity of psychosis.

Cognition and movement in PD

There is an intricate relationship between cognition and movement in PD. Studies of specific goal-directed movements show that PD patients can produce rapid movements, but these tend to be inaccurate. This inaccuracy is counteracted in most circumstances by utilizing visual direction, which causes slowing of movement. It has been postulated that some of the slowness of movement and hypokinesia in PD may be due to the adoption of a cautious cognitive strategy, in order to overcome the inaccuracy of movement.[71] In increasingly complex grasping tasks, however, PD patients do not adopt the normal cautious strategy of widening the hand with increasingly demanding tasks, but persist with hypometric hand grasp movements.[72] In simple tasks, difficulty in initiating movements is due to cortical under-activation or poor preparation for movement. In more complex tasks poor performance is due to a cognitive deficit in set shifting, with an inability to adopt appropriate strategies.[73] Increasingly severe cognitive deficits are associated with increasing motor disability and abnormal latency of P$_{300}$ on ERP due to prolonged processing time.[74] PET scan studies have shown that impairment of self-initiated movement is associated with under-activation of the dorsolateral prefrontal cortex.[13] With increasing motor severity, patients demonstrate frontal dysfunction, with poor verbal fluency and difficulty with divided attention. This can be seen in practice with patients demonstrating difficulty walking and talking at the same time.

In PD there are deficits of set shifting in both cognitive and motor tasks, with set shifting being the primary role of the basal ganglia. Movement may be a consequence of constant shifting of postural sets.[75] Regulation of the force of muscles is necessary in order to control the point at which opposing muscle groups reach equilibrium, and shifting this equilibrium point along a desired trajectory produces movement. A deficit of set shifting, and consequent force regulation, may be responsible for some of the motor syndrome of PD. Movement may be divided into separate sensory-motor-cognitive actions, with the basal ganglia playing a critical role in preparing, initiating and suppressing these actions.[75] Such theories unify cognition and movement, and explain the interaction between the cognitive and motor syndromes seen in PD.

This relationship between cognition and movement in PD has important implications for therapy (see Chapter 15). Function may be improved by encouraging attentional strategies to anticipate movement.[76] These strategies may allow movement to be produced by less automatic and more conscious attentional motor pathways,[76] such as the cerebellar-lateral premotor cortex pathways which develop compensatory over-activity in PD.[25]

Driving is one of the best examples of a complex psychomotor task which can be impaired by cognitive deficits in PD. Poor performance on some psychological tests can predict driving errors.[6] The best predictor is slowing of visual processing speed,[6] which is supported by the finding that in older adults without PD visual processing speed is a predictor of accident risk.[24] Specific tests have been developed which measure the limitations of useful visual field as a predictor of poor driving performance.

Extrapyramidal syndrome in AD

It is important to distinguish AD from DLB and PD with dementia. DLB has a male preponderance, with more fluctuation, hallucinosis and attentional deficits. Extrapyramidal signs occur early in DLB and late in AD. In both AD and DLB rigidity and bradykinesia are symmetrical and rest tremor is uncommon. The latter is due to the different pattern of striatal cell loss in the putamen, in these conditions, compared with PD. Extrapyramidal signs are much more common in AD than in age-matched controls, are more common in older patients, and tend to predict a worse prognosis, with increased mortality. The pathological basis for extrapyramidal signs is heterogeneous, but is most probably associated with the presence of subcortical Lewy bodies.[77]

Psychiatry of other multisystem degenerations

The psychopathology of other conditions causing parkinsonism reflects the relative distribution of pathological changes in the basal ganglia, frontal, limbic and cortical regions of the brain.

Multiple system atrophy (MSA) causes extensive cell loss and gliosis in the striatum, basal ganglia, brainstem and cerebellum. There are no clear cognitive differences between patients with MSA and PD. One study has suggested that PD patients have more depression and anxiety, with MSA patients having more blunting of affect. The latter may reflect neuronal loss in the caudate and ventral striatum which are part of the lateral orbitofrontal and limbic circuits.[78]

Patients with PSP present with subjective complaints of forgetfulness and loss of concentration. They develop a dysexecutive syndrome, with marked planning difficulties, reflecting extensive involvement of subcorticofrontal circuits. Bilateral involvement of these pathways may cause apathy, but relative sparing of the *raphé nucleus* and *locus ceruleus* may reduce the occurrence of depression compared with PD. Emotional liability is common, but psychosis is rare in PSP. Subcorticofrontal dementia leads to a delay in initiation of thoughts, perseveration, reduced verbal fluency and a dissociation between normal storage and impaired retrieval of information. Patients with PSP are more reliant on external environmental stimuli for behaviour (environmental dependence), which may be due to a lack of frontal control.[79] Patients need to be given adequate time to respond to questions, and may respond to cueing to improve memory.

Patients with corticobasal degeneration (CBD) have more depression and irritability, but less apathy than in PSP.[80] Patients may demonstrate cognitive abnormalities reflecting cortical disease including apraxias, alien hand, visual and sensory neglect. Gesture problems are said to be specific for CBD. Corticobasal syndrome can be rarely due to motor neurone disease (MND), which itself can be associated with parkinsonism. MND may prove to be a multisystem disease and a common cause of frontotemporal dementia .

Movement disorders in psychiatric illness

Movement disorders in psychiatric conditions can be primary, due to the disease itself, or secondary to treatment. Primary abnormalities are now difficult to separate from the effects of drug treatment. Patients with untreated schizophrenia can demonstrate dyskinesias (15 per cent), extrapyramidal signs (10 per cent), catatonia (rare) and abnormalities of voluntary movement such as mannerisms and stereotypic movements.[81] Catatonic patients become immobile, rigid, mute, resist movement and refuse nutrition. Catatonia can rarely be a feature of severe depression. Stereotypies and mannerisms including repetitive hand rubbing and rocking can be seen in depressed elderly patients and in dementia. Most commonly, movement disorders are secondary to drug treatment, particularly neuroleptics. Increasing age, female sex, organic brain disease, long-term treatment and rapid withdrawal can predispose to the development of tardive movement disorders, the most common of which is tardive dyskinesia. This condition can be very difficult to treat, and the best treatment is prevention by avoidance of precipitating medications. Atypical neuroleptics, used as alternative agents, may occasionally reduce the dyskinesia. With continued withdrawal of the causative drug, 33 per cent of patients will improve over 2 years. Only rarely, with severe disability, should dopamine-depleting agents be used (tetrabenazine, starting with 12.5 mg). The routine use of anticholinergic agents for patients on neuroleptics is not recommended. In elderly patients prochlorperazine and metaclopramide, used for nausea and dizziness, are common causes of tardive dyskinesia. Other drug-induced movements include dystonia, akathisia, parkinsonism and rarely tics and myoclonus. Drug-induced parkinsonism may require the use of levodopa, occasionally in association with continued low-dose neuroleptics, in patients with continuing psychosis. Tremors, dystonias and extrapyramidal signs have also been reported with antidepressants, including TCA and SSRI agents.[82] Close liaison between the physician and psychiatrist is essential in the management of these disorders in order to avoid conflicting advice.

Conclusions

Professionals, carers and patients need to be aware of the intimate relationship between the cognitive, emotional and motor components of PD and related disorders. The recognition, assessment and management of psychiatric problems in PD are important in order to improve the quality of life of both patients and carers. Brief assessments of mood, cognition and executive function may aid management, and help patients, carers and families to adjust to impairments in these areas.[83] Close cooperation between the primary healthcare team and specialist interdisciplinary team is important at all stages of the disease.

References

1. Parkinson J. *An essay on the shaking palsy*. 1817. Published by Macmillan magazines and the Parkinson's Disease Society of the United Kingdom. London, 1992.
2. Berrios GE. *The History of Mental Symptoms*. Cambridge: Cambridge University Press, 1996.
3. Hobson P, Holden A, Meara J. Measuring the impact of Parkinson's disease with the Parkinson's disease quality of life questionnaire. *Age Ageing* 1999; **28**: 341–6.
4. Meara J, Mitchelmore E, Hobson P. Use of the GDS-15 geriatric depression scale as a screening instrument for depressive symptomatology in patients with Parkinson's disease and their carers in the community. *Age Ageing* 1999; **28**: 35–8.
5. Goetz CG, Stebbins GT. Mortality and hallucinations in nursing home patients with advanced Parkinson's disease. *Neurology* 1995; **45**: 669–71.
6. Heikkila VM, Turkka J, Karpelanen J, Kallanrunta T, Summala H. Decreased driving ability in people with Parkinson's disease. *J. Neurol. Neurosurg. Psychiatry* 1998; **64**: 325–30.

7. De la Fuente-Fernandez R, Calne D. What do Lewy bodies tell us about dementia and parkinsonism? In: Perry R, McKeith I, Perry E (eds). *Dementia with Lewy bodies.* Cambridge: Cambridge University Press, 1996: 287–301.

8. Goetz CG. Historical background of behavioural studies in Parkinson's disease. In: Huber SJ, Cummings JL (eds). *Parkinson's disease – Neurobehavioural aspects.* New York & Oxford: Oxford University Press, 1992: 3–9.

9. Stern GM. Pre-morbid personality structure of patients with Parkinson's disease. In: Wolters EC, Scheltens P (eds). *Mental Dysfunction in Parkinson's disease.* Vrije Universiteit Amsterdam, 1993: 103–17.

10. Heberlein I, Ludin HP, Scholz J, Vieregge P. Personality depression and premorbid lifestyle in twin pairs discordant for Parkinson's disease. *J. Neurol. Neurosurg. Psychiatry* 1998; **64**: 262–6.

11. Williams DT, Ford B, Fahn S. Phenomenology and psychopathology related to psychogenic movement disorders. In: Weiner WJ, Lang AE (eds). *Behavioural Neurology of Movement Disorders.* Advances in Neurology, Vol. 65. New York: Raven Press, 1995: 231–58.

12. Lishman WA. *Organic psychiatry – The psychological consequences of cerebral disorder.* Oxford: Blackwell Science, 1998.

13. Jahanshahi M, Jenkins H, Brown R, Marsden D, Passingham RE, Brooks DJ. Self initiated versus externally triggered movements – An investigation using measurement of regional cerebral blood flow with PET and movement-related potentials in normal and Parkinson's disease subjects. *Brain* 1995; **118**: 913–33.

14. Ben Amer H, Grosset D. SPECT imaging in the diagnosis and staging of parkinsonism. *CNS* 1999; **2**: 9–12.

15. Hu MTM, Taylor-Robertson SD, Ray Chaudhuri K, Bell JD, Morris RG, Clough C, Brooks DJ, Turjanski N. Evidence for a cortical dysfunction in clinically non-demented patients with Parkinson's disease: a proton MR spectroscopy study. *J. Neurol. Neurosurg. Psychiatry* 1999; **67**: 20–6.

16. Saint-Cyr JA, Taylor AE, Nicholson K. Behaviour and the basal ganglia. In : Weiner WJ, Lang AE (eds). *Behavioural Neurology of Movement Disorders.* Advances in Neurology, Vol. 65. New York: Raven Press, 1995: 1–28.

17. Hodges JR. *Cognitive assessment for clinicians.* Oxford: Oxford University Press, 1994.

18. Savage CR. Neuropsychology of subcortical dementias. *Psychiatr. Clin. North Am.* 1997; **20**: 911–31.

19. Rinne JO, Rummukainen J, Paljarvi L, *et al.* Dementia in Parkinson's disease is related to neuronal loss in the medial substantia nigra. *Ann. Neurol.* 1989; **26**: 47–50.

20. Rascol O, Sabatini U, Fabre N, Brefel C, Loubinoux I, Celsis P, Senard JM, Montastruc JL, Chollet F. The ipsilateral cerebellar hemisphere is overactive during hand movements in akinetic parkinsonian patients. *Brain* 1997; **12**(Pt.1): 103–10.

21. Dubois B, Defontaines B, Deweer B, Malapani C, Pillon B. Cognitive and behavioural changes in patients with focal lesions of the basal ganglia. In: Weiner WJ, Lang AE (eds). *Behavioural Neurology of Movement Disorders.* Advances in Neurology, Vol. 65. New York: Raven Press, 1995: 29–42.

22. Dubois B, Pillon B. Cognitive deficits in Parkinson's disease. *J. Neurol.* 1997; **224**: 2–8.

23. Hunt LA, Sadun AA, Bassi CJ. Review of the visual system in Parkinson's disease. *Optometry Vis. Sci.* 1995; **72**: 92–9.

24. Owsley C, Ball K, McGwin G, Sloane ME, Roenker D, White MF, Owsley T. Visual processing impairment and risk of motor vehicle crash among older adults. *JAMA* 1998; **279**: 1083–8.

25. Brooks DJ. Practical problems in Parkinson's disease – insights from PET scanning.

Presented at: The science and practice of multidisciplinary care in Parkinson's disease and parkinsonism. British Geriatrics Society Special Interest Group in Parkinson's disease. July 9th 1999. Royal College of Physicians.

26. Katzen HL, Levin BE, Llabre ML. Age of disease onset influences cognition in Parkinson's disease. *J. Int. Neuropsychol. Soc.* 1998; **4**: 285–90.

27. Vingerhoets G, Van der Linden C, Lannoo E, Vandewalle V, Caemaert J, Wolters M, Van den Abeele D. Cognitive outcome after unilateral pallidal stimulation in Parkinson's disease. *J. Neurol. Neurosurg. Psychiatry* 1999; **66**: 297–304.

28. Mahieux F, Fenelon G, Flahault A, Manifanicier M, Michelot D, Boller F. Neuro-psychological prediction of dementia in Parkinson's disease. *J. Neurol. Neurosurg. Psychiatry* 1998; **64**: 178–83.

29. Hobson P, Meara J. The detection of dementia and cognitive impairment in a community population of elderly people with Parkinson's disease by use of the CAMCOG neuro-psychological test. *Age Ageing* 1999; **28**: 39–43.

30. Hurtig HI, Trojanowski JQ, Galvin J, *et al*. Alpha-synuclein cortical Lewy bodies correlate with dementia in Parkinson's disease. *Neurology* 2000; **54**: 1916–21.

31. McKeith IG, Galasko D, Kosaka K, *et al*. Consensus criteria for the clinical diagnosis of dementia with Lewy bodies (DLB). In: Perry R, McKeith I, Perry E (eds). *Dementia with Lewy bodies*. Cambridge: Cambridge University Press, 1996: 491–492.

32. Ballard CG, O'Brien J, Lowery K, Ayre GA, Harrison R, Perry R, Ince P, Neill D, McKeith IG. A prospective study of dementia with Lewy bodies. *Age Ageing* 1998; **27**: 631–6.

33. Gananalingham KK, Byrne EJ, Thornton A, Sambrook MA, Bannister P. Motor and cognitive function in Lewy body dementia: comparison with Alzheimer's and Parkinson's diseases. *J. Neurol. Neurosurg. Psychiatry* 1997; **62**: 243–52.

34. Holmes C, Cairns N, Lantos P, Mann A. Validity of current clinical criteria for Alzheimer's disease, vascular dementia and dementia with Lewy bodies. *Br. J. Psychiatry* 1999; **174**: 45–50.

35. De Vos RAI, Jansen ENH, Yilmazer D, Braak H, Braak E. Pathological and clinical features of Parkinson's disease with and without dementia. In: Perry R, McKeith I, Perry E (eds). *Dementia with Lewy bodies*. Cambridge: Cambridge University Press, 1996: 255–67.

36. Newhouse PE, Potter A, Levin ED. Nicotinic system involvement in Alzheimer's and Parkinson's diseases. *Drugs Ageing* 1997; **11**: 206–28.

37. Riekkinen M, Kejonen K, Jakala P, Soininen H, Riekkinen P, Jr. Reduction of noradrenaline impairs attention and dopamine depletion slows responses in Parkinson's disease. *Eur. J. Neurosci.* 1998; **10**: 1492–35.

38. Tandberg E, Larsen JP, Aarsland D, Cummings JL. The occurrence of depression in Parkinson's disease – a community based study. *Arch. Neurol.* 1996; **53**: 175–9.

39. Miyawaki E, Meah T, Kormos D, Tarsy D. Depression in Parkinson's disease: a meta-analysis regarding severity. Poster 588. Presented at 4th international congress on movement disorders. Vienna, Austria. June 1996.

40. Pluck GC, Brown RG. Neuropsychological aspects of apathy in Parkinson's disease. Abstracts on disc. Poster presented at XIIIth International Congress on Parkinson's disease. Vancouver, Canada. July 1999.

41. Tom T, Cummings JL. Depression in Parkinson's disease. Pharmacological characteristics and treatment. *Drugs Ageing* 1998; **12**: 55–74.

42. Shajahan P, Ebmeier K. Transcranial magnetic stimulation: a treatment of the future? *Prog. Neurol. Psychiatry* 1998; **2**: 19–22.

43. Kuzis G, Sabe L, Tiberti C, Leiguarda R, Starkstein SE. Cognitive functions in major depression and Parkinson's disease. *Arch. Neurol.* 1997; **54**: 982–6.

44. Coen RF, Kirby M, Swanwick GR, Maguire CP, Walsh JB, Coakley D, O'Neill D,

Lawlor BA. Distinguishing between patients with depression or very mild Alzheimer's disease using the delayed word recall test. *Dementia Geriatr. Cogn. Disord.* 1997; **8**: 244–7.

45. Devos D, Bordet R, Brique S, Touitou Y, Guieu JD, Libersa C, Destee A. Changes in circadian secretion patterns of melatonin in Parkinsonian patients with levo-dopa induced motor complications. Abstracts on disc. Poster presented at XIIIth International Congress on Parkinson's disease. Vancouver, Canada. July 1999.
46. Fahim S, van Duijn CM, Baker FM, Launer L, Breteler MM, Schudler WJ, Hofman A. A study of familial aggregation of depression, dementia and Parkinson's disease. *Eur. J. Epidemiol.* 1998; **14**: 233–8.
47. Pohjasvaara T, Leppavuori A, Siira I, Vataja R, Kaste M, Erkinjuntti T. Frequency and clinical determinants of post stroke depression. *Stroke* 1998; **29**: 2311–17.
48. Bejjani BP, Damier P, Arnulf I, Thivard L, Bonnet A, Dormont D, Cornu P, Pidoux B, Samson Y, Agid Y. Transient acute depression induced by high-frequency deep-brain stimulation. *N. Engl. J. Med.* 1999; **340**: 1476–80.
49. Yudofsky SC. Parkinson's disease depression and electrical stimulation of the brain. *N. Engl. J. Med.* 1999; **340**: 1500–2.
50. Brown R, Jahanshahi M. Depression in Parkinson's disease a psychosocial viewpoint. In: Weiner WJ, Lang AE (eds). *Behavioural Neurology of Movement Disorders.* Advances in Neurology, Vol. 65. New York: Raven Press, 1995: 61–84.
51. Maricle RA, Nutt JG, Valentine RJ, Carter JH. Dose response relationship of levodopa with mood and anxiety in fluctuating Parkinson's disease: a double-blind placebo-controlled study. *Neurology* 1995; **45**: 1757–60.
52. Lynd LD, Gerber PE. Selective serotonin reuptake inhibitor induced movement disorders. *Ann. Pharmacother.* 1998; **32**: 692–8.
53. Meara RJ, Bhowmick BK, Hobson JP. Safety and efficacy of sertraline in the treatment of depression concomitant to Parkinson's disease. *J. Psychopharmacol.* 1998; **12**(3 suppl. A):A19.
54. Silver JM, Yudofsky SC. Drug treatment of depression in Parkinson's disease. In: Huber SJ, Cummings JL (eds). *Parkinson's Disease – Neurobehavioural Aspects.* New York & Oxford: Oxford University Press, 1992: 240–54.
55. Montgomery SA. New developments in the treatment of depression. *J. Clin. Psychiatry* 1999; **60** (suppl. 14): 10–15; discussion 31–5.
56. Bierbrauer J. Motor signs in Parkinson's disease are altered by serotonergic and noradrenergic transmission levels. *Movement Disord.* 1998; **13** (suppl. 2): P1.155.
57. Normann C, Hesslinger B, Frauenknecht S, Berger M, Walden J. Psychosis during chronic levodopa therapy triggered by the new antidepressive drug mirtazapine. *Pharmacopsychiatry* 1997; **30**: 263–5.
58. Steur ENHJ, Ballering LAP. Moclobamide and selegeline in the treatment of depression in Parkinson's disease. *J. Neurol. Neurosurg. Psychiatry* 1997; **63**: 547.
59. Moellentine C, Rummans T, Ahlskog JE, Harmsen WS, Suman VJ, O'Connor MK, Black JL, Pileggi T. Effectiveness of ECT in patients with parkinsonism. *J. Neuropsychiatr. Clin. Neurosci.* 1998; **10**: 187–93.
60. Factor SA, Molho ES, Podskalny GD, Brown D. Parkinson's disease: drug induced psychiatric states. In: Weiner WJ, Lang AE (eds). *Behavioural Neurology of Movement Disorders.* Advances in Neurology, Vol. 65. New York: Raven Press, 1995: 115–38.
61. Harvey NS. Serial cognitive profiles in levodopa-induced hypersexuality. *Br. J. Psychiatry* 1988; **153**: 833–6.
62. Wermuth L, Stenager E. Sexual problems in young patients with Parkinson's disease. *Acta Neurol. Scand.* 1995; **91**: 453–5.
63. Graham JM, Grunwald RA, Sagar HJ. Hallucinosis in idiopathic Parkinson's disease. *J. Neurol. Neurosurg. Psychiatry* 1997; **63**: 434–40.

64. Roane DM, Rogers JD, Robinson JH, Feinberg TE. Delusional misidentification associated with parkinsonism. *J. Neuropsychiatr. Clin. Neurosc.* 1998; **10**: 194–8.

65. Inzelberg R, Kiperwasser S, Korczyn AD. Auditory hallucinations in Parkinson's disease. *J. Neurol. Neurosurg. Psychiatry* 1998; **64**: 533–5.

66. Hindle JV. Psychiatric problems in Parkinson's disease. *Geriatr. Med.* 1999; **29**: 37–43.

67. Graham JM, Sussman JD, Ford KS, Sagar HJ. Olanzapine in the treatment of hallucinosis in idiopathic Parkinson's disease: a cautionary note. *J. Neurol. Neurosurg. Psychiatry* 1998; **65**: 774–7.

68. Parsa MA, Bastani B. Quetiapine in the treatment of psychosis in patients with Parkinson's disease. *J. Neuropsychiatr. Clin. Neurosci.* 1998; **10**: 216–19.

69. Trosch RM, Frioedman JH, Lannon MC, Pahwa R, Smith D, Seeberger LC, O'Brien CF, LeWitt PA, Koller WC. Clozapine use in Parkinson's disease: a retrospective analysis of a large multicentred clinical experience. *Movement Disord.* 1998; **13**: 377–82.

70. Reading PJ, Luce AK, McKeith IG. Rivastigmine in the treatment of Parkinsonian hallucinosis. Abstracts on disc. Poster presented at XIIIth International Congress on Parkinson's disease. Vancouver, Canada. July 1999.

71. Brown RG, Jahanshahi M. Cognitive motor dysfunction in Parkinson's disease. *Neurology* 1996; **36** (suppl.1): 24–31.

72. Jackson GM, Jackson SR, Hindle JV. The control of bimanual reach-to-grasp movements in hemi-parkinsonian patients. *Experimental Brain Research* 2000; **132(3)**: 390–8.

73. Wascher E, Verlanger R, Vieregge P, Jaskeowoski P, Compf D. Responses to cued signals in Parkinson's disease – distinguishing between disorders of cognition and activation. *Brain* 1997; **120**: 1355–75.

74. Hayashi R, Hanya N, Kurashima T, Tokutake T. Relationship between cognitive impairments, event related potentials and motor disability scores in Parkinson's disease. *J. Neurol. Sci.* 1996; **141**: 45–8.

75. Hayes AE, Matthew CD, Keele SW, Rafal RD. Towards a functional analysis of the basal ganglia. *J. Cogn. Neurosci.* 1998; **10**: 178–98.

76. Cunnington R, Iansek R, Bradshaw JL. Movement related potentials in Parkinson's disease: external cues and attentional strategies. *Movement Disord.* 1999; **14**: 63–8.

77. Mitchell S. Extrapyramidal features in Alzheimer's disease. *Age Ageing* 1999; **28**: 401–9.

78. Fetoni V, Soliveri P, Testa D, Girotti F. Affective symptoms in multiple system atrophy and Parkinson's disease: response to levodopa therapy. *J. Neurol. Neurosurg. Psychiatry* 1999; **66**: 541–4.

79. Personal communication from Prof. Robert Rafal, University College of Wales, Bangor, Wales, UK. From: Litvan I, *et al.* Research needed in progressive supranuclear palsy: Statement of the brainstorming conference on PSP. Bethesda MD. March 18-19, 1999. Statement submitted *Annals of Neurology* August, 1999.

80. Litvan I, Cummings JL, Mega M. Neuropsychiatric features of corticobasal degeneration. *J. Neurol. Neurosurg. Psychiatry* 1998; **65**: 717–21.

81. Marsden CD. Motor disorders in schizophrenia. *Psychol. Med.* 1982; **12**: 13–15.

82. Kompoliti K. Drug induced and iatrogenic neurological disorders. In: Goetz CG, Pappert EJ (eds). *Textbook of Clinical Neurology*. Philadelphia: WB Saunders, 1999: 1123–52.

83. Elias JW, Treland JE. Executive function in Parkinson's disease and subcortical disorders. *Semin. Clin. Neuropsychiatry* 1999; **4**: 34–40.

9

Oral considerations: Communication and swallowing problems*, diet⁺ and oral care⁺

*L. Marks, ⁺K.M. Hyland and ⁺J. Fiske

Introduction

The purpose of this chapter is to highlight the importance of the roles of the speech and language therapist, dietician and dentist in the team approach to the management of the person with Parkinson's disease.

Communication problems*

Clinical relevance

Speech, swallowing and drooling difficulties are responsible for some of the most embarrassing, upsetting and socially isolating effects of Parkinson's disease (PD). The first section of this chapter will address practical aspects of assessment and management of these difficulties from the speech and language therapist's viewpoint.

Incidence

In a study of 261 people with PD, Oxtoby[1] found that 49 per cent of those surveyed reported speech disturbances of a significant degree. Speech symptoms become more prevalent as the disease progresses. Speech and language therapists commonly report that people with PD tend to seek advice only when the deficits markedly interfere with everyday life. Unfortunately, however, the greater the speech difficulty the greater the cognitive change, and this makes it more difficult for the person not only to learn new skills and strategies in the therapy situation, but also to carry over these skills into consciously controlled speech production in everyday conversations.

Features and assessment

In 1969, Darley et al.[2] analysed the dysarthric speech of PD and defined it in terms of problems with respiration, phonation (voice), articulation, and prosody (the variations in rate, pitch and loudness that lend the individual their unique emphasis and interest in verbal expression).

More recently Marigliani et al.[3] described four groups of speech deficits:

1. Voice
2. Fluency
3. Articulation
4. Language

The characteristics of the four main groups are detailed below, and can be used to identify the predominant communication disorder as part of a functional assessment.

VOICE

At least 89 per cent of people with PD have voice deficits,[4] the main features of which include:

- reduced respiratory support for speech;
- reduced voice volume;
- harsh, breathy, whispery or gurgly voice quality;
- limited or reduced ability to signal intonation; and
- disturbed resonance, often hypernasal.

Additional clinical observations include: (i) reduced attempts to communicate due to poor initiation, motivation and the degree of effort required; and (ii) a lack of awareness of a soft voice.

FLUENCY

The main features of fluency include:

- a 'stuttering-like' speech pattern;
- a large number of pauses;

- the listener's impression of hurried speech;
- inaccurate articulatory movements for intended speech;
- sound, syllable or word repetitions;
- initial word blocks and initiation difficulties; and
- difficulty in sustaining airflow, with poor respiratory control.

Additional clinical observations of fluency are that: (i) it can result in non-functional communication; and (ii) effort, anxiety and frustration are exhibited by the patient.

ARTICULATION

The main features of articulation include:

- a listener's impression of 'undershooting' of articulatory movements;
- disturbed intonation; and
- a listener's impression of a progressive reduction in volume, but an increase in rate.

Additional clinical observations of articulation are that: (i) it can result in non-functional communication; and (ii) the patient has poor perception of his/her own speech pattern.

LANGUAGE AND COGNITION

The main features of language and cognition include:

- a reduction in general cognitive function;
- disturbed auditory comprehension;
- poor topic maintenance;
- reduced initiation of conversation;
- inappropriate cessation of sentences;
- disrupted thought sequencing, which is reflected in the content of the conversation;
- limited eye contact, facial expression and body language;
- decreased insight and self-monitoring skills; and
- an increased dependence on the support person in conversation.

Additional clinical observations of language and cognition are that: (i) the support person reports an altered quality of conversation, and sometimes also 'personality changes'; they also report an impression of reduced motivation to converse on the part of the patient; and (iii) high levels of support person stress related to the altered conversational skills.

ASSESSMENT

Formal dysarthria assessments available include, the *Frenchay Dysarthria Assessments* (Pamela Enderby, College Hill Press, San Diego, CA, USA, 1980), and the *Assessment of Intelligibility of Dysarthric Speech* (Yorkston and Beukleman, 1981; available from Taskmaster Ltd, Morris Road, Leicester, LE2 6BR, UK: Taskmaster@webleicester.co.uk). Ramig *et al.*,[5] in the *Lee Silverman Voice*

Treatment Guide, provide various reproducible forms for assessment including a visual analogue scale (VAS) which can be completed by patients and/or carers, or by the speech and language therapist (see Appendix 1).

The coexistence of other age-related factors can influence assessment,[6] the ability to participate in therapy, and it's outcome. Examples include reduced vision, hearing, respiratory and laryngeal control, resonance and articulation. Some individuals may have been diagnosed as having had a right and/or left hemisphere stroke in addition to their PD.

Management of communication problems

The primary aim is to teach straightforward strategies to encourage conscious attention to speech production.[3] The speech and language therapist starts by explaining the mechanism of speech production and how it is affected by PD, using diagrams of the vocal tract. The goals will be made explicit and focus attention on a specific aspect of communication, for example to produce a voice that is loud enough for a person to hear from a distance. External cueing is often used successfully in the management of other aspects of PD. A cue card with the words 'I must speak LOUDER', 'Think LOUD' or 'Think SHOUT' can be used to prompt the goal.

For fluency difficulties, the strategy to 'Think and speak in short phrases' or 'One-word-at-a-time' can be helpful.

Teaching methods of slowing down the rate of speech can help articulation difficulties. This may include cue cards with 'SS LL OO WW DD OO WW NN', 'Exaggerate beginnings, middles and ends of words', or teaching pausing between words and phrases. Some patients report benefit from sucking sweets or lozenges while speaking. This may be due to an increase in conscious attention to speech, caused by the presence of an object in the mouth. However, any sweets used in this way must be sugar free, or they will jeopardise oral health.

The individual's speech and swallowing may be affected by the timings of medication. Patients may need to consider seeing people and making telephone calls when they know they will be at their best, in order to avoid fatigue and frustration.

Performing two tasks simultaneously – such as walking and speaking – may be problematic as one or both activities can become compromised. This is likely to be due to conscious attention being directed mainly to the content of the spoken message.

Teaching the family and/or carer what is taught to the patient is central to ensuring improved carry-over of the strategy provided in the clinical setting. The majority of patients require constant prompting and this support is crucial to the therapy outcome.

Research has demonstrated that repetition, reinforcement and follow-up have a positive impact on outcome of speech and language therapy. Intensive therapy (a minimum of twice weekly) is of more benefit than once weekly, fortnightly or monthly therapy.[7]

AUGMENTATIVE AND ALTERNATIVE COMMUNICATION SYSTEMS

Some individuals may benefit from equipment to facilitate their speech and writing. Such equipment can be costly, and patients needs also change over time.[7] A speech and language therapist can offer advice on where to go for assessment, advice and funding or loaning of equipment, as well as the appropriate support to use the aid.

Commonly used aids include the following:

- A pacing board may be used to assist people with dysfluent speech to break the message into smaller units. This is a rectangular wooden block, measuring approximately 35 cm × 9 cm, which is divided into five equal blocks. The individual points to each section in turn while speaking, so as to break the phrase down into manageable units.
- A voice amplifier for use in conversations and on the telephone. For further information, see suppliers such as Kapitex Healthcare Ltd, Kapitex House, 1 Sandbeck Way, Wetherby, West Yorkshire, LS22 7GH (Tel: 01937-580211)
- A communication board to clarify words or specific letters. This can be provided by the therapist and made in conjunction with the patient and their family and/or carers, tailored to the individual's needs.
- A portable computer with speech output. For example, the Lightwriter SL35 has optional features of a 'keyguard' for those with tremor and a portable printer (Fig. 9.1). For further information, contact Toby Churchill Ltd, 20 Panton Street, Cambridge, CB2 1HP (Tel: 01223-576117).
- A metronome can be used to overcome initiation difficulties and problems with festinant speech.

Swallowing problems*

The following section focuses on the practical issues relating to the investigation and management of swallowing disorders in PD.

Clinical relevance

Research shows that 50–80 per cent of people with PD experience a degree of dysphagia.[8] Swallowing problems in PD may result in one or more of the following:

- weight loss;
- high levels of anxiety during each meal for both the patient and carer;
- disturbed intake of medication(s);
- reduced social contact; and
- bronchopneumonia, which is a common cause of death in PD.

Additional complications in managing the patient may be that: (i) the presence of dysphagia is not always apparent to either the person with PD, the caregiver or the team; and (ii) aspiration may be silent, with no obvious signs

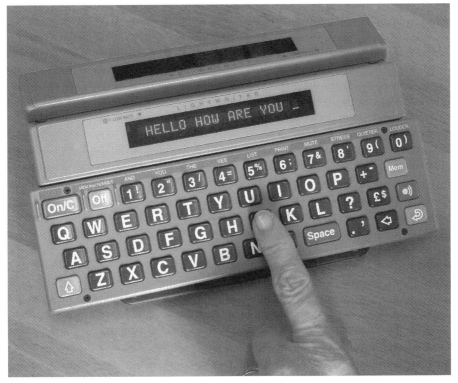

Fig.9.1 'Lightwriter' communication aid with speech synthesis.

of coughing or choking post swallow.[3] Thus, the speech and language therapist's detailed evaluation is an important element of the team's assessment.

Assessment

Assessment needs to be tailored to the individual's needs, and among the various methods of investigation that may be used, the following merit discussion.

DETAILED CASE HISTORY

A detailed case history is normally obtained from the patient and/or the caregiver by the speech and language therapist. In 1965, Eadie and Tyrer[9] identified that only 2 per cent of patients reported dysphagic problems, even though specific questioning revealed that 50 per cent of them experienced dysphagic symptoms. Therefore, it is important to ask the right questions to elicit information regarding oro-motor and associated features.

Oro-motor features[3]

These include:

- drooling of saliva; this may occur when the person opens their mouth to eat or drink, or it may be constant.
- difficulty swallowing tablets or capsules.
- a 'gurgly' voice quality; this is the strongest indicator of risk of aspiration.
- coughing before, during or after swallowing.
- 'choking' episodes.
- 'discomfort' or 'sticking' with swallowing.
- regurgitation of food via the nose.
- oesophageal reflux; if present, this may lead to increased pharyngeal secretions and hence aspiration.

Associated features

These include:

- an increased time taken to complete a meal.
- nocturnal coughing or choking; this is indicative of difficulty in managing saliva.
- an ability to self-feed. A note should be made of how much assistance is needed, and when.
- whether the patient prefers to be 'on' (active) or 'off' (inactive) phase of fluctuating parkinsonian symptoms while eating.
- whether there is any weight loss. If the patients do not have weighing scales, they should be asked if their trousers or skirt is loose.
- whether the food needs to be cut up into smaller pieces.
- a 'fear' of swallowing.
- a reduced appetite; this may be exacerbated by reduced oesophageal motility.
- 'forgetting' how to swallow.
- a history of chest infections.

OBSERVATION OF EATING/DRINKING

Observation should be made of eating habits, especially meal duration. If the patient is taking more than 45 min to complete his/her due to fatigue, the food may become unappetising when cold. The presence of drooling should also be noted.

Prepharyngeal symptoms

Symptoms to be identified include:

- impaired head and neck posture;
- upper limb dysmotility;
- jaw rigidity;

- impulsive feeding behaviour;
- impaired amount regulation; and
- fatigue

Oral features

These include tongue tremor, repetitive 'tongue pumping', poor bolus formation or control and an increased time being taken for manipulation of the food bolus in the mouth.

Pharyngeal features

These include difficulty initiating the swallow reflex, delay in triggering of the swallow reflex, and pooling in the pyriform sinuses or valleculae.

Laryngeal features

These include reductions in laryngeal closure and laryngeal elevation, as well as reduced or slow epiglottal lowering. Penetration and/or aspiration (sometimes silent) is indicated by voice change or coughing, which may occur a number of minutes after swallowing.

VIDEOFLUOROSCOPY

A modified barium videofluoroscopy might be performed: first, to identify the specific areas of breakdown in the swallowing process; second, to try out rehabilitation strategies; and third, to demonstrate the effectiveness of these treatments. All patients must undertake a 'bedside or clinical' evaluation before a videofluoroscopy is performed. There are several points to consider before performing a videofluoroscopy.[10]

- It involves transport and/or porters to get to the videofluoroscopy suite, and therefore also the potential for waiting and fatigue.
- It takes place in an unfamiliar setting; these artificial conditions are unlike any other 'meal'.
- Do you want to assess the patient while 'on' or 'off' or both? This can create additional stress.
- Positioning can be difficult; it is often uncomfortable for the patient.
- The taste of barium is not overly pleasant, and this can affect the swallow.
- There are few data available to demonstrate that it is representative of an entire meal.
- The duration of exposure to radiation may be several minutes.
- The total time for the investigation. Videofluoroscopy can take about 2 h to set up, perform, analyse the video, write the report, and then inform the patient and team of the results and recommendations.
- The cost of an investigation that potentially involves many professionals.

Videofluoroscopy can be helpful in some instances, particularly for research purposes. However, it only offers a snapshot in time and the patient may be more likely to aspirate due to the stress of the situation, which may switch them 'off' as they walk into the room, and so the results are not representative of their abilities.

FIBREOPTIC ENDOSCOPIC EVALUATION OF SWALLOWING SAFETY (FEESS)

This may be carried out jointly by a speech and language therapist and an ear, nose and throat surgeon, either in the out-patient department or at the bed-side. Use of the technique has been clearly described.[11] A nasoendoscope is passed through the nose and down into the pharynx, to hover above the lar-ynx. This permits a direct view of the larynx and pharynx while the patient is swallowing food and drink. Penetration and aspiration of the food or drink through the vocal cords can be observed, and any pooling or residue above the cords is commented on, as this may lead to potential aspiration. FEESS also permits the identification of any defects in the larynx, pooling of saliva in the hypopharynx, and any mass lesions that may be causing obstruction. The technique is not appropriate for people with dyskinesia, due to the delicate nature of the nasoendoscope's fibres.

CERVICAL AUSCULTATION

This non-invasive, highly portable, low-cost technique uses a stethoscope held against the neck at the junction of the cricoid cartilage and the trachea, to help detect aspiration for the occurrence of the breath and the swallow sounds before and after swallowing, by listening. Bosma[12] described the signals from the normal swallow as being associated with two discrete and perceptually distinct sounds – the 'Initial Discrete Sound' and the 'Final Discrete Sound'. Abnormal sounds would be:

- Change in respiratory rate
- No/delayed/weak expiratory puff
- No/early apnoea
- No swallow sounds
- Only one 'click' or 'burst'
- Indistinct sound
- Sound out of place

Many other investigators have explored this approach.[13-16] The technique requires training, and is an adjunct to the speech and language therapist's assessment.

PULSE OXIMETRY

The oxygen saturation of the blood stream is measured with a probe attached to the patient's fingertip. Measurements can be taken before, during and after swallowing. If aspiration is occurring, the respiratory rate will increase and the percentage of oxygen in the blood will fall.[17]

This technique is particularly helpful in a ward environment as an adjunct to the speech and language therapist's clinical evaluation, and also as a management strategy for monitoring swallowing function.

DRAWING THE RESULTS TOGETHER

The members of the multidisciplinary team need to use each other's skills during the ongoing assessment period, and also ensure that they share results. Next, they explain the results and their implications to the patient and his/her carer. From here, they formulate an agreed management plan with the patient and caregiver and offer consistent reinforcement of each other's advice, as well as monitoring its effectiveness.

Management

The prime considerations in the management of swallowing problems in PD are as follows:

1. Airway protection – that is, the ability to prevent food or drink entering the trachea as safety is a paramount consideration.
2. Nutrition – can the person take in sufficient calories?
3. Hydration – can the person take in sufficient fluid?
4. Raising the patient's and carer's awareness of their problems.
5. Management strategies to address specific problems experienced by each individual patient.
6. Regular monitoring and modifying advice as appropriate by all members of the multidisciplinary team.

EXPLANATION OF DYSPHAGIA

The starting point for management of dysphagia is an explanation of the normal swallowing mechanism, using pictures of oral, pharyngeal and oesophageal stages, and how PD affects swallowing.

POSITIONING AND POSTURE

The characteristic stooped posture of PD, combined with impaired lip seal and tongue movement, leads to reduced oral retention of food and saliva.[18] In more advanced disease, positioning the person upright and then maintaining this during a meal is not always easy. Speech and language therapists need to work closely with physiotherapists and occupational therapists on mealtime seating. Tilting chairs, which allow the head and neck to be maintained in an upright position, may be helpful.

Another strategy during swallowing is the chin tuck towards the chest. This widens the vallecular space and increases the chance that the bolus will hesitate in the valleculae while waiting for the swallow to be fully triggered, rather than falling into the airway. Posterior spoon placement may help to reduce oral transit times.

CONSISTENCY AND TEMPERATURE OF FOOD AND FLUIDS

To reduce the problem of the bolus dissipating in the oral and pharyngeal cavities, the food should be cohesive and require only two to three chews before swallowing. It is vital to consider 'lubricity' and aesthetics when helping people modify their diet. Purée is generally not recommended, as it is nutritionally less beneficial, gives insufficient sensory feedback, and is aesthetically less pleasing.

Other recommendations include avoiding mixed textures, anything with pips, seeds, bones, skin or that is stringy. Thickened fluids have a slower rate of flow than thin fluids; they are therefore easier to control and less likely to spill into the pharynx before triggering of the swallow reflex. Thickening powder is often more palatable in fruit juice and squash rather than in tea or plain water. A chilled bolus is found to trigger a swallow reflex more promptly as it adds stimulation to the sensory receptors in the mouth.[19]

RATE

Self-feeding – when physically feasible – is the main goal for most people, using adapted cutlery if indicated. If not allowed to self-feed, the person loses out on kinaesthetic feedback obtained when lifting the cup or spoon to the lips. Self-feeding may help initiation and rhythm, which is disrupted if fed by another person.

If the patient tends to overfill his/her mouth and forget to swallow, then loading the spoon and then passing it to them to feed themself is often helpful. Verbal cueing is an extremely important strategy. If there is a similar problem with drinks, verbal cues to take one small sip at a time and assisting the patient to put the glass down between mouthfuls, is of benefit. Saying, '1-2-3-SWALLOW' may assist those with problems initiating.

Having smaller portions more frequently, for example six per day, is psychologically advantageous and motivating. This is because: (i) patients feel under less pressure to finish a large portion in the same length of time, and therefore can enjoy the meal more; and (ii) they will not be left feeling hungry if they do not finish one large meal in a fixed time segment.[19]

REFLUX AND OESOPHAGEAL DYSFUNCTION

In 1965, Eadie and Tyrer[20] found that 54 per cent of people with PD over a 2-year period reported oesophageal reflux. The irritation caused by reflux may lead to an increase in oral and pharyngeal secretions, and hence aspiration. Similarly, reduced oesophageal motility may contribute to reduced appetite. Remaining upright for 30 min after a meal is therefore desirable.

MEDICATION

The timing of meals shortly after administration of levodopa/carbidopa medications may also improve swallowing and prevent aspiration.[21] Generally, it is true that patients prefer to be 'on' rather than 'off', and this may be at the expense of their swallowing function especially if they are very dyskinetic.

For difficulties swallowing tablets, it may help to:

- place the tablet on the centre of the tongue;
- reduce distractions;
- use verbal cues, such as '. . .1-2-3-SWALLOW';
- take several mouthfuls of thickened fluid to moisten the mouth and pharynx before taking the medication; and
- have medication that is dispersible or in a sugar-free elixir or as a subcutaneous injection.

INSIGHT AND CUEING

The basis of self-modification is insight and the ability to self-monitor. Management needs to include carer education, as patients may not be able to modify their swallowing behaviour reliably, and may require external cueing.

This ensures that the task is given conscious attention. For example, a cue card (Fig. 9.2) showing the instructions can be read silently by the person with PD, or mentally rehearsed.[3] Alternatively, a carer or staff member can read the card.[3]

DIFFICULTY MANAGING SIMULTANEOUS TASKS

Meal times should be sociable, but it is also necessary to encourage the person with PD to concentrate on swallowing, when pausing between conversational turns, such as talking and listening.

REDUCING ENVIRONMENTAL DISTRACTIONS

This is also beneficial, particularly for people with cognitive change. For example, turn off the radio or television during meals.

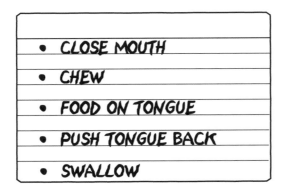

- CLOSE MOUTH
- CHEW
- FOOD ON TONGUE
- PUSH TONGUE BACK
- SWALLOW

Fig. 9.2   Cue card to help swallowing.

WEIGHT LOSS

Dysphagia does not account for the weight loss completely. Jankovic *et al.*[22] stated that it may be related to hypothalamic dysfunction, though there may be other reasons. A dietician may recommend oral supplements, e.g. Fortifresh™, Enlive™, Ensure™, Maxijul™, or non-oral routes such as naso-gastric or gastrostomy feeding tubes.

The decision to start alternative feeding regimens must be based on a range of factors. These include the patient's and carer's wishes, docu-mented evidence of the need for alternative feeding, and also a risk/bene-fit analysis (if it is recommended). In some cases it may be recommended that oral feeding be combined with gastrostomy feeding if the individual is either not meeting their nutrition and hydration needs orally, spending the majority of the day trying to eat and drink, and experiencing recurrent chest infections.

The timing of the introduction of this strategy needs to be discussed as a team. If the patient and carer opt for this treatment they will require coun-selling pre-insertion from a nutrition link nurse and/or dietician regarding management of the tube at home, as well as training to manage it confidently. A discharge planning meeting with all involved can smooth the transition from hospital to home.

OTHER USEFUL EQUIPMENT

The 'swallow reminder'

This is a simple brooch-style device that 'beeps' at regular intervals to remind the user to swallow. Measuring 37 mm diameter by 22 mm thick, it is powered by a watch-style battery, and is available from the Bath Institute of Medical Engineering The Woolfson Centre, RUH, Combe Park, Bath, BA1 3NG (Tel: 01225 824 103).

The Pat Saunders straw

This has a valve that prevents the liquid form falling to the bottom of the straw once it has been sucked up. It is useful in reducing fatigue and ingestion of excessive quantities of air through a straw, which causes pain and discomfort. It is available from Nottingham Rehab Supplies, 17 Ludlow Hill Road, Melton Road, West Bridgford, Nottingham, NG2 6HD (Tel: 0115 945 2345).

The 'Flexicup'

This is a lightweight cup that is shaped to allow drinking, without having to tilt the head back. The nose cut-out enables easy delivery, allowing the chin tuck position (Fig. 9.3). It is available from Kapitex Healthcare Ltd, Kapitex House, 1 Sandbeck Way, Wetherby, West Yorkshire, LS22 7GH (Tel: 01937-580211).

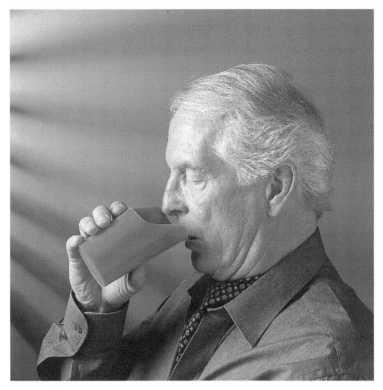

Fig. 9.3 Use of the 'Flexicup', with chin tuck position.

Parkinson's disease and diet[+]

Clinical relevance

Parkinson's disease can have a major effect on food intake and nutritional status. The key issues with regard to achieving and maintaining optimal nutrition are outlined, and appropriate remedial action described.

Getting correct nourishment is an important part of looking after the health of a person with PD. An individual requires advice on how to balance nutrients from different food groups in order to achieve a healthy diet.

A healthy weight

It is important for everybody to maintain an optimum body weight. Being overweight – or more commonly in PD, underweight – can have adverse effects on health. If a PD patient becomes less active and still has a 'healthy appetite', but continues to eat the same amount of food, then weight gain can occur. It is important to eat a variety of foods, and to have regular meals, yet at the same time reduce the energy content of the diet sensibly by eating fewer fried foods, cakes, puddings and confectionery. Unfortunately, weight loss

Table 9.1   Factors affecting weight loss – reduced energy intake

- poor appetite (often associated with medication)
- sensory change (loss of food smell and taste)
- nausea/vomiting
- dysphagia
- feeling full
- poorly fitting dentures
- dementia
- depression

Physical and social factors
- difficulty in accessing food, i.e. shopping when mobility is affected
- difficulty in cooking
- difficulty in handling eating utensils
- increased length of time to eat a meal, which goes cold and becomes unappetizing
- increased anxieties about eating and drinking, i.e. conveying food from the plate to the mouth, food scattering, loss of lip seal causing drooling, excess salivation, and inability to retain fluids and semi-solids in the mouth

Table 9.2   Factors affecting weight loss: increased energy expenditure

As a result of:
- dyskinesia (primarily associated with loss of body fat rather than muscle bulk)
- tremor
- jerky movements

appears to be a common feature of PD. In 1992, significant malnutrition was found among elderly individuals with PD,[23] while in 1995 Beyer et al.[24] reported that patients with PD appear to be at greater nutritional risk than a matched population. PD patients have lower body mass index (BMI), lower triceps skinfold thickness (TSF), and lower percentage ideal body-weight (IBW). The weight loss may result from reduced energy intake (Table 9.1), an increased energy expenditure (Table 9.2), or a combination of both factors. Research carried out in 1993 showed that under-nutrition is present in people with PD, and becomes more prevalent in the later stages of the disease.[25]

By virtue of its effect on muscular movement, PD has widespread effects on eating, swallowing and bowel function; and consequently also affects the nutritional status and oral health of the individual. Social isolation, loss of self esteem and depression increase the risk of developing malnutrition and dental disease, especially when high-sugar snacks and drinks replace well-balanced meals.

Nutrition

Nutrition is increasingly recognized as having an important role to play in the management of PD. Careful attention to nutritional and dietary elements of treatment can lessen the associated symptoms of the disease, and may also improve nutritional status and (possibly) the efficacy of drug therapy. The key issues in the dietary management of PD are to achieve optimal nutrition and energy balance, address swallowing difficulties in collaboration with other multidisciplinary team members, maintain good oral health, and reduce the problems of constipation. To assist patients and their carers to understand the diet-related problems associated with PD, the Dieticians in Neurological Therapy (DINT) and Nutrition Advisory Group for the Elderly (NAGE) Special Interest Groups of the British Dietetic Association have collaborated with the Parkinson's Disease Society to produce the 'Parkinson's and Diet' booklet. Effective multidisciplinary treatment with constant review of patients' needs can improve the quality of life and delay the needs for institutional care. Simple screening and assessment tools can be used to detect and quantify nutritional status and identify persons at risk of malnutrition. The information gathered is assessed against specific criteria (Table 9.3), and a 'score' is calculated. This process can be part of any screening strategy used by healthcare professionals working in hospitals, out-patient departments, day hospitals and community or home settings. Such an assessment identifies people who require nutrition support, thus facilitating appropriate referrals to the multidisciplinary team. The optimal multidisciplinary team includes doctor, nurse(s), physiotherapist, occupational therapist, speech and language therapist, dietician, dentist and pharmacist, together with the support of catering services and carers who are the providers of food and nourishment.[26]

Malnutrition can occur in individuals with PD, often as a deficiency of a particular nutrient or perhaps after a period of inadequate eating due to the physical problems related to the disease. The consequences of malnutrition include depression, apathy, fatigue, weakness, anorexia and anxiety, and these can be experienced by someone whose appearance is not significantly abnormal. Weight loss with muscle wasting and a loss of subcutaneous fat are typical physical signs of malnutrition. Vulnerable individuals have an increased risk of pressure sores with the loss of lean body mass and increased immobility; there is also an increased risk of general infection due to depressed cellular immunity.

Social isolation, physical disability, lack of good dentition and reduction of mobility, as well as dysphagia, all affect food intake and can lead to malnutrition. A lack of mobility may mean that it is difficult to purchase, carry and prepare food. A restricted income with competing demands will affect the type, quantity and quality of food purchased.

Table 9.3   Main elements of a nutrition risk assessment tool

- eating patterns and habits, including ethnic and cultural behaviour
- food likes and dislikes, with any known digestive problems and current appetite
- height, weight and trends in weight, i.e. loss/gain usually over the past 3–12 months
- activity (dyskinesia/akinesia) and rest patterns
- medical and physical condition
- dental and oral health
- swallowing and chewing difficulties, and mouth condition
- other risk factors and socioeconomic circumstances

NUTRITIONAL SUPPORT

Most persons identified as nutritionally at-risk will require an individually prescribed regime, which is regularly monitored, reviewed and communicated between the patient, carers, dietician and other healthcare professionals.

The simplest way of providing nutrition support is to encourage the person to eat more. The provision of and access to small snacks and meals is not always easy. Patients should be advised to:

- eat little and often – try to have something to eat or a nourishing drink every 2–3 h;
- have snacks between meals, such as nibbles of cheese and crackers, a sandwich, or cereal and milk.

Although dieticians recommend three to four intakes of food each day, PD patients must try to achieve three meals and three snacks per day. Suggested between-meal snacks include:

- full-cream milk with plain biscuits such as cream crackers, or digestive;
- milky tea or coffee with plain biscuits (e.g. rich tea);
- fresh or dried fruit such as satsuma, banana, prunes, apricots, with a milky drink;
- high-fibre breakfast cereal with full-cream milk (and fresh or dried fruit);
- cubed or grated cheese with buttered crackers; and
- smooth peanut butter with or without buttered crackers.

Patients who are not able to eat or drink quantities sufficient to match their identified nutritional needs require nutritional supplements. A nutritional supplement is any item given in addition to the ordinary or usual diet in order to increase energy and/or nutrient intake of an inadequately nourished person. Nutrition support can be varied and diverse, and includes:

- food enrichment;
- the addition of energy, e.g. glucose polymer;
- the addition of nutritional supplements, e.g. energy-dense, protein-enriched beverages and desserts; and
- artificial feeding, e.g. enteral nutrition, nasogastric/gastrostomy feeding for partial or total nutrition.

Enrichment of an ordinary food with another energy- and/or nutrient-dense food that does not increase the volume of the meal might include:

- milk powder added to ordinary milk, and used for drinks, cereals, puddings and soups;
- cream or grated cheese added to soup, potatoes, vegetables; or
- butter/margarine added to potatoes and vegetables.

If these feeds no longer improve the nutritional status of patients, prescription food or nutritional supplements are recommended in the short-term, and diet therapy should be started. There is a wide range of nutrition support products, ranging from a 100 per cent energy source (i.e. glucose polymer powder or syrup) to fruit juice or milk-based protein and energy-enhanced drinks with additional vitamins and minerals and milk-based desserts. The range of nutrition support products is extensive, and information on them and their use is easily obtained from dieticians.

To add variety, many of the manufacturers provide recipes and tips on use. The use of nutritional supplements needs to be monitored and is subject to regular review, particularly with regard to their impact on other food and fluid consumption, overall nutrition and dental health.

ENHANCEMENT OF NUTRITION: SUPPLEMENT USE

This can be achieved in several ways, including:

- sipping milk-based food supplement drinks (rather than more acidic fruit juice-based drinks) with food, at main meal times, or perhaps serving them frozen as 'ice-cream' dessert or sorbet.
- adding Scandishake™ to full-cream milk and sipping this with meals; alternatively, it can be added to desserts such as custard, trifle, milk pudding or full-cream yoghurt.
- encouraging savoury food supplements, such as Ensure, Complan, Buildup, as soup with meals, or added to sauces on meat or fish dishes.

Other suggestions include thickening drinks, i.e. with Thick & Easy™ – remember it is easier to use a thickener in fluids such as milky drinks, rather than fluid/food supplements such as Ensure or Entera™. It is also possible to add cream and fats (e.g. oil, butter, margarine) to foods and drinks. Patients should also be encouraged to consume 2 litres of fluid every day, for example boiled, cooled water with lemon juice rather than sugar or honey first thing in the morning, or at night.

CHANGES IN THE TEXTURE OF FOOD

The texture of food is very important to its palatability, and in general meals should consist of a variety of different textures. The texture of food needs to be modified if the person has:

- problems in the mouth, e.g. ill-fitting dentures; or
- problems with swallowing reflex, e.g. dysphagia.

Food textures are classified according to their ease of consumption (Table 9.4).[27]

A patient with progressively worsening levels of dysphagia should be assessed for the following staged dysphagia diets:

- a soft diet, e.g. using minced meat, flaked fish, soft fruit, vegetables and mashed potato (with food enrichment, i.e. butter/margarine, milk powder)
- a soft, smooth diet where food is soft and mashed, e.g. puréed meat with gravy, fish in sauce, mashed soft vegetables, soft mashed potatoes, milk pudding, fruit yoghurts (with food enrichment)

Table 9.4 A classification of food textures, with food examples[27]

Texture classification	Example of food
Hard	apple
Chewy	cooked meat
Soft	cake, bread/butter (no crust)
Liquid hard lump	muesli
Liquid soft lump	cornflakes and milk
Thickened soft lump	plain yoghurt and banana
Thickened hard lump	stew with chewy meat
Liquid	milk, water and orange juice
Slides down easily	butter, peanut butter, mousse

- a puréed diet (homogenized) where food is puréed using a blender and additional fluid is added, e.g. puréed meat, potato, vegetables and fruit, smooth yoghurt, mousse, ground rice pudding.

In some centres these dysphagia diets are staged for use with other neurological causes of dysphagia, particularly recovery from stroke, with the first stage diet for the most severe dysphagia.[28] These staged diets can also be adapted for PD.

- 3rd stage diet – bitesize – for people with difficulty biting or chewing, but with some strength to chew and move food around the mouth, as well as effective cough and swallow reflexes.
- 2nd stage diet – easychew/soft diet – lacking the chewing or swallowing ability for harder or mixed texture but still able to manage moderate variation in texture.
- 1st stage diet – smooth/thick purée – for people with chewing and swallowing disorders.

As the degree of restriction increases, so too does the likelihood of an inadequate intake. Puréed food becomes more dilute with added fluid, and often has a watery taste and unacceptable appearance. If a whole meal is liquidized together, the resulting mixture is often revolting, bearing little resemblance in appearance or taste to the original, and this is not recommended. Commercial food moulds can be used to shape puréed vegetables, potatoes, meat and fish separately when being served. Some puréed foods benefit from being prepared with a little thickening agent, e.g. cornflour, potato flour or arrowroot. As the puréed diet is generally inadequate in energy (even if consumed), food and nutrition supplements are required to prevent malnutrition.

FIBRE

Constipation

Many people with PD find constipation a problem, but this can be helped by: (i) increasing fluid intake; (ii) taking exercise; and (iii) increasing the intake of fibre-rich food.

Fibre works by absorbing fluid as it moves through the bowel, forming a soft stool that can be passed more easily. However, too much bulk with little fluid can increase constipation.

Increasing fibre intake

Fibre is found in cereal grains, seeds, nuts, fruit, vegetables and pulses, e.g. peas, beans and lentils. Loose bran, which can be added to food, is not recommended as it can lead to bloating and also reduces the absorption of vitamins and minerals. Increased fibre intake should be achieved by:

- including high-fibre varieties of foods, e.g. wholemeal bread, whole-wheat pasta and brown rice; recipes can be adapted to use some wholemeal flour instead of all white.
- including a breakfast cereal containing wheat, wheatbran or oats, e.g. Weetabix, porridge or branflakes.
- increasing the intake of all kinds of vegetables – raw/cooked, fresh/frozen; also, more peas, beans or lentils should be used.
- increasing the intake of fruit – fresh, stewed, tinned or dried, e.g. prunes, bananas or oranges.

When increasing fibre intake it is important to do so gradually in order to avoid bloating or flatulence. As a rule, one new fibre food should be introduced every 3 days.

FLUIDS

It is essential to drink plenty throughout the day, in order to help the fibre to do its work. The aim should be to drink 8–10 cups (6–8 mugs) every day. Any fluid is suitable, e.g. tea, coffee, fruit juice, squashes, fizzy drinks, milk or water. (Note: fizzy drinks can make some people feel bloated.)

PROTEIN

High-protein diets can reduce the clinical response to levodopa because of their influence on drug absorption in the gastrointestinal mucosa. In addition, large amounts of neutral amino acids (e.g. phenylalanine, tryptophan, tyrosine) compete with levodopa and reducing its uptake at the blood–brain barrier. Decreasing dietary protein and therefore neutral amino acids may improve clinical response to medication, by decreasing competition at both absorption sites. When symptom control on medication is not adequate, dietary manipulation is a viable option. Any dietary manipulation should be carried out under controlled conditions, since in some cases it is not in the patient's best interest to alter existing dietary patterns as it could result in malnutrition.

Healthy, motivated individuals can maintain an adequate intake of nutrients, yet restrict their dietary protein intake, if they are educated, supported and advised by their state-registered dietician and PD team.

VITAMINS, MINERALS AND ANTIOXIDANTS

Eating a well-balanced diet will provide adequate levels of the vitamin and minerals for most people. It is generally advised to increase the intake of foods containing fibre, valuable nutrients, vitamins and minerals, rather than buying expensive vitamin supplements. Some vitamins, when taken in large doses can cause severe side effects. If a person is taking supplements with high doses of vitamin and minerals, or requires further advice on this matter generally, it is highly recommended that they see a state-registered dietician.

The production of free radicals may cause cellular damage, and is thought to play a part in the development of PD. Antioxidants, including vitamins A, C and E, can (in theory) inhibit free radical production. Although many patients take supplementary anti-oxidants, there is no current evidence to suggest that they will alter the progression of PD. In a well-balanced diet, antioxidant intake should be adequate.

Teamwork

Comprehensive nutritional screening through referral to a multidisciplinary team will identify those individuals who require further assessment and possible nutritional support. Effective interdisciplinary working can improve nutrition. Each profession has its own knowledge base, skills and expertise, though this is not always recognized by other occupations. Working 'interprofessionally' across occupational boundaries will enable dieticians to share knowledge and experience of nutrition in PD, and also enable other team members to identify problems at an early stage.

Oral care[+]

Clinical relevance

Parkinson's disease can have a profoundly adverse effect on oral health and oral healthcare. A number of factors act together to compound the overall detrimental effect. An understanding of the issues concerned prepare both the individual with PD and the dental team to work together to minimize actual and potential oral problems. Poor oral health can endanger health, as the aspiration of saliva containing oral pathogens can cause bronchopneumonia.[29]

Access to dental services

In a review of the dental awareness and needs of PD patients, 71 per cent of people with PD felt that dental care was extremely, or very, important.[30] The reviewers identified three major factors as barriers to obtaining dental care. The first two factors – cost and anxiety – are common to the general population. The third factor – access to dental premises – is related to the mobility problems of PD. Dental services need to take into account the current mobility of the individual and their likely mobility throughout the life of their disease process. This requires the consideration of: (i) the individual's access to the dental surgery while they remain ambulant and if they become confined to a wheelchair; (ii) the individual's best times of day for coping with dental care (often dictated by the pattern of their PD symptoms and medication); and (iii) the possible, eventual need for domiciliary (home-based) dental care.

People with PD need to be made aware of the importance of good oral healthcare as early as possible after their diagnosis. Those people who already have a general dental practitioner (GDP) should alert the dentist to their diagnosis and continue with regular dental care. People without a GDP need to be put in contact with a dentist in the general dental service, the community dental service (CDS), or the hospital dental service, as appropriate. In the event, that a local dentist cannot be found the British Society for Disability and Oral Health (BSDH) may be able to advise.

Individuals are more amenable to dental treatment in the early stages of PD. At this point, they require the provision of high-quality, low-maintenance dental care. It is especially pertinent to put long-term preventive measures in place to minimize the need for further invasive dental treatment. It is important for the individual with PD and/or their carer to realize that the dental team understands both the process of PD and the problems associated with it; and that they are a part of their multidisciplinary care team.

Within this context, dental team members will find it particularly useful to liaise with the dietician, speech and language therapist and the PD nurse.

Communication

The progressive, communication difficulties associated with PD can affect the ability to access dental services and to voice individual needs and wants. Aspects of the condition which affect communication include:

- the characteristic 'mask-like', expressionless face which robs the individual of much of their non-verbal communication;
- the monotone, quiet speech which makes a person both difficult to hear and to listen to; and
- the slowness of response which can lead to the person being labelled as having a learning disability.

Depression or Alzheimer's disease can further erode the individual's ability to communicate with the dental team and further affect their ability to cooperate for dental treatment.

Oral problems

The oral problems associated with PD have been described as:[26]

- xerostomia (dry mouth);

- burning mouth;
- dental caries (decay);
- drooling of saliva;
- muscle control over dentures;
- periodontal (gum) disease; and
- maintenance of oral hygiene.

XEROSTOMIA

Dry mouth, due to a decreased quantity or quality (thick, ropey or frothy) of saliva, is commonly associated with PD and its associated drug treatment. Up to 55 per cent of people with PD complain of a dry mouth. This compares with 3–5 per cent of the total population and 20 per cent of the elderly population.[30] Xerostomia is disadvantageous to:

- oral health, as it leads to an increased risk of caries, exacerbation of periodontal disease and poor denture control;
- oral comfort, as it causes difficulty in talking, eating and swallowing, as well as burning mouth, and denture discomfort;
- general health, due to dysphagia, reduced nutritional status and oesophageal injury from dietary acid; and
- quality of life, as a result of the combined effects of all of the above factors.

BURNING MOUTH

Burning mouth (BM) is five times as commonly reported by people with PD (24 per cent) than it is by the general population.[31] Within the general population, the associated continuous, burning sensation of the oral mucosa and/or tongue has been attributed to vitamin and mineral deficiencies; hormonal imbalances; xerostomia; candidal infections; denture design faults; parafunctional activity; depression and alexithymia (feelings of powerlessness to cope with circumstances or problems in dealing with feelings).[31]

In PD, BM seems to be associated with medication, depression and alexithymia. Clifford *et al.* believe that BM in PD could be particularly associated with levodopa medication which promotes parafunctional, purposeless chewing.[31] In their study, 77 per cent of respondents and 96 per cent of people with BM were taking levodopa and none of them had experienced BM before the onset of PD. BM is a distressing complaint, but is treatable in 70 per cent of cases by identifying and treating the underlying cause. Where levodopa is the prime cause of BM, treatment is only possible if this medication can be changed. A high proportion of PD people have BM that seems to go largely unreported and, consequently, untreated – possibly because people assume that it is a symptom of their condition which cannot be treated.[31] It is recommended that dentists and dieticians enquire about BM when taking a history from anyone with PD.

DENTAL CARIES (DECAY)

Elderly people with PD have been described as having significantly more teeth and less caries than a control group of corresponding age.[32] However, this statement is based on a sample of only 30 elderly, Swedish people with PD and cannot be considered representative of people with PD as a whole. Indeed, it is the author's (J.F.) experience and subjective opinion that elderly people with PD have an increased incidence of dental decay, particularly root caries which occurs at the necks of the teeth. While tooth loss can have profound emotional effects on people,[33] for the person with PD it can also jeopardise their general health by compromising dietary selection and intake.

Aetiology of dental caries

This is determined by host factors, including susceptibility of the enamel, and also the flow rate and composition of the saliva, which has buffering, washing and remineralization functions. Diet and plaque microorganisms are also involved.[34] There is a direct relationship between dental caries and the intake of carbohydrates, particularly sucrose. The frequency of carbohydrate/sugar intake, rather than the amount consumed, is the important factor. The greater the number of intakes, the greater the risk of developing caries. Also, the stickiness and concentration of the sugars consumed have an influence. The main source of nutrition for oral bacteria, which adhere to the teeth as plaque, is carbohydrate in the saliva. The interaction between bacterial plaque and carbohydrate results in a fall in pH which causes demineralization of the dental enamel and initiates the process of dental caries.

A number of factors put people with PD at greater risk of developing dental caries. These include xerostomia; eating little and often, the long-term consumption of energy-enriched foods/drinks and the use of high-calorie dietary supplements to maintain body weight; dietary manipulation to increase the efficacy of levodopa as the restricted protein intake can lead to increased consumption of carbohydrate; the retention of pooled high-sugar foods and drinks in the mouth for long periods of time depending on the degree of dysphagia; and the difficulty of achieving good standards of daily oral hygiene.

It is important that the dietician and the dental team work together with the aim of achieving an improved nutritional intake and maintaining good oral health. Without collaboration, the dietary and dental advice given to the person with PD and their carer can be conflicting and confusing. There will be times when prioritising is necessary as part of the person's individual care plan.

Root caries

This occurs at the necks of the teeth; it can develop rapidly and is also very destructive (Fig. 9.4). The condition is often painless, and the first indication of its presence can be when an undermined crown of a tooth breaks off. The best treatment is to prevent it in the first place. For the person with PD, this involves advice about:

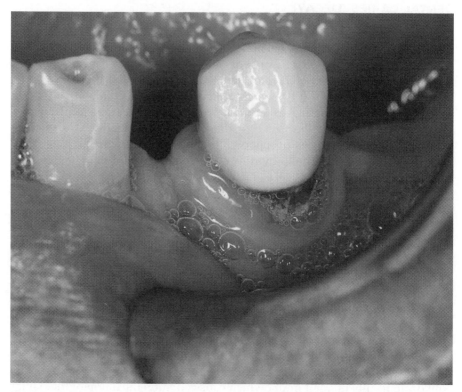

Fig. 9.4   Root caries and associated 'frothy' saliva in a person with Parkinson's disease.

- alleviating xerostomia by sipping water and avoiding acidic or fizzy drinks and encouraging the use of sugar-free or xylitol-containing chewing gum. Additionally, artificial saliva may be helpful for some people, particularly at meal times.[35]
- ensuring measures to prevent dental disease are in place. This requires a partnership between the dental team, the person with PD and (if appropriate) their carer. The dental team can provide advice, support and the professional application of fluoride and chlorhexidine varnishes. The individual and/or the carer have to take responsibility for daily regimes such as the use of fluoride or chlorhexidine gels and tooth-brushing.
- providing dietary advice which is compatible with national, nutritional guidelines for healthy eating in general and for maintaining body weight in particular. This is consistent with good oral health.

DROOLING

It is a paradox that, in a condition where xerostomia is a common complaint, drooling of saliva is a common symptom. Bateson *et al.* [36] found that drooling and difficulty swallowing saliva are reported by 78 per cent of people with PD. Initially drooling is attributed to 'hypersalivation', studies have shown that people with PD secrete similar amounts of saliva to age-matched controls.

The cause of the problem is pooling of saliva in the mouth due to the impaired swallowing mechanism associated with PD, coupled with a head-down posture and poor oral muscular control.

Dribbling is embarrassing to the individual. It contributes to low self-esteem and social unacceptability, as well as causing angular chelitis (sore cracks at the corners of the mouth) due to candidal infection. Drooling can be exacerbated by oral and dental problems, and recent onset may be associated with an acute problem. Continuing dental care can help to avoid this situation. Referral to a speech and language therapist for training in swallowing techniques may also be beneficial.

Strategies which have been used in an effort to reduce drooling include:

- external cueing – this is a useful and non-invasive technique.
- a timed beeper brooch (the 'swallow reminder; see p. 148) – this can act as an auditory cue to swallowing.
- verbally cueing – 'Big swallow' before each turn at talking.
- regular chewing of sugar-free gum; this can stimulate the swallowing reflex and may help to assist with the problem in the long term.
- sucking on a sweet or lozenge helps; patients indicate that this helps, although the sweets must be sugar-free in order to avoid tooth decay and subsequent loss.
- botulinum toxin injections into the parotid salivary gland; these appear helpful, but there is a risk of producing permanent dry mouth.
- parotid radiotherapy (unilateral or bilateral); this technique is not recommended as it can lead to a dry mouth and all its associated problems. Additionally, irreversible damage to the blood vessels of bone in the irradiated area occurs. If, at a later date, it is necessary to extract teeth in this area, there is a major risk of osteoradionecrosis (a form of osteomyelitis).

MUSCLE CONTROL OVER DENTURES

The success of wearing dentures depends, to a large extent, on the wearer's ability to control the dentures with their oral musculature. It also relies on the presence of an adequate amount and quality of saliva. Thick, 'ropey' or 'frothy' saliva in an abundant quantity (which sometimes occurs in PD) has the same detrimental effect on denture retention as does dry mouth. The muscle incoordination, rigid facial muscles and xerostomia of PD conspire to jeopardise denture retention and control. This is particularly so in the case of complete upper and lower dentures and some acrylic (plastic) partial dentures. For some people this will mean they are not able to cope with dentures. Other people will require the use of a denture fixative/adhesive to increase denture retention and denture-wearing confidence.

A dentist providing a person with PD with replacement dentures would be prudent to consider using one of the copy/duplication techniques in order to retain the learned muscle control of familiar dentures. The individual should keep their old dentures as, even if they no longer fit well, they can provide the dentist with useful information which may contribute to easier adaptation to the new dentures.

Dentists planning to provide a person with PD with complete dentures for the first time might consider the use of overdentures (where strategic roots of teeth are left in the jaw bone and the denture sits over them) as they help to retain proprioception and maintain jaw control. For the person with early PD who requires dentures, consideration should be given to the possible role of dental implants or implant retained overdentures. Although, this is an expensive option it may well be cost-effective in the long term, providing the individual with security and helping to preserve their self-esteem and social contacts.

PERIODONTAL (GUM) DISEASE

Poor oral hygiene leads to plaque accumulation. In the long term this can lead to periodontal disease, which has been categorized as:

- gingivitis – inflammation of the gums, giving them a red, swollen appearance and causing bleeding when they are brushed; and
- periodontitis – this develops from a pre-existing gingivitis, to destroy the supporting bone of the teeth, and leads to gum recession, loose teeth and tooth loss. Not every gingivitis develops into periodontitis.[34]

The degree of susceptibility of the individual and adequate removal of dental plaque on a daily basis are integral to the process. Xerostomia and refined carbohydrate intake contribute by reducing the capacity for oral clearance of food.

Maintenance of oral hygiene

The prevention of dental disease is the most important aspect of dental care for people with PD. Reduced muscle coordination, muscle rigidity and tremors mitigate against the individual's ability to achieve adequate plaque control. Maintaining independence for as long as possible is an important part of the general management of PD, and is to be encouraged in oral care wherever possible. Toothbrush handle adaptations, to improve the grip and manipulation of the brush, can help retain independence for teeth or denture cleaning (Fig. 9.5).

An electric toothbrush can facilitate cleaning, particularly where manual dexterity is compromised. Some people find the extra weight of an electric toothbrush helps to reduce hand and arm tremors. Dental gels, such as chlorhexidine and fluoride, and toothpastes can be used as normal. The use of mouthrinses should be avoided due to the increased risk of silent aspiration.

The recruitment of a family member or carer to supervise and provide support for daily oral hygiene measures is pertinent. If PD reaches the stage where the individual can no longer provide self-care, this person can be trained to take over the task. With advice and support from an empathic dental team, many of the anxieties that carers experience in providing mouth care can be allayed. Finnerty, in association with the Parkinson's Disease Society of the UK, has addressed the issue of oral awareness in a useful booklet 'Parkinson's and Dental Health'.[37]

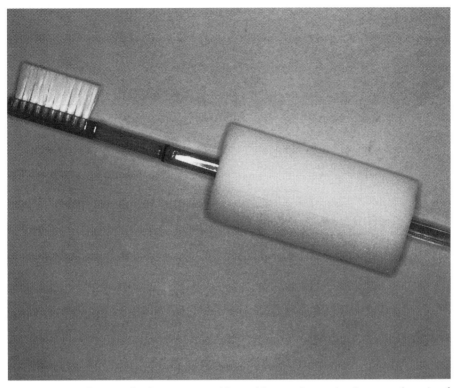

Fig. 9.5 A small piece of polystyrene or rubber tubing can be used to improve the grip of a toothbrush handle.

Dental management

Appointments should be scheduled for the individual's best time of day. They should be as short and stress-free as possible, as anxiety and stress tend to increase tremors and random movements. Asking the person to relax or to sit sill is likely to increase involuntary movements, and is best avoided.

Individuals with PD should be assisted to the dental chair only as needed; however, the path to the chair should be cleared of obstacles. The person should be seated in and raised slowly from the dental chair in order to avoid problems with loss of balance or postural hypotension. On leaving the dental chair, the characteristic slow movements and shuffling gait of PD can make it difficult for the person to get moving. Reminding the person to '. . . take big steps' helps to initiate the walking process.

During operative dentistry, the control of the person's movements can be difficult. Jolly *et al.* advocate the use of mouth props (such as rubber bite blocks) during restorative procedures.[35] Additionally, these authors suggest that the person's head might be cradled in the operator's arm at the elbow to control head movements. This practice can help, though on occasion movements can be severe and this practice may lead to bruised ribs! Some days it may be best to abandon the treatment – which can be challenging to all concerned – in the hope that the next appointment will be on a 'less mobile' day.

While inhalational sedation using relative analgesia or intravenous sedation may help to control tremor, they may exacerbate the risk of aspiration as they depress the (already impaired) swallow reflex. Care is required in the administration of local anaesthetic agents in order to avoid either damage to the patient or needle-stick injury to the operator as a result of random movements.

The person should not be reclined more than 45° in the dental chair because of the poor swallowing reflex and the risk of pulmonary aspiration of saliva and debris. Rubber dam, with additional suction behind the dam to cope with salivary secretions, is recommended for restorative dentistry. The use of 'four-handed' (denatal nurse assisted) dentistry and high-volume suction are advocated.

General principles for oral healthcare

The following guidelines are suggested as a way of attaining optimal oral healthcare for people with PD:

- Contact with a dentist as early as possible after the diagnosis of PD.
- Advise the person with PD of potential oral and denture problems and make available information on how to avoid or minimize these problems.
- Aim to maintain comfort, independence and self-esteem.
- Provide information and support to improve/maintain oral hygiene and oral comfort.
- Put rigorous preventive regimes in place.
- Provide high-quality, low-maintenance dental care in the early stages of the disease.
- Organize continuing care by arranging regular reviews at intervals tailored to meet the individual's needs.

The Parkinson's Disease Society leaflet carries the title 'Just a little more time'. This is one of the main requirements of people with PD in the dental setting. Good time management is an important feature of a successful dental practice. Sufficient time needs to be allocated for appointments to avoid the sense of rushing which will only delay communication further. The use of questions which require yes/no responses can both aid the flow of information and reduce the time taken to obtain it. The time required by some people with PD, is best accommodated by the use of a salaried dental service.

Conclusions

A carefully taken case history and observation of eating and drinking are helpful forms of investigation for patients with PD. Management plans need to be formulated with the patients and carers, who benefit from awareness raising, regular support, reinforcement of strategies and monitoring, particularly within their own environments. Effective swallowing therapy has the potential to reduce the morbidity seen in PD.

The dietician is the resource to assess, advise and monitor the nutritional status and dietary intake of people with PD, while the dental team advises on preventing dental disease, maintaining oral comfort and managing oral problems.

The speech and language therapist, the dietician and the dental staff are all important members of the PD multidisciplinary care team. They contribute unique and complementary aspects of care associated with PD and help to maintain the individual's self-esteem and quality of life.

References

1. Oxtoby M. *Parkinson's Disease Patients and their Social Needs*. London: Parkinson's Disease Society, 1982.
2. Darley F, Aronson A, Brown J. Differential diagnostic patterns of dysarthria. *J. Speech Hearing Res.* 1969; **12**: 246–69.
3. Marigliani C, Gates S, Jacks D. Speech pathology and Parkinson's disease. In: Morris M, Iansek R (eds). *Parkinson's Disease: A Team Approach*. Australia: Southern Health Care Network, 1998; Chapter 7.
4. Logemann J, Fisher H, Boshes B, Blonsky E. Frequency and concurrence of vocal tract dysfunctions in the speech of a large sample of Parkinson patients. *J. Speech Hearing Disord.* 1978; **42**: 47–57.
5. Ramig L, Pawlas A, Countryman S. *The Lee Silverman Voice Treatment*. National Center for Voice and Speech, USA, 1995.
6. Scott S, Caird F, Williams B. *Communication in Parkinson's Disease*. London, Sydney: Croom Helm, 1985.
7. *Parkinson's and the Speech and Language Therapist*. The Parkinson's Disease Society, 215 Vauxhall Bridge Road, London, SW1V 1EJ, UK.
8. Leopald N, Kagel M. Pre-pharyngeal dysphagia in Parkinson's disease. *Dysphagia* 1996; **11**: 14–22.
9. Eadie M, Tyrer J. Alimentary disorders in parkinsonism. *Austr. Ann. Med.* 1965; **14**: 13–22.
10. Groher M, Crary M. Glan Hafren NHS Trust, Dysphagia Conference. National Museum of Wales, Cardiff, May 1997.
11. Langmore S, Schat K, Olson N. Fibreoptic endoscopic examination of swallowing safety: a new procedure. *Dysphagia* 1988; **2**: 216–19
12. Bosma J. Introduction to the Cervical Auscultation Workshop. Department of Paediatrics, University of Maryland, Baltimore, Maryland, April 22, 1992.
13. Takahashi K, Groher M, Michi K. Methodology for detecting swallowing sounds. *Dysphagia* 1994; **9**: 54–62.
14. Hamlet S, Penney D, Formolo J. Stethoscope acoustics and cervical auscultation of swallowing. *Dysphagia* 1994; **9**: 63–8.
15. Chichero J, Murdoch B. The physiologic cause of swallowing sounds: answers from heart sounds and vocal tract acoustics. *Dysphagia* 1998; **13**: 39–52.
16. Zenner P, Losinski D, Mills R. Using cervical auscultation in the clinical dysphagia examination in long-term care. *Dysphagia* 1995; **10**: 27–31.
17. Sellars C, Dunnet C, Carter R. A preliminary comparison of videofluoroscopy of

swallow and pulse oximetry in the identification of aspiration in dysphagic patients. *Dysphagia* 1998; **13**: 82–6.

18. Scott A. The management of dysphagia in Parkinson's disease. *Austr. Commun. Q.* 1997; **Winter**: 30–1.

19. Groher M. *Dysphagia Diagnosis and Management*. 2nd edn. Boston: Butterworth-Heinemann, 1992.

20. Eadie M, Tyrer J. Radiological abnormalities of the upper part of the alimentary tract in parkinsonism. *Austr. Ann. Med.* 1965; **14**: 23–7.

21. Kirshner H. Disorders of the pharyngeal and esophageal stages of swallowing in Parkinson's disease. *Dysphagia* 1997; **12**: 19-20.

22. Jankovic J, Wooten M, Van der Linden C, Jansson B. Low body weight in Parkinson's disease. *South. Med. J.* 1992; **85**: 351–4.

23. Durrieu G, Llau M, Rascol D, Denard J, Rascol A, Montastruc J. Parkinson's disease and weight loss: a study with anthropometric and nutritional status. *Clin. Autonom. Res.* 1992; **2**: 153–7.

24. Beyer PL, Palarino MY, Michalek D, Buscubavik K, Keller W. Weight change and body composition in patients with Parkinson's disease. *J. Am. Dietet. Assoc.* 1995; **95**: 979–83.

25. Markus HS, Tomkins AM, Stern GM. Increased prevalence of undernutrition in Parkinson's disease and its relationship to clinical disease parameters. *J. Neural Transm.* 1993; **5**: 117–25.

26. Hyland K, Fiske J, Mathews N. Nutritional and dental health management in Parkinson's disease. *Community Nurs.* 2000; **14**: 28–32.

27. Webb G, Copeman C. *The Nutrition of Older Adults*. London, Arnold, 1996.

28. Staged dysphagia diet. Department of Nutrition and Dietetics. North West Wales Trust. Ysbyty Gwynedd. Bangor, 1998.

29. Curtis J, Langmore S. Respiratory function and complications related to deglutition. In: Perlman A, Schulze-Delrieu K (eds). *Deglutition and its Disorders: Anatomy, Physiology, Clinical Diagnosis and Management*. San Diego, CA: Singular Publishing, 1997; Chapter 4.

30. Clifford T, Finnerty J. The dental awareness and needs of a Parkinson's disease population. *Gerodontology* 1995; **12**: 99–103.

31. Clifford TJ, Warsi MJ, Burnett CA, Lamey PJ. Burning mouth in Parkinson's disease sufferers. *Gerodontology* 1998; **15**: 73–8.

32. Persson M, Sterberg T, Granrus A-K, Karlsson S. The influence of Parkinson's disease on oral health. *Acta Odontol. Scand.* 1992; **50**: 37–42.

33. Fiske J, Davis D, Frances C, Gelbier S. The emotional effects of tooth loss in edentulous people. *Br. Dent. J.* 1998; **184**: 90–3.

34. Samaranayake LP. *Essential Microbiology for Dentistry*. London: Churchill Livingstone, 1996.

35. Jolly DE, Paulson RB, Paulson GW, Pike JA. Parkinson's disease: a review and recommendations for dental management. *Special Care in Dentistry* 1989; **9**: 74–8.

36. Bateson M, Gibberd F, Wilson R. Salivary symptoms in Parkinson's disease. *Arch. Neurol.* 1989; **39**: 1309–14.

37. Finnerty J. Parkinson's and dental health. Parkinson's Disease Society, code B45, 1996.

Autonomic problems

R.A. Kenny and L. Allcock

Introduction

Autonomic symptoms in Parkinson's disease (PD) were first reported in 1817 by James Parkinson himself,[1] who described abnormalities of salivation and sweating, and dysfunction of the alimentary tract and urinary bladder. Since then, a number of autonomic symptoms have become well-known clinical features of PD, including dysphagia, heartburn, constipation, sialorrhoea, postural hypotension and urinary disturbances.

The signs of autonomic dysfunction are rarely elicited in the standard clinical examination. A more detailed assessment of heart rate and blood pressure variability in response to standing, deep breathing, Valsalva manoeuvre and cold stimulus or isometric exercise will yield a more definitive statement of a patient's autonomic status. Urodynamic investigations and urinary sphincter electromyography are among other tests which can yield evidence of autonomic dysfunction.

The prevalence of autonomic dysfunction in idiopathic PD is controversial,[2–5] varying from 23 per cent to 80 per cent in selected hospital attendees.[6,7] Difficulty in distinguishing true PD from other parkinsonian syndromes constitutes the major problem in accurately defining prevalence. Early studies have been criticised for the heterogeneity of patients studied. We now know that idiopathic PD, Shy–Drager syndrome, Lewy body dementia and vascular Parkinson's are distinct disease entities with an overlap of clinical symptoms and signs. The introduction of standardized diagnostic criteria for PD[8] has improved diagnostic accuracy,[9,10] but no reports have been published of the community prevalence of autonomic dysfunction in idiopathic PD since the introduction of these guidelines.

Classification of autonomic dysfunction in parkinsonian patients

Autonomic disorders can be divided into primary disorders – where the aetiology is not known, and secondary disorders – where the lesion has been defined or where there are definite associations with other diseases, syndromes or medications. The primary and secondary causes of autonomic dysfunction in parkinsonian patients are listed in Table 10.1.

Primary autonomic disturbance

There are three primary causes of autonomic dysfunction in patients with definite extrapyramidal signs: multiple system atrophy (MSA); idiopathic Parkinson's disease (IPD) with autonomic failure; and Lewy body dementia. It is important to distinguish between these syndromes as treatment and prognosis differs markedly between them.

MSA

A syndrome of chronic autonomic failure associated with the parkinsonian features of rigidity, tremor and akinesia was first described by Shy and Drager in 1960.[11] There are three major clinical groups within the definition of MSA:[12]

1. A parkinsonian form, comprising 20 per cent of cases: there are extrapyramidal features, with autonomic failure, perhaps indicating striatoniral degeneration.
2. A cerebellar form, also comprising 20 per cent of cases: there are cerebellar and/or pyramidal features, and the pathology indicates olivopontocerebellar atrophy.
3. A multiple form, comprising 60 per cent of cases: there is a combination of parkinsonian and cerebellar or pyramidal features, and multiple neuronal system degeneration.

MSA is difficult to distinguish from PD, as between 7 per cent and 22 per cent of patients considered to have PD in life have neuropathological features of MSA on post-mortem examination.[13,14]

Patients with MSA are often not responsive to dopaminergic therapy, and have a median life expectancy of only 6 years from diagnosis.[15]

IPD WITH AUTONOMIC FAILURE

Patients with true IPD and autonomic failure are a recognized group.[16] These patients are often elderly, have usually been parkinsonian for a substantial period of time, and are responsive to dopaminergic therapy. Available studies on mortality in PD provide heterogeneous mortality rates, probably because of discrepancies between patient populations with respect to co-morbidity, disease stage at study entry and diagnostic accuracy. However, the most recent follow-up from the DATATOP cohort suggests normal life expectancy

Table 10.1   Drugs, chemicals and toxins that cause or exacerbate autonomic symptoms in Parkinson's disease

---

I. DECREASING SYMPATHETIC ACTIVITY

Centrally acting

    Clonidine
    Methyldopa, Reserpine
    Barbiturates, Anaesthetics

Peripherally acting

    Sympathetic neurone (guanethidine, bethanidine)
    α-Adrenoceptor blockade (phenoxybenzamine, prazosin)
    β-Adrenoceptor blockade (propranolol, timolol)

II. INCREASING SYMPATHETIC ACTIVITY

    Amphetamines
    Releasing norepinephrine (tyramine)
    Uptake blockers (imipramine)
    Monoamine oxidase inhibitors (trancypromine)
    β-Adrenoceptor stimulants (isoproterenol)

III. DECREASING PARASYMPATHETIC ACTIVITY

    Antidepressants (imipramine)
    Tranquillizers (phenothiazines)
    Antidysrhythmics (disopyramide)
    Anticholinergics (atropine, probanthine), toxins (botulinum)

IV. INCREASING PARASYMPATHETIC ACTIVITY

Cholinomimetics (carbachol, bethanechol, pilocarpine, mushroom poisoning)
Anticholinesterases
    Reversible carbonate inhibitors (pyridostigmine, neostigmine)
    Organophosphorus inhibitors (parathion)

V. MISCELLANEOUS

    Alcohol, thiamine (vitamin B$_1$) deficiency
    Vincristine
    Perhexilene maleate
    Thallium, arsenic, mercury, Cyclosporin

Adapted from Mathias[76]

in carefully selected patients without significant co-morbidity and with adequate treatment and expert follow-up.[17]

LEWY BODY DEMENTIA

This clinical syndrome was originally described by the Newcastle group in 1989,[18] and accounts for 5–10 per cent of patients in PD 'brain banks'[19] and 12–27 per cent of dementia in the elderly.

Guidelines for clinical and pathological diagnosis were published in 1996.[21] The majority of patients have a dominant syndrome of cognitive impairment, frequently characterized by fluctuations in cognitive performance, episodic confusion, visual (and less often) auditory hallucinations and delusions. The extrapyramidal features tend to be mild and occur late, although they are usually levodopa responsive. Less often, patients present with classical levodopa-responsive PD, often followed by early development of dementia.[22] Other features are unexplained falls, early gait impairment, myoclonus, weight loss, rapid eye movement (REM) sleep disorders, supranuclear gaze palsy and marked sensitivity to neuroleptics.

Pathologically, widespread Lewy bodies are seen in the brainstem and other cortical areas. Diffuse amyloid plaques are found in two-thirds of cases, while neurofibrillary tangles are seen less often.

Recent investigation in our unit has shown that 77 per cent of LBD patients had evidence of carotid sinus hypersensitivity, orthostatic hypotension or vasovagal syncope.[23] Overall, patients with LBD have a six-fold higher prevalence of neurocardiovascular instability than the normal elderly population,[24] though this cannot be explained by medication or co-existent heart disease. It is currently unclear whether this neurocardiovascular instability represents a cause, or a consequence, of the neurodegenerative process.

The type and extent of autonomic dysfunction in LBD is currently unknown. The high prevalence of abnormal asystolic responses to carotid sinus stimulation suggests that the prevalence of autonomic dysfunction is high.

Secondary causes of autonomic failure

Antiparkinsonian medications and other drugs may interfere with autonomic function (see Table 10.1). Since the introduction of levodopa during the 1970s, it has become accepted clinical dogma that dopaminergic medications are the cause of orthostatic hypotension in PD. There is certainly evidence that levodopa,[25] or levodopa in combination with selegeline,[26] exacerbates the tendency towards orthostatic hypotension, but recent investigators have demonstrated that disease duration, severity and patient age are more important factors in the development of autonomic dysfunction than the dose of levodopa given.[27,28]

Autonomic dysfunction in parkinsonian patients may also result from an associated disorder known to cause autonomic neuropathy, for example amyloidosis or diabetes mellitus (Table 10.2).

A careful assessment of secondary causes is an important component of the investigation and management of parkinsonian patients with autonomic symptoms.

Table 10.2 Classification or autonomic disorders in the elderly

---

I. PRIMARY AUTONOMIC FAILURE

A) Chronic
Pure autonomic failure
Multiple System Atrophy
- with parkinsonian features
- with cerebellar and pyramidal features
- with multiple features (combination of above) Parkinson's disease with autonomic failure Lewy body Dementia

B) Acute or subacute dysautonomias

II. SECONDARY AUTONOMIC FAILURE OR DYSFUNCTION

A) Central
Brain tumours, especially of the third ventricle or posterior fossa
Multiple sclerosis
Syringobulbia

B) Spinal
Spinal transverse myelitis
Transverse myelitis
Syringomyelia
Spinal tumours

C) Peripheral
Afferent
    Guillain–Barré syndrome
    Tabes dorsalis
    Holmes–Adie syndrome
Efferent
    Diabetes mellitus
    Amyloidosis
    Surgery (such as splanchnicectomy)

D) Miscellaneous
Autoimmune and collagen disorders
Renal failure
Neoplasia
Human immunodeficiency virus infection

III. DRUGS (see Table 10.1)

IV. NEURALLY MEDIATED SYNCOPE

Vasovagal syncope
Carotid sinus hypersensitivity
Swallow syncope
Situational syncope

Adapted and modified from Mathias.[76,77]

Features of autonomic dysfunction

Table 10.3 Reported frequency of autonomic symptoms in patients with Parkinson's disease derived from two studies ($n = 178$)

Symptoms	% of frequency
Orthostatic hypotension	21–58
Urgency	14–45
Urinary incontinence	2
Sialorroea	55
Dysphagia	9–22
Constipation	43–72
Seborrhoea	61
Sweating	13
Heat/cold intolerance	22
Impotence	20–60

From Martignoni *et al.*[29] and Singer *et al.*[30]

Whilst difficulties distinguishing PD with autonomic failure from MSA confound prevalence studies, available data suggest a significant co-morbidity related to autonomic dysfunction in PD[29,30] (Table 10.3).

Cardiovascular features

Orthostatic hypotension (OH) is a cardinal feature of autonomic dysfunction. Symptoms may be non-specific, with generalized weakness and lethargy. Dizziness, syncope and falls may result from cerebral ischaemia. Between 10 per cent and 58 per cent of patients with PD have OH,[31] and up to 80 per cent of these suffer with dizziness and falls.[32] Drop attacks and seizures may occasionally occur. The characteristic 'coathanger' ache is a common symptom,[33] while chest discomfort, spinal cord ischaemia and calf claudication may also occur.

Patients with long-standing OH may have fewer symptoms because of compensatory changes in cerebrovascular autoregulation.[34] Preliminary studies suggest that patients with PD maintain normal middle cerebral artery perfusion during head-up tilt.[35] The relationship between cerebral perfusion and orthostatic hypotension in patients with PD has yet to be documented.

Patients with age-related OH show a reduction in cognitive function compared with age-matched controls.[36] The presence of OH may accelerate or exaggerate cognitive decline, or it may occur secondary to the neurodegenerative process. A causal association between OH, cognitive dysfunction and dementia requires further study.

Gastrointestinal features

Sialorrhoea and dysphagia, although common in late PD, are not regarded as features of true autonomic dysfunction. They are thought to be manifestations of hypokinesia, with resultant poverty of automatic swallowing. Both symptoms respond to dopaminergic therapy.

Constipation is seen in 61–73 per cent of patients compared with 28 per cent of age-matched controls.[37] In 46 per cent of patients, constipation predates the first motor manifestations. It is probably multifactorial in origin, though reduced motor activity, poor oral food and fluid intake, and anticholinergic medications may all contribute to the problem. Specific abnormalities of intestinal motility have been assumed, and case report studies have reported diminution in fibres and ganglion cells, with Lewy bodies in the visceral autonomic nervous system of PD patients,[38] though definitive evidence of PD-induced gastrointestinal autonomic degeneration/dysfunction has yet to be provided.

The constipation in PD will usually respond to dietary and drug manipulations, including mild laxatives, but some patients depend on enemas.

Genitourinary features

The function of the urinary tract is often impaired in MSA at an early stage.[39] This is caused by a combination of detrusor hyperreflexia and sphincter denervation/re-innervation, leading to urgency, frequency, incontinence and difficulty in initiating voiding. Sphincteric denervation is caused by progressive cell loss in the motor nuclei of the striated sphincters in segments S2–S4 of the spinal cord,[40] part of the widespread degeneration and gliosis characteristic of MSA. This cell loss causes denervation and re-innervation of motor units, with resultant characteristic changes in urethral and anal sphincteric electromyography (EMG). Since idiopathic PD does not involve sacral motor neurone damage, urethral sphincter EMG is useful in distinguishing PD from MSA.[41]

Isolated detrusor hyperreflexia is more common in PD than MSA,[42,43] and this can be treated with anticholinergic medication. In older patients, other factors – including prostatic hypertrophy in the male and pelvic floor dysfunction in the female – are often initially and erroneously considered to cause urinary urgency and frequency.

Erectile and ejaculatory failure occurs in 20–60 per cent of patients with PD,[29,30] with psychogenic and other factors each possibly contributing to the problem.

Thermoregulatory disturbance

While hyperhydrosis or excessive sweating is frequently cited as a feature of autonomic disturbance in PD, it is related to 'off' periods with tremor, and is felt by many authors to represent an appropriate thermoregulatory response to increased muscle activity. Patients with true autonomic failure exhibit hypohidrosis and anhidrosis with defective temperature regulation.[44]

Investigation of autonomic function

A battery of tests which may be performed to investigate the patient with autonomic failure is listed in Table 10.4. In practice, extensive testing will only be required in a few patients, as most of the tests necessary to confirm autonomic dysfunction are non-invasive and relatively simple to carry out. The tests most frequently used will be discussed, with particular emphasis on the

Table 10.4 Investigations of autonomic dysfunction in Parkinson's disease

Cardiovascular	
Physiological	Head-up tilt; Active stand; Valsalva manoeuvre Pressor stimuli-isometric exercise, cold pressor, mental arithmetic Heart rate responses – deep breathing, hyperventilation, standing, head-up tilt, 30:15 ratio. Carotid sinus massage Liquid meal
Biochemical	Plasma noradrenaline – supine and standing; urinary catecholamines; plasma renin activity and aldosterone
Pharmacological	Noradrenaline: α receptors, vascular Isoprenaline: f3 receptors, vascular and cardiac Tyramine: pressor and noradrenaline response Edrophonium: noradrenaline response Atropine: parasympathetic cardiac blockade
Sweating	Central regulation – increase of core temperature by 10°C Sweat gland response – intradermal acetylcholine, quantitative sudomotor axon reflex test (Q-SART), spot test
Gastrointestinal	Barium studies, video cinefluoroscopy, endoscopy, gastric emptying studies
Renal function	Day and night urine volumes, sodium and potassium excretion
Urinary tract	Urodynamic studies, intravenous urography, ultrasound examination, sphincter lectromyography
Sexual function	Penile plethysmography Intracavernosal papaverine
Respiratory	Laryngoscopy Sleep studies to assess apnea/oxygen desaturation
Eye	Schirmer's test Pupil function – pharmacological and physiological

Source: Adapted from Mathias and Bannister.[78]

effects that ageing might have upon their outcome, after which details will be provided of investigations that are particularly relevant to current research into the pathophysiology underlying autonomic dysfunction in PD.

Essential investigations

POSTURAL CHALLENGE TESTING: ACTIVE STAND AND HEAD-UP TILT

Orthostatic hypotension is defined as a 20 mmHg fall in systolic blood pressure, or a fall to <90 mmHg on standing for 3 min.[45] A 2-min stand is adequate to demonstrate reproducible OH in elderly subjects. Some definitions of OH have included a 10 mmHg fall in diastolic blood pressure in the diagnostic criteria, but in practice there is no correlation between falls in diastolic pressure and orthostatic symptoms. Thus, the principal focus remains systolic blood pressure change.

While manual blood pressure measurement may be a useful screening test in a busy clinic, phasic beat-to-beat blood pressure recording using digital photoplethysmography (Portapres®) is more accurate in detecting transient, but symptomatic, orthostatic change. Care must be taken to ensure that the arm (sphygmomanometer) or hand (Portapres®) is maintained at the level of the heart on standing in order to avoid the hydrostatic effect of a column of blood giving a falsely elevated reading.

Orthostatic blood pressure changes are not always reproducible. The effect of recumbent posture on the renin–angiotensin system and atrial natriuretic pepide levels, with resultant decrease in plasma volume, results in a higher level of reproducibility of OH with repeated morning recordings. Postprandial hypotension may coexist with OH,[46] thus measurements taken between 30 and 90 min after a meal or a glucose load may also have a higher diagnostic yield. Measurements are more likely to be reproducible in patients with abnormal autonomic function.[47]

Failure of the heart rate to rise in the presence of a substantial fall in blood pressure is indicative of a baroreflex abnormality, as in sympathetic or parasympathetic failure.

CARDIOVASCULAR AUTONOMIC FUNCTION TEST BATTERY[48]

Resting heart rate is determined mainly by vagal tone, which decreases on standing with a consequent increase in the heart rate of 11–29 beats/min. There is a biphasic response, with maximum heart rate reached at around the 15th beat after standing, slowing to a relatively stable rate at around the 30th beat. A comparison of the R-R intervals measured at these times yields a 30:15 ratio. A reduction in the 30:15 ratio is indicative of parasympathetic dysfunction. The integrity of vagal outflow is further assessed by the variability of the heart rate to deep breathing.

Placing one hand in ice water, mental stress (e.g. serial seven test) and isometric exercise such as sustained hand grip, result in increased systemic blood pressure. The afferent pathways involved in these stresses (pain, central command, muscle receptors) are distinct from the afferent pathways of the arterial baroreflex. In subjects with evidence of disturbances in control of systemic blood pressure during orthostatic stress or Valsalva straining, a rise suggests that efferent sympathetic pathways are functioning.

The cold pressor test is most easy to apply to elderly subjects. Subjects are rested in the semi-recumbent position. Responses are measured before and during immersion of one hand in ice water for 1 min. The changes in blood pressure during the last 10 s of the test are compared with baseline values. A blood pressure rise of 10–15 mmHg in systolic blood pressure and of 10 mmHg in diastolic blood pressure is considered to be a normal response.

The response to isometric exercise can be assessed using sustained hand grip. The maximum voluntary contraction is first determined using a hand-grip dynamometer, or measuring the maximum pressure of mercury attained when squeezing the bulb of a sphygmomanometer. Hand grip is then maintained at 30 per cent of that maximum for as long as possible up to 5 min. Blood pressure is measured three times before and at 1-min intervals during handgrip. The result is expressed as the difference between the highest diastolic blood pressure during hand grip exercise and the mean of the three resting diastolic blood pressure readings. A rise in diastolic blood pressure of <10 mmHg is regarded as abnormal.

The Valsalva manoeuvre tests the integrity of the entire baroreflex pathway. The heart rate is recorded with an electrocardiogram at the bedside as the patient breathes forcibly into a mercury manometer, sufficient to elevate the

Table 10.5 Cardiovascular autonomic function tests: age-related normal values

	Normal values age < 65 years	Normal values age > 65 years
Valsalva ratio (ratio of longest R-R interval with 20 beats after the manoeuvre and shortest R-R interval during the manoeuvre)	>1.10	>1.12
Phase 4 Valsalva SBP overshoot		>5 mmHg
30:15 ratio (heart rate variability following standing)	>1.00	>1.06
Heart rate variability with deep breathing (5 seconds inspiration, 5 seconds expiration: difference between mean maximum and minimum heart rates over six cycles)	>10 beats per minute	>1 beat per minute
Cold pressor test (DBP rise following contact with ice)	>10 mmHg rise	>4 mmHg rise

Source: Ewing and Clarke[48] and Stout and Kenny.[51]

column to 40 mmHg for 10–15 s. This allows the ratio of the longest R-R interval during the manoeuvre to the shortest R-R interval after the manoeuvre to be calculated.

There is an age-related decline in the heart rate and blood pressure variability as measured with this test battery.[49,50] We have defined 'age-related' normal values for subjects aged over 65 years, taking a normal range as within two standard deviations of the mean for healthy elderly controls.[5] These values are listed in Table 10.5. The American Diabetic Association requires the presence of only one abnormal value on two occasions to diagnose autonomic dysfunction.[5] The high, but unexplained, number of abnormal tests in asymptomatic healthy elderly volunteers has led us to use more stringent criteria for those aged over 65 years, requiring three or more abnormal tests before a diagnosis of autonomic failure is made.

In a recent series in our unit, 78 per cent of patients with PD and OH had autonomic failure using age-related parameters of cardiovascular control.[53] Despite making allowances for age, practical difficulties can cause problems in the interpretation of cardiovascular autonomic function tests in parkinsonian patients. Bradykinetic subjects may take longer to stand, complicating interpretation of the 30:15 ratio, and standardization of depth of breathing and Valsalva effort can be difficult in frail individuals.

BIOCHEMICAL, PHARMACOLOGICAL AND IMAGING TECHNIQUES

The resting plasma noradrenaline level and its response to head-up tilt may be used to investigate the nature of autonomic failure. Resting values of blood pressure, heart rate and plasma noradrenaline and adrenaline are normal in both lying and standing positions in newly diagnosed untreated patients with PD.[54,55] This suggests that efferent orthosympathetic fibres and baroreceptor adaptation to orthostasis are normal in the early stages of the disease. Pharmacological studies have found evidence of down-regulation of post-synaptic α_2-adrenoceptors in *de novo* PD subjects.[56,57] Treatment with dopaminergic drugs increases platelet α_2-adrenoceptors up to normal values, without any change in plasma catecholamine levels.[58] There does not appear to be any change in α_1- or β_1-receptor function in early PD.[59] During the course of their disease some patients with PD develop OH. These subjects have reduced baseline plasma noradrenaline levels with supersensitivity to exogenous noradrenaline and up-regulation of peripheral α-receptors.[60] Some authors suggest that decreased noradrenaline release from peripheral sympathetic different nerves as a result of peripheral autonomic dysfunction may underlie these findings. This is supported by reduction in yohimbine (presynaptic α_2-receptor antagonist) -induced noradrenaline release in patients with PD and OH compared with those without OH and controls.[61]

The growth hormone (GH) response to the central α-receptor agonist clonidine has attracted recent attention for those interested in the pathophysiology underlying autonomic dysfunction in PD. Normal subjects and those with pure autonomic failure show an 8–10 mU/l rise in OH following a 2 μg/kg dose of intravenous clonidine.[62] This response is lost in subjects with MSA, and has led to the conclusion that failure of the OH response indicates central autonomic dysfunction.[63] Early reports suggested that the response is preserved in idiopathic PD,[64] thereby supporting the suggestion of a predominantly peripheral autonomic disturbance in PD. Recent investigators have failed to reproduce the early findings in older patients with more advanced PD.[53,65] Until the effects of ageing and disease progression on OH secretion in response to clonidine are more completely documented, the significance of the GH/clonidine response in relation to autonomic pathophysiology, and its potential as an investigation to differentiate PD from SDS, must be viewed with some caution.

As already mentioned, urethral and anal sphincter EMG has some role in the differential diagnosis of PD from Shy–Drager syndrome, but is limited by the invasive nature of the test. Neuroimaging techniques such as positron emission tomography (PET) have shown some promise in helping distinguish Shy–Drager syndrome from PD.[66,67] Subtle differences in putaminal intensity may be seen, though this is still primarily a research investigation and limited to only a few centres.

Post-mortem studies on parkinsonian subjects do not support the 'peripheral hypothesis' of autonomic dysfunction generated by the biochemical and pharmacological data. There is strong evidence for the presence of Lewy bodies in the central brainstem nuclei and hypothalamus,[68,69] but only limited documentation exists of degenerative pathology in the peripheral autonomic ganglia.[70,71]

Management of symptomatic autonomic dysfunction

Orthostatic hypotension is probably the most common and disruptive symptom of autonomic dysfunction in the parkinsonian patient. Although impressive falls in blood pressure may be recorded during autonomic assessment, currently the treatment of OH is not thought necessary unless the patient is symptomatic. If future studies confirm a relationship between repeated hypotensive insults and cognitive decline, then this approach to asymptomatic OH may change.

Initial treatment of OH is non-pharmacological, and includes 'conservative' advice to avoid sudden postural change, elastic stockings and elevation of the head of the bed at night – all can be surprisingly effective (Table 10.6). The patient's medication chart should be carefully reviewed, and medications which exacerbate a hypotensive tendency withdrawn if possible.

Fludrocortisone is often the initial drug of choice when treating OH. It has multiple pharmacological actions, including plasma volume expansion, reduction of natriuresis and sensitization of remaining α-adrenoceptors to noradrenaline. A dose of 0.1–0.2 mg is the usual starting dose. A study of six parkinsonian patients with symptomatic OH showed effective reduction in orthostatic symptoms with 0.05–0.2 mg fludrocortisone.[72] Unfortunately,

Table 10.6 'Conservative' methods for the control of orthostatic hypotension in parkinsonian patients

Method	Comment
Avoidance of sudden head-up positional change, and straining at stool	Most likely to be effective in the morning following nocturnal polyuria
Avoidance of large meals and alcohol	Postprandial hypotension may aggravate problems Alcohol vasodilates
Adequate fluid and salt intake	Maintenance of plasma volume
Avoidance of excessive heat	Loss of intravascular volume and cutaneous vasodilatation
Elevation of bed-head 20–30 degrees at night	Reduces salt and water loss, via reduced renal arterial pressure and increased renin
Elastic stockings, abdominal binders	Attempt to reduce venous pooling. Many patients find them uncomfortable
Awareness of vasoactive/hypotensive drug side-effects when prescribing	Even minor changes of an agent may cause major changes via supersensitivity. The combination of levodopa with selegeline may have particularly potent hypotensive effects and should be avoided. Psychotropic drugs may also have significant cardiovascular effects.

fludrocortisone is poorly tolerated in the long term in older patients with hypotensive disorders, and up to 33 per cent discontinue treatment within 5 months of commencement.[73] Supine hypertension, peripheral oedema and hypokalaemia are common side effects.

α-Receptor agonists such as midodrine may have some role in the treatment of debilitating OH.[74] Supine hypertension and peripheral vasoconstriction are particular problems in the elderly. Midodrine can be prescribed under general licence in the USA, but is prescribed on a named patient basis only in the UK.

DDAVP (desmopressin) is a synthetic antidiuretic hormone analogue which can be given via intramuscular or intranasal routes. It acts on the renal tubules as a potent antidiuretic, reducing nocturnal polyuria and thereby raising morning blood pressure. Treatment requires careful monitoring, with water intoxication and hyponatraemia a problematic side effect, especially in the elderly. A pilot trial of triglycl-lysine-vasopressin in patients with PD and OH resulted in a 25 per cent increase in supine blood pressure, but only minimal reduction in blood pressure during head-up tilt.

Recommended drug treatments in the treatment of OH are listed in Table 10.7.

Further manifestations of autonomic failure may be managed as outlined

Table 10.7 Drug treatments used in the management of orthostatic hypotension

Proposed mode of action/class	Drugs used
Sympathomimetic vasoconstrictor	
Direct-acting	Midodrine, phenylephrine, clonidine
Indirect acting	Tyramine with monoamine oxidase type A inhibitors (e.g. tranylcypramine)
Preventing vasodilatation	
Prostaglandin synthetase inhibitors	Indomethacin, flurbiprofen
Dopamine receptor blockade	Metoclopramide, domperidone
Beta$_2$-adrenoceptor blockade	Propranolol
Increasing cardiac output	Pindolol, prenalterol
Reducing salt loss/blood volume expansion	Fludrocortisone, erythropoietin
Reducing nocturnal polyuria – vasopressin V2 receptor agonists	Demopressin (DDAVP)
Reducing postprandial hypotension	
Adenosine receptor blockade	Caffeine
Gut peptide release inhibitors	Octreotide (SMS 201-94~5)

Table 10.8 The management of non-cardiovascular symptoms of autonomic failure

System/disorder	Treatment
Hyperhidrosis	Anticholinergic drugs; local astringents containing glutaraldehyde
Thermoregulation	
Hypothermia	Space blanket and warm drinks
Hyperthermia	Cold drinks, tepid sponging, cold fan
Gastrointestinal	
Gastroparesis	Domperidone/metoclopramide
Achalasia	Surgery
Diarrhoea	Broad-spectrum antibiotics/codeine phosphate
Constipation	High-fibre diet and aperients
Urinary tract	Anticholinergics/phenoxylbenzamine; intermittent or permanent catheterization
Impotence	Papaverine injections; implanted prosthesis; electroejaculatory procedures
Inspiratory stridor	Tracheostomy, if due to laryngeal abductor paralysis
Xerophthalmia and xerostomia	Hypomellose-based substitutes

Source: Burn and Bates.[79]

in Table 10.8. Treatment of these problems is usually more successful than that of OH, and may lead to significant improvement of the patient's quality of life.

Conclusions

The autonomic problems associated with PD can be summarized as follows:

- Autonomic dysfunction accounts for significant cardiovascular, gastrointestinal and genitourinary co-morbidity in PD.

- Difficulty in distinguishing patients with Shy–Drager syndrome makes ascertainment of the prevalence of autonomic dysfunction in PD difficult
- Drugs and coexistent diseases may contribute to autonomic symptoms.
- Numerous tests are available to investigate the presence and severity of autonomic dysfunction in parkinsonian patients. In practice, simple and non-invasive tests of cardiovascular function such as active stand, autonomic function test battery and head-up tilt are easiest to interpret and to incorporate into the PD clinic assessment. The effect of ageing on these parameters should be carefully considered.
- Biochemical, pharmacological and imaging techniques are still primarily research tools.
- Current evidence supports a predominantly peripheral autonomic disturbance in PD with autonomic failure; neuropathological studies do not support this view. Further documentation of the effect of ageing on the dynamic biochemical and pharmacological tests is required before we can interpret the current data with more certainty.

References

1. Parkinson J. *An essay on the shaking palsy.* Neely A, Jones D (eds). London: Sherwood, 1817.
2. Gross M, Bannister R, Godwin-Austin R. Orthostatic hypotension in Parkinson's disease. *Lancet* 1972; **1**: 174–6.
3. Aminoff MJ, Wilcox CS. Assessment of autonomic function in patients with a parkinsonian syndrome. *Br. Med. J.* 1971; **4**: 80–4.
4. Piha SJ, Rinne JOT, Rinne UK, Seppares A. Autonomic dysfunction in recent onset and advanced Parkinson's disease. *Clin. Neurol. Neurosurg.* 1988; **90**: 221–6.
5. Ludin SM, Steiger UH, Ludin HP. Autonomic disturbances and cardiovascular reflexes in idiopathic Parkinson's disease. *J. Neurol.* 1987; **235**: 10–15.
6. Netten PM, de Vos K, Horstink MW, Hoefnagels WH. Autonomic dysfunction in Parkinson's disease, tested with a computerised method using a Finapres device. *Clin. Auton. Res.* 1995; **5**: 85–9.
7. Werbuch GJ, Sandyk R. Autonomic functions in the early stages of Parkinson's disease. *Int. J. Neurosci.* 1994; **74**: 9–16.
8. Ward CD, Gibb WR. Research diagnostic criteria for Parkinson's disease. *Adv. Neurol.* 1990; **53**: 245–9.
9. Jellinger KA. The neuropathologic diagnosis of secondary parkinsonian syndromes. In: Battistin L, Scarlato G, Caraceni T, Ruggieri S (eds). *Parkinson's Disease. Advances in Neurology, Vol. 169.* Philadelphia: Lippincott-Raven Press, 1996: 293–303.
10. Ansorge O, Lees AJT Daniel SE. Update on the accuracy of clinical diagnosis of idiopathic Parkinson's disease (abstract). *Movement Disord.* 1997; **12** (suppl.): 96.
11. Shy GM, Drager GA. A neurological syndrome associated with orthostatic hypotension. *Arch. Neurol.* 1960; **3**: 511–27.
12. Bannister R, Mathias CJ, Polinsky R. Autonomic failure: a comparison between UK and US experiences. In: Bannister R (ed.). *Autonomic Failure – A Textbook of Clinical Disorders of the Autonomic Nervous System*, 2nd edn. Oxford: Oxford University Press, 1988: 281–8.

13. Rajput AH, Rozdilsky B, Rajput A, Ang L. Levodopa efficacy and pathological basis of Parkinson's syndrome. *Clin. Neuropharmacol.* 1990; **13**: 553–8.
14. Hughes AJ, Daniel SE, Kilford L, Lees AJ. The accuracy of clinical diagnosis of idiopathic Parkinson's disease: a clinico-pathological study of 100 cases. *J. Neurol. Neurosurg. Psychiatry* 1992; **55**: 181–2.
15. Ben-Shlomo Y, Wenning GK, Tison F, Quinn NP. Survival of patients with pathologically proven multiple system atrophy: a meta-analysis. *Neurology* 1997; **48**: 384–93.
16. Mathias O. Disorders affecting autonomic function in parkinsonian patients. *Adv. Neurol.* 1996; **69**: 383–91.
17. Poewe WH, Wenning GK. The natural history of Parkinson's disease. *Ann. Neurol.* 1998; **44** (3 Suppl.): S1–9.
18. Perry RH, Irving D, Blessed A, Perry EK, Fairburn AF. Clinically and neuropathologically distinct form of dementia in the elderly. *Lancet* 1989; **i**: 166.
19. Hughes AJ, Daniel SE, Blanston S, Lees AJ. The clinical features of Parkinson's disease: a clinicopathological study of 100 cases. *Arch. Neurol.* 1993; **50**: 140–8.
20. Kalra S, Bergeron C, Lang AE. Lewy body disease and dementia. *Arch. Intern. Med.* 1996; **156**: 487–93.
21. McKeith LA, Aalasko D, Kosaka K, *et al.* Consensus guidelines for the clinical and pathologic diagnosis of dementia with Lewy bodies (DLB). *Neurology* 1996; **47**: 1113–24.
22. Kosaka K. Diffuse Lewy body disease in Japan. *J. Neurol.* 1990; **237**: 197–204.
23. Ballard C, Shaw F, McKeith I, Kenny RA. High prevalence of neurocardiovascular instability in neurodegenerative dementias. *Neurology* 1998; **51**: 1760–2.
24. Wentink JRM, Jansen RWMM, Hoefnagel WHL. The influence of age on the response of blood pressure and heart rate to carotid sinus massage in healthy volunteers. *Cardiol. Elderly* 1993; **1**: 453–9.
25. Calne DB, Brennan J, Spiers ASD, Stem OM. Hypotension caused by L-Dopa. *Br. Med. J.* 1970; **i**: 474–5.
26. Churchyard A, Mathias CJ, Boonkongcheun P, Lees AJ .Autonomic effects of selegeline: possible cardiovascular toxicity in Parkinson's disease. *J. Neurol. Neurosurg. Psychiatry* 199'7; **63**: 228–34.
27. Orskov L, Jakobsen J, Dupont E, de Fine Olivarius B, Christensen NJ. Autonomic function in parkinsonian patients relates to duration of disease. *Neurology* 1987; **37**: 1173–8.
28. Wilson JA, Smith RA. The prevalence and aetiology of long-term L-dopa side-effects in elderly Parkinsonian patients. *Age Ageing* 1989; **18**; 11–16.
29. Martignoni E, Pacchetti C, Aodi L, Micieli A, Nappi A. Autonomic disorders in Parkinson's disease. *J. Neural Transm.* 1995; **45** (Suppl.): 11–19.
30. Singer C, Weiner WJ, Sanchez-Ramos JR. Autonomic dysfunction in men with Parkinson's disease. *Eur. Neurol.* 1992; **32**: 134–40.
31. Senard JM, Rai S, Lapeyre-Mestre M, Brefel C, Rascol O, Rascol A, Montastruc JL. Prevalence of orthostatic hypotension in Parkinson's disease. *J. Neurol. Neurosurg. Psychiatry* 1997; **63**: 584–9.
32. Koller W, Glatt S, Vetere-Overfield B, *et al.* Falls and Parkinson's disease. *Clin. Neuropharmacol.* 1989; **12**: 98.
33. Bleasdale-Barr K, Mathias CJ. Suboccipital (coathanger) and other muscular pains – frequency in autonomic failure and other neurological problems, and association with postural hypotension. *Clin. Autonom. Res.* 1994; **4**: 82.
34. Brooks CJ, Redmond S, Mathias CJ, Bannister R, Symon L. The effect of orthostatic hypotension on cerebral blood flow and middle cerebral artery velocity in auto-

nomic failure, with observations on the action of ephedrine. *J. Neurol. Neurosurg. Psychiatry* 1989; **52**: 962–6.

35. Angeli S, Marchese A, Focacci A, Del Sette M, Abbruzzese A. Middle cerebral arteries monitoring during tilt test in Parkinson's disease and MSA. *Movement Disord.* 1998; **13**: 116.

36. Stout NR, Galloway SW, Ayre A, Wesnes K, Kenny RA. Cognitive impairment in elderly patients with orthostatic hypotension. *Age Ageing* 2000; in press.

37. Korczyn AD. Autonomic nervous system screening in patients with early Parkinson's disease. In: Przuntek H, Riederer P (eds). *Early diagnosis and preventive therapy in Parkinson's disease.* Vienna, New York: Springer, 1989: 41–8.

38. Wakabayashi K, Takahashi H, Ohama E, Takeda E, Ikuta F. Lewy bodies in the visceral autonomic nervous system in Parkinson's disease. *Adv. Neurol.* 1993; **60**: 609–12.

39. Beck RO, Fowler CJ, Mathias CJ. Genito-urinary dysfunction in disorders of the autonomic nervous system. In: Rushton DN (ed.) *Handbook of Neuro-Urology.* New York: Marcel Dekker, 1994: 281–301.

40. Konno H, Yamamoto T, Iwasaki Y, *et al.* Shy-Drager syndrome and amyotrophic lateral sclerosis. Cytoarchitecture and morphometric studies of sacral autonomic neurones. *J. Neurol. Sci.* 1986; **73**: 193–204.

41. Eardley I, Quinn NP, Fowler CJ, Kirby RS, Parkhouse HF, Marsden CD, Bannister R. The value of urethral sphincter electromyography in the differential diagnosis of parkinsonism. *Br. J. Urol.* 1989; **64**: 360–2.

42. Mumagham OF. Neurogenic disorders of the bladder in parkinsonism. *Br. J. Urol.* 1961; **33**: 403.

43. Pavlakis AJ, Siroky MB, Goldstein I, Krane RJ. Neurologic finding in Parkinson's disease. *J. Urol.* 1983; **129**: 80.

44. De Marinis M, Stocchi F, Testa SR, De Pandis F, Agnoli A. Alterations of thermoregulation in Parkinson's disease. *Funct. Neurol.* 1991; **6**: 279–83.

45. Atkins D, Hanusa B, Sefcik T, Kapoor W. Syncope and orthostatic hypotension. *Am. J. Med.* 1991; **91**: 179–84.

46. Robinson BJ, Johnson RH, Lambie DO, Palmer KT. Autonomic responses to glucose ingestion in elderly subjects with orthostatic hypotension. *Age Ageing* 1985; **14**: 168–73.

41. Ward C, Kenny RA. The reproducibility of orthostatic hypotension in the elderly presenting with postural symptoms. *Age Ageing* 1994; **23**: 19.

48. Ewing DJ, Carke BF. Diagnosis and management of diabetic autonomic neuropathy. *Br. Med. J.* **285**: 916–98.

49. Low PA, Opferoerhrking TL, Proper CJ, Zimmerman I. The effect of aging on cardiac autonomic and postganglionic sudomotor function. *Muscle Nerve* 1990; **13**: 152–7.

50. Kaijser L, Sachs C. Autonomic cardiovascular responses in old age. *Clin. Physiol.* 1985; **5**: 347–57.

51. Stout N, Kenny RA. Reference ranges for clinical autonomic function testing in healthy elderly. *Clin. Auton. Res.* 1999; (in press)

52. American Diabetic Association. Report and recommendations of the San Antonio Conference on diabetic neuropathy. *Diabetes* 1988; **37**: 1000–4.

53. Allcock LM, Dey AB, Gibb I, Bum DJ, Kenny RA. Neurohumoral responses: to cardiovascular and pharmacological stimuli in Parkinson's disease with orthostatic hypotension and age-related orthostatic hypotension. *Age Ageing* 1999 (in press).

54. Durrieu G, Senard IM, Rascol O, Tran MA, Lataste X, Rascol A, Montastruc IL. Blood pressure and plasma catecholamines in never-treated parkinsonian patients: effect of a D1 agonist (CY 208-243). *Neurology* 1990; **40**: 707–9.

55. Durriue G, Senard IM, Tran MA, Rascol A, Montastruc IL. Effects of levodopa and bromocriptine on blood pressure and plasma catecholamines in Parkinsonians. *Clin. Neuropharmacol.* 1991; **14**: 84–90.
56. Montastruc IL, Villeneuve A, Berlan M, Lafontan M, Caranobe C, Boneu B, Rascol A. Study of platelet alpha2-adrenoceptors in Parkinson's disease. *Adv. Neurol.* 1986; **45**: 253–8.
57. Villeneuve A, Berlan M, Lafontan M, Caranobe C, Boneu B, Rascol A, Montastruc IL. Platelet alpha2- adrenoceptors in Parkinson's disease: decreased number in untreated patients and recovery after treatment. *Eur. J. Clin. Invest.* 1985; **15**: 403–7.
58. Durrieu G, Valet P, Berlan M, Villeneuve A, Montastruc IL. Levodopa up-regulation of platelet alpha2- adrenoceptors. *Eur. J. Pharmacol.* 1990; **182**: 597–601.
59. Zoukos Y, Thomaides T, Pavitt DV, Cuzner ML, Mathias CI. Beta-adrenergic expression on circulating mononuclear cells of idiopathic Parkinson's disease and autonomic failure patients before and after reduction of central sympathetic outflow by clonidine. *Neurology* 1993; **43**: 1181–7.
60. Senard IM, Valet P, Durrieu G, *et al.* Adrenergic supersensitivity in parkinsonians with orthostatic hypotension. *Eur. J. Clin. Invest.* 1990; **20**: 613–19.
61. Senard IM, Rascol O, Durrieu G, Tran MA, Berlan M, Rasol A, Montastruc IL. Effects of yohimbine on plasma catecholamine levels in orthostatic hypotension related to Parkinson's disease or multiple system atrophy. *Clin. Neuropharmacol.* 1993; **16**: 70–6.
62. Alba-Roth I, Losa M, Speiss Y, Schopohl I, Muller OA, Von Weder C. Interaction of clonidine and GHRH on OH secretion in vivo and in vitro. *Clin. Endocrinol.* 1989; **30**: 485–91.
63. Thomaides TN, Ray Chaudhiri K, Maule S, Watson L, Marsden CD, Mathias CI. Growth hormone response to clonidine in central and peripheral autonomic failure. *Lancet* 1992; **340**: 263–6.
64. Kimber IR, Watson L, Mathias CI. Distinction of idiopathic Parkinson's disease from multiple-system atrophy by stimulation of growth-hormone release with clonidine. *Lancet* 1997; **349**: 1877–81.
65. Clarke CE, Ray PS, Speller IM. Failure of the clonidine growth hormone stimulation test to differentiate multiple system atrophy from early or advanced idiopathic Parkinson's disease. *Lancet* 1999; **353**: 1329–30.
66. Bum DI, Sawle GV, Brooks DI. Differential diagnosis of Parkinson's disease, multiple system atrophy, and Stelle-Richardson-Olszewski syndrome: discriminant analysis of striatal 18F-dopa PET data. *J. Neurol. Neurosurg. Psychiatry* 1994; **57**: 278–84.
67. Brooks DI, Ibanez V, Sawle GV, Quinn N, Lees AI, Mathias CI, Bannister R, Marsed CD, Frackowiak SI. Differing patterns of striatal 18F-Dopa uptake in Parkinson's disease, multiple system atrophy, and progressive supranuclear palsy. *Ann. Neurol.* 1990; **28**: 547–55.
68. Ohama E, Ikuta F. Parkinson's disease: distribution of Lewy bodies and monoamine neuron system. *Acta Neuropathol.* 1976; **34**: 311–19.
69. Lanston IW, Forno LS. The hypothalamus in Parkinson's disease. *Ann. Neurol.* 1977; 3: 129–33.
70. Rajput AH, Rozdilsky B. Dysautonomia in parkinsonism: a clinicopathological study. *J. Neurol. Neurosurg. Psychiatry* 1976; **39**: 1092–100.
71. Fomo LS, Norville RL. Ultrastructure of Lewy bodies in the stellate ganglion. *Acta Neuropathol.* 1976; **34**: 183–97.
72. Hoehn MM. Levodopa-induced postural hypotension. Treatment with fludrocortisone. *Arch. Neurol.* 1975; **32**: 50–1.

73. Hussain RM, McIntosh SJ, Lawson J, Kenny RA. Fludrocortisone in the treatment of hypotensive disorders in the elderly. *Heart* 1996; **76**: 507–9.

74. Low PA, Gilden JL, Freeman R, Sheng KN, McElliott MA. Efficacy of midodrine vs. placebo in neurogenic orthostatic hypotension. A randomized, double blind multicenter study. Midodrine Study Group. *JAMA* 1997; **277**: 1046–51.

75. Rittig S, Arentensen J, Sorenson K, Matthiesen T, Dupont E. The hemodynamic effects of triglycyl-lysine-vasopressin (Glypressin) in patients with parkinsonism and orthostatic hypotension. *Movement Disord.* 1991; **6**: 21–8.

76. Mathias CJ. Disorders of the autonomic nervous system. In: Bradley WG, Dlirroff RB, Fenichel OM, Marsden CD (eds). *Neurology in Clinical Practice, Vol. 2.* Stoneham, MA: Butterworths, 1991: 1661–85.

77. Mathias CJ. Orthostatic hypotension – causes, mechanisms and influencing factors. *Neurology* 1995; **45** (Suppl. 5): S6–11.

78. Mathias CJ, Bannister R. Investigation of autonomic disorders. In: Bannister R, Mathias C (eds). *Autonomic Failure: A Textbook of Disorders of the Autonomic Nervous System.* Oxford: Oxford University Press, 1992: 255–90.

79. Burn DJ, Bates D. Primary and secondary autonomic dysfunction. In: Kenny RA (ed.). *Syncope in the Older Patient.* Chapman & Hall, 1996.

11 Motor problems

P.W. Overstall

Introduction

Postural instability causing unsteadiness when standing and walking is a cardinal feature of Parkinson's disease (PD), and is particularly associated with disease onset after the age of 70 years. Older patients are more likely to have balance impairment, both at onset and after 5 years of treatment, and its presence as the major criterion for Hoehn and Yahr stage 3 marks a significant shift from mild to more disabling disease. Mobility and independence are threatened, and the risk of serious injury from a fall increases. Patients with imbalance appear to have a more rapidly progressive form of the disease, and the presence of a gait disorder in a parkinsonian patient doubles the relative risk of death.[1,2] Whether or not these patients have a different underlying pathology is still unclear, although co-morbidity – in particular cerebrovascular disease – is likely to be the explanation in at least some of these patients.

The challenge therefore for clinicians is two-fold: first, to decide whether the patient with the all too common presentation of falls and 'off his/her legs' really does have idiopathic PD; and second – having made the diagnosis – to determine the best form of treatment. Unfortunately, gait continues to deteriorate despite levodopa treatment.[3] However, modern gait laboratories, which can measure balance using force platforms and surface electromyography (EMG), both during quiet standing and following perturbations and when walking using three-dimensional (3D) motion analysing systems, have provided important information on the kinetics and kinematics of PD and possible physical therapies.

Normal standing balance

During normal quiet standing, balance is maintained when the vertical projection of the centre of mass (COM) on the ground (often called the centre of gravity, COG) is kept within the support base provided by the feet. Maintenance of this upright position is associated with body sway mainly in the anterior/posterior (A/P) direction, and this sway may be measured either as degrees of angular movement or using force platforms as the excursions of the centre of pressure (COP). The COP is independent of the COM and represents the pressure over the surface of the feet in contact with the ground. There are separate COPs under each foot, and when both feet are in contact with the ground the net COP lies somewhere between the two feet, depending on the relative weight taken by each foot.[4] Both A/P sway velocity and area increase in normal elderly subjects (i.e. those who report that their balance is normal and are functionally independent), and this difference is more obvious if the difficulty of the test is increased by using a moving platform or when the eyes are closed.[5] Further increases in A/P sway have been correlated with spontaneous falls, but a better predictor of falls is mediolateral sway.[6]

In contrast to this increased sway that is seen in normal elderly subjects, PD patients have an unusually small sway area – about half that seen in elderly controls. They do not appear to have any difficulty using visual, somatosensory or vestibular information, and the sway areas remain small even under challenging sensory conditions.[7] This reduced sway may be due to higher intrinsic musculoskeletal stiffness, or it may be compensation for inadequate postural control when the COM is displaced. The result is an overall increase in stiffness, which offers a certain advantage in resisting minor displacements. However, because postural responses to perturbations are impaired, the PD patient is like a tin-soldier in that although there is increased stability during quiet standing, stable equilibrium can be maintained only over a very small area, and loss of balance follows even modest displacements. Interestingly, an increase in mediolateral sway has been noted in PD patients – especially those who have fallen – and this may be a response to the postural inflexibility seen in the A/P direction. PD patients are unable to achieve extremes of forward or backward leaning, and this has been blamed on their reduced sway: the increased sway seen in these extreme positions in controls reflects not insta-bility but rather a deliberate action aimed at reducing further displacement. The increased mediolateral sway may thus be a compensatory strategy which introduces the necessary slight shifts and postural adjustments to counteract the restricted A/P movement.[8, 9].

Senile gait

There has been a long-running debate on what constitutes a normal gait in old age, and the cause of the senile gait (idiopathic gait disorder). There are undoubtedly some elderly people who maintain a normal gait with a speed greater than 1 m/s,[10] and a normal gait has been observed in 18 per cent of a community living sample aged between 88 and 96 years.[11] However, gait lab-oratory studies show subtle changes even in carefully screened healthy elderly subjects. Gait slowing is due to a decreased stride length, and cadence (steps per minute) remains unaltered. Stance time and double support time increase, and there is a less vigorous push-off. Whether this represents an early degeneration of the balance control system or an adaptation to make the gait safer is unclear.[12]

It is now apparent that the senile gait disorder, which is characterized by caution and shorter and more frequent strides (for which there is no apparent cause) and said to occur in 15–24 per cent of the elderly, is not due to age but to underlying neurodegenerative syndromes and stroke.[13] These patients have a two-fold increased risk of cardiovascular death compared with age-matched subjects with a normal gait, further supporting the view that senile gait is caused by subclinical cerebrovascular disease.[14] The considerable confusion over the aetiology of different gait disorders in the elderly has been clarified by the classification suggested by Nutt et al.[15] These authors proposed three broad categories of gait disorder: (i) the lowest level due to peripheral skele-tomuscular or sensory problems; (ii) a middle level causing distortion of appropriate postural and locomotor synergies (early Parkinsonism could be included in this category); and (iii) highest level disorders, which are those most commonly seen by geriatricians. This last category includes five gait types of which subcortical dysequilibrium, frontal dysequilibrium and frontal gait disorder are the most relevant, since all of these gaits may include an ele-ment of parkinsonism.

In deciding whether or not a patient with impaired balance and gait has PD, it should be remembered that for postural instability to be regarded as a cardinal sign of PD it must be unrelated to primary visual, cerebellar, vestibu-lar or proprioceptive dysfunction. In practical terms, the important diagnoses to exclude are a frontal gait disorder due to cerebrovascular disease or normal pressure hydrocephalus, and a cervical myelopathy. For further discussion of the differential diagnosis, see Chapter 4.

Differential diagnosis

Arteriosclerotic parkinsonism

This is also called lower-half parkinsonism, and the gait is sometimes described as *marche à petits pas*. It is characteristically a frontal gait disorder. The gait tends to be wider than in idiopathic PD, the steps are short and shuffling, and there is start and turn hesitation.[15] Dysequilibrium can be more marked than in idiopathic PD, and in both conditions there is increased reliance on visual cues. A possible explanation is that the multiple vascular lesions produce a disconnection of cortical modulation rather than an impairment of the functions of the basal ganglia. If the periventricular lesions affect the afferent loop between the basal ganglia and the supplementary motor area, there will be a loss of internally triggered movements and increased reliance on visually triggered external movements.[16] Other clues that distinguish it from idiopathic PD are the upright trunk and leg posture and the preservation of arm swing. Pyramidal tract signs and pseudobulbar palsy are common in arteriosclerotic parkinsonism, but not in PD. Although it is sometimes said that the upper limbs are normal in arteriosclerotic parkinsonism, it is not uncommon in elderly patients to find both bradykinesia and rigidity (and even occasionally tremor), although the limb rigidity is more likely to be symmetrical than in idiopathic PD. A good response to levodopa would make one question the diagnosis of arteriosclerotic parkinsonism, but a modest improvement in symptoms (<50 per cent) is occasionally seen.[17]

Computed tomography (CT) scanning of patients with arteriosclerotic parkinsonism and gait abnormalities shows leuko-araiosis and ventricular enlargement in 90 per cent of cases.[18] Lacunar strokes and white matter lesions on CT are better predictors of the development of parkinsonism than territorial strokes. White matter lesions are more likely to be found in patients with idiopathic PD than in healthy subjects, and are a marker for more severe disease, particularly bradykinesia, postural instability and gait difficulties. These patients have a shorter disease duration and their bradykinesia responds less well to levodopa.[19]

Cervical myelopathy

This is a common cause of gait disorder in the elderly, and is due to degenerative arthritis of the cervical spine. In advanced cases there is spasticity and hyper-reflexia in the legs, with dorsal column signs and urinary urgency. The patient has a spastic gait and often there are lower motor neurone signs in the upper limbs, with reduced neck movements. However, before these patients develop the typical stiff-legged para-spastic gait there is impairment of balance apparent to the patient, who compensates by producing a protective gait pattern. Gait velocity, step length and cadence are reduced, and step width is increased. Improvement follows decompressive surgery.[20]

Alzheimer's disease

Parkinsonian signs are more likely to occur in Alzheimer's disease (AD) patients than in the general population. There are similarities (but also differences) between AD with parkinsonism and diffuse Lewy body disease. In both, the parkinsonism is typically symmetrical, and rest tremor is uncommon. However, in diffuse Lewy body disease there is a male predominance and the parkinsonian signs – and particularly the gait abnormalities – occur early, whereas in AD dementia is the presenting feature and the parkinsonian signs occur late. The neuropathological findings in patients with AD and parkinsonism are variable, but most cases are associated with subcortical Lewy bodies.[21]

Normal gait initiation

In order to understand what is happening in start hesitation, it is helpful to recall normal gait initiation. This begins with anticipatory postural adjustments (APA), the first of which is inhibition of the swing limb gastrocnemius-soleus, causing the COP to move posteriorly. Simultaneously, the tensor fascia lata is inhibited on the stance limb and activated on the swing limb, resulting in the COP moving towards the swing limb with loading of the swing limb and unloading of the stance limb. There is then rapid unloading of the swing limb and loading of the stance limb as the COP shifts to the stance limb. The COM accelerates forwards and towards the stance limb and, at the point of toe-off of the swing limb, the entire body weight is over the stance limb. The body falls forwards, and the COM moves towards where the heel of the swing foot will land.[4] The APA are programmed in advance of the intended voluntary movement, and shifting the COM allows a step to be taken.

Gait initiation in Parkinson's disease

In 1961, Purdon Martin conducted a famous study of 130 post-encephalitic parkinsonian patients cared for at Highlands Hospital in north London. He observed that some patients, although able to stand, were unable to either walk forwards or backwards, but if they were tilted slightly forwards and rocked from side to side, they could walk more or less normally. He concluded that the stepping mechanism as such is not disordered, and that the fault lies in disturbance of the APA, essential for the initiation and continuation of regular stepping.[22] This observation has remained at the heart of PD gait research ever since. In essence, in PD patients the APA and the forward velocity of the COM at heel-off are significantly reduced, but are improved by levodopa.[23] The APA show several changes, the initial standing posture is abnormal with increased likelihood of activation of quadriceps, hamstrings and tibialis anterior. This change in the postural set appears to prolong the time interval between gastrocnemius-soleus inhibition and heel-off of the swing limb. Even when standing EMG activity is normal, the APA may be slowed by prolonged recruitment of tibialis anterior before heel-off, but the most common abnormality is a loss of effectiveness of the APA. The initial inhibition of gastrocnemius-soleus may either be repeated several times, or be incomplete or even completely absent. Activation of tibialis anterior is desynchronized or absent and where soleus inhibition is present, there can be marked delay before activation of tibialis anterior. The defective APA means that the initial posterior shift of the COP is reduced (proportional to the degree of disability of the patient), and this in turn reduces the force of forward propulsion.[24–26]

Stepping in response to an external cutaneous cue improves both force and velocity of the APA,[23] and is consistent with the observation that external stimuli – such as visual and auditory cues – assist gait initiation. Although the precise function of the basal ganglia is unclear, it has been suggested that one important role is to provide an internal non-specific cue to trigger switching from one sequential movement to the next. Automatic predictable movement sequences appear to be particularly impaired in PD.[27]

Motor fluctuations

These eventually trouble most patients, and appear to be related to the length of time that the patient has been on levodopa. The fluctuations can be divided into short duration (which last seconds to minutes and consist of sudden, transient freezing episodes), medium duration and diurnal (minutes to hours) and long duration (days).[28]

Medium duration fluctuation begins as gradual end-of-dose deterioration. The patient's increasing awareness of this reflects an increased amplitude of the 'on–off' difference. Eventually, the development of sudden dramatic fluctuations indicates that a threshold level of dopaminergic stimulation has been reached, where the patient is either 'on' or 'off', with very little useful time in between. Frequent small doses may mean that the patient does not turn on at all, or has unpredictable fluctuations, and there is a more predictable response with larger, less frequent doses. Although this may improve the quality of the 'on' time, the 'off' time is subsequently worse. Diurnal variations are often noted, typically the patient being better in the morning than in the afternoon and evening

Freezing

Freezing tends to be a later feature of PD. It can occur in both the 'on' and 'off' states, and even in the absence of levodopa treatment. It is influenced by the patient's attention and sensory input, and although it usually affects both legs it is often asymmetrical. Turning hesitation is often noted to be worse in one direction more than another. Although freezing is most apparent in gait it is also observed in speech, the eyelids, hand writing and tasks such as shaving.

Freezing is not pathognomonic of PD, and indeed it occurs more commonly in progressive supranuclear palsy (PSP), arteriosclerotic parkinsonism and normal-pressure hydrocephalus. It is rare in multisystem atrophy and very rare in drug-induced parkinsonism. Early severe freezing is unusual in PD, and would suggest a diagnosis of PSP. The most common type of freezing is start hesitation (gait ignition failure). The patient attempts to start walking, but the feet remain stuck to the ground. Several short incomplete steps may be made before the patient is able to move forwards. Other typical situations where patients freeze are turning in a confined space or when passing through doorways.[29] The most important predictor for freezing is not disease duration, but progression of disease as measured by the Hoehn and Yahr scale. Duration of levodopa treatment is the second most significant factor, followed by duration of treatment with agonists. Treatment with amantadine, selegiline and anticholinergic drugs does not affect freezing, but there is a significant association between freezing and the presence of dyskinesia, early morning foot dystonia, postural instability and dementia.[30]

Freezing has been described as a feature of pure akinesia, a syndrome marked by the presence of postural instability and akinesia but the absence of rigidity or tremor. It is now known that many of these patients go on to develop PSP.[31]

Deficient force production during gait initiation does not explain freezing;[23] rather, it appears that during freezing the 'gain', i.e. velocity of the forward movement, reduces to zero[4] and is associated with a total absence of any APA. Freezing is notoriously resistant to treatment with levodopa, and yet both the delayed APA and the reduced force production for a self-generated step can be improved with levodopa. In other words, gait initiation – but not freezing – improves with levodopa, suggesting that in freezing either the levodopa fails to produce a normal response or else other non-dopaminergic pathways are involved. Impaired serotonin (5HT) neurotransmission has been suggested as a possible candidate.[32]

PATHOPHYSIOLOGY

The pathophysiology underlying freezing remains unclear. Frontal lobe disease and, more specifically, frontal white matter lesions, have been suggested.[15,17] However, patients with severe freezing due either to idiopathic PD or to isolated gait ignition failure, have not been shown to have significant frontal hypoperfusion (using single photon emission computed tomography, SPECT), although hypoperfusion can be demonstrated in patients with PSP. Interestingly, only 5 per cent of this PSP group had freezing, so the frontal lobe hypoperfusion that was observed may be related to other deficits, such as cognitive impairment, rather than to gait ignition failure.[33]

TREATMENT

Treatment of freezing depends crucially on distinguishing between episodes occurring when the patient is 'off' or is starting to develop end of dose deterioration and those patients whose episodes are unpredictable and unrelated to their 'on' or 'off' state. 'Off' freezing improves with levodopa, apomorphine or surgery to the sub-thalamic nucleus. Botulinum toxin injected into the calf muscles can be particularly helpful for patients with dystonic posturing. Up to five injections may be required. Improvement may not be noticed for a week, but the benefit lasts for about six weeks. 'On' freezing is rare and improves with a reduced dose. Patients with unpredictable freezing, who are taking frequent small doses of levodopa may be helped by a change to less frequent larger doses. Physical measures to overcome freezing include advice from the physiotherapist on how to turn, various trick manoeuvres such as marching on the spot to command or stepping over an object, a small electronic metronome worn on the belt and strips of white tape on the floor in parts of the house such as the WC where freezing tends to occur.

Dyskinesias

About 10 per cent of PD patients on levodopa treatment develop dyskinesias each year, and eventually virtually all patients are affected. The most common type is peak-dose dyskinesia, which appears earlier in patients with more severe disease. Typically, it is choreiform and painless and appears first on the most affected side, although in the elderly the lips, mouth or head are frequently involved. High doses of levodopa and long duration of treatment increase the risk, whereas agonist monotherapy reduces it. These dyskinesias can significantly interfere with the patient's gait and balance and, if the legs are severely affected, the dyskinesias must be controlled by reducing the levodopa dosage before the physiotherapist can start work on the patient. Unfortunately, for many patients turning 'on' becomes synonymous with dyskinesias. A variety of strategies can be tried, including controlled release preparations of levodopa, agonists, apomorphine and amantadine. Apomorphine can remain effective for at least 5 years,[34] and some patients can be weaned off levodopa altogether, provided that the dosage reduction is very gradual (50 mg per week). Patients with severe dyskinesias who have had PD for at least 4 years and are under 75 years of age are increasingly being considered for surgery. Lesioning (or stimulation) of globus pallidus interna or the subthalamic nucleus are the most promising operations at present.

'Off'-period dystonias may occur at the beginning or end of dose, during 'off' periods, or in the early morning.[28] Typically, the patient wakes in the morning with the foot distorted and painful, usually on the least affected side. The patient can be advised to stay in bed until the first dose of levodopa starts to work. Apomorphine or an injection of botulinum toxin can also be effective.

Biphasic dyskinesias (occurring at the onset and end of Levodopa action) are more common in young-onset patients and are best managed by larger and less frequent doses of levodopa and, if this is unsuccessful, by neurosurgery.

Gait

In most patients, PD first becomes apparent in the arms and trunk, and it may be months (or even years) before any abnormality is noted in the legs. Initial symptoms affecting only the legs is unusual. One 66-year-old patient whose first symptoms began in the legs complained of 'incoordination' when putting his left foot into a wellington boot or when using the clutch on his car, and described his walking as being like 'Robocop'. The only clinical abnormalities were a slight reduction in step length and increased tone in the left leg.

For most patients, the first sign of gait impairment is a reduction in step length and changes in the swing phase. A reduction both in knee flexion and heel elevation causes the heel to scuff as the foot moves forwards. Further progression of the disease is shown by slowing of walking speed, a tendency to take smaller steps and slow down when turning, and increasing flexion of arms, neck and trunk. In advanced disease the patient is severely flexed forwards and there is complete loss of the normal toe raise at the end of leg swing, so that the patient takes short quick steps by sliding his/her toes along the floor.

Gait analysis shows that PD patients have increased stride-to-stride variability, and they walk slowly because they are unable automatically to regulate their stride length. If asked to walk faster, they normally increase cadence (steps per minute) but not step length unless trained to do so.[35,36] Why patients can maintain or increase their cadence yet are unable accurately to regulate stride-to-stride gait is unknown, but it may represent a loss of automaticity in smoothly maintaining sequential movements so that walking becomes a matter of separate steps rather than a continuous flowing motion. Inability to generate adequate muscle force may also be a factor.[23]

Current views on the role of the basal ganglia suggest two main functions. First, they contribute to cortical motor set (i.e. the tonic discharge in motor cortical neurones that keeps the motor plans in a state of readiness). Motor set allows initiation of the motor plan and enables it to run with the correct amplitude, to completion and without attention. The second function is to provide internal cues to ensure that the motor plans, which are thought to be a predetermined set of submovements, run precisely and accurately with correct timing between the submovements. The basal ganglia, supplementary motor area and motor cortex form a loop and it is thought that the basal ganglia provides internal cues to the supplementary motor area that allows the correct submovement, in well-learned automatic movement sequences, to occur smoothly. Abnormal internal cues would impair submovement preparation and interrupt habitual movements such as walking. Another possibility is that the gait disturbance could be due to a disorder of motor set for the entire movement sequence. A series of experiments has shown that PD patients are able to generate normal stride length, not only with visual cues, but also with attentional strategies where the patient is asked to form a mental picture of the correct step size.[36] Furthermore, patients maintain the ability to produce rhythmic steps in response to a metronome cue, suggesting that it is not a loss of movement timing that causes the reduced stride length, but rather a defective scaling of stride size. This has been attributed to the reduced contribution of the basal ganglia to cortical motor set. Attention enhances this cortical motor set possibly via prefrontal regions of the brain and compensates for the defective basal ganglia output. Levodopa improves stride length and velocity,[37] indicating that dopamine regulates the amplitude of the whole gait plan.[38]

Axial movements

Rigidity of the shoulder, neck and trunk can be detected early in the course of PD. The arms swing less when the trunk is rotated by the examiner. Increased neck rigidity is felt when the head is passively flexed and extended. The head and shoulders are thrust slightly forwards, the trunk appears stiff when walking, and when the patient turns the body is seen to turn en bloc instead of the normal smooth sequential movement of pelvis, lumbar and thoracic spine. Disordered axial movement also shows up as difficulty in turning over in bed, and its presence appears to be related more to the duration of disease than the age of onset.[39] Although difficulty in turning in bed is regarded as a characteristic feature of PD it is not diagnostic, as it can be found in 9 per cent of healthy elderly subjects and 38 per cent of elderly patients without neurological disease attending a geriatric day hospital.[40] Difficulty in turning over in bed is not an apraxia, but is due to bradykinesia and disruption of the normal limb and trunk synergies. Thus it can be regarded, along with disordered gait and loss of arm swing when walking, as another example of basal ganglia disease causing loss of sequencing of a well-practised, automatic movement. Difficulty in turning in bed is significantly associated with disturbed gait, postural instability, difficulty in rising from a chair, whole-body bradykinesia and axial rigidity. All of these axial motor impairments respond to levodopa.[39]

Falls

Falls are not usually a presenting feature of idiopathic PD, and their early presence raises the possibility of one of the parkinsonian plus syndromes, such as PSP. Falls are recurrent in up to 40 per cent of patients, so a history of previous falls is an important predictor of further falls. Up to 90 per cent of patients will eventually become fallers, but the fall frequency probably declines in late-stage disease because of the patient's immobility.[41] Most PD patients fall indoors, and injuries are uncommon; however, the loss of confidence and effect on quality of life is considerable.

Falls correlate with increasing PD duration, the patient's age, severity of disease, rigidity, bradykinesia, gait impairment and postural instability. Tremor, orthostatic hypotension and cognitive impairment are not associated with falling in PD.[42] The main determinant of whether or not a PD patient will fall is postural instability, particularly impairment in the response to perturbations and in the anticipatory postural adjustments. Although the increased stiffness of the PD patient improves standing balance, the loss of flexibility increases the risk of falls. Other important factors are the reduced height of the foot from the ground during the swing phase; this increases the risk of tripping, and the tendency to walk on the balls of the feet also reduces postural stability. Many patients describe falling when they freeze; when turning, their feet remain rooted to the ground while their upper body continues with the turn.

The fall rates in PD undoubtedly depend very much on the age of the group studied, since in the normal elderly population falls increase linearly with age, reaching 50 per cent in those aged 85 years and over. Thus, postural instability due to PD may not be the only explanation for falls in older patients. Other relevant factors include the presence of small-vessel disease,[19] visual impairment, vestibular disease, cutaneous and proprioceptive loss in the feet, cervical spondylosis, muscle weakness and a general slowing of central information processing.[43–45]

Response to perturbation

Laboratory studies of PD patients who are deliberately thrown off balance by a sudden movement of the platform they are standing on has shown that the main deficit is an inability to produce a postural response, both quickly enough and of sufficient force.[46,47]

Responses to an external perturbation consist of corrective responses, such as the ankle and hip strategies, muscle stiffening and co-contraction, which do not require any change in the base of support provided by the feet and protective responses where one or more steps are taken or an arm is thrown out to grab hold of an external support.[48] Although the timing of the onset of corrective responses in PD has variously been described as normal or delayed, the main abnormalities in addition to inadequate force are an inappropriate sequencing of postural strategies. These result in co-contraction and joint stiffness, which interferes with the rapid corrective movements needed to prevent a fall. There are also changes in reflex amplitude, with an increased medium latency reflex and decreased long latency reflexes. As a result, PD patients sway further backwards than controls following toe-up tilt of the platform, and this cannot be corrected by levodopa. Furthermore, the inappropriately large medium latency reflexes to the stretched gastrocnemius soleus muscles – which destabilizes the response to the toe-up perturbation – is unresponsive to levodopa. This suggests that non-dopaminergic lesions contribute to the postural instability seen in PD.[49]

The protective responses are characterized by changes in support strategies (CIS), and involve stepping and grasping reactions. These are not reactions of last resort and are often initiated very early after the onset of an unexpected perturbation. Indeed, these CIS reactions are much more rapid than even the fastest voluntary limb movements. In contrast to a voluntary step, which is invariably preceded by a large APA, the APA is small or even absent during

CIS reactions. The lack of APA shortens the time to unload the limb, but at the cost of increasing mediolateral instability.[50] The typical CIS strategy of a young subject is a single step, but older subjects take more steps and the second step is often a lateral one, suggesting that they have difficulty controlling the tendency of the COM to fall to the unsupported side during stepping. Rather than using a cross-over step, elderly subjects take a sequence of small side steps.[51] Why there is this change in strategy is not clear, but it is probably related to reductions in muscle strength, especially of the quadriceps, slowing in psychomotor speed and reduced plantar sensation due to loss of pressure receptors in the sole of the foot. In the control of compensatory stepping there appears to be a trade-off between speed and stability. A single-step reaction offers maximum stability, but where stability is already compromised, additional steps will be required.[52]

In PD, the compensatory step made in response to a platform perturbation produces perseveration of the APA. Instead of one weight shift over the stance foot before foot-off, the weight shifts between left and right foot several times with gradually increasing force until the last one is larger than in controls. As a result, the time to foot-off is significantly prolonged. This perseveration may be due to an inability either to trigger a step or to sequence stepping and posture quickly enough to maintain balance. Patients with PD frequently fall during these perturbations, especially when off levodopa and when distracted by a cognitive task. levodopa improves both voluntary and compensatory stepping and reduces perseveration of the APAs.[53]

Some aspects of the APAs are actually impaired by levodopa. The normal baseline tone particularly in tibialis anterior and quadriceps in PD patients is reduced by levodopa, so there is a reduction in the normal stiffness that resists perturbation and patients are unable to produce adequate bursts of muscle activity to correct the displacement.[47]

Testing postural control is an important part of the clinical examination, but the usual retropulsion test – where the examiner stands behind the patient and gives a gentle tug on the shoulders – is a poor predictor of falls. The first time the test is done is usually the most reliable, as patients learn what is expected. For research purposes a battery of four tests – tandem stance, single limb stance, functional reach, and external perturbation – distinguishes between fallers and non-fallers.[54]

Effect of attention on posture

Postural control, even during quiet standing, is not entirely automatic and requires cognitive input. Certainly it appears that greater attention needs to be paid to balance when sensory information is impaired either as a result of ageing or peripheral vestibular disease,[55] or in posturally challenging laboratory conditions.[56] Patients with chronic dizziness due to a peripheral vestibular disorder have worse balance than controls, but the stability (i.e. sway) of both patients and controls improves as the mental tasks increase.[57]

The response differs with the task: visuospatial tasks reduce sway, while verbal tasks increase it.[58] This suggests that another motor task, i.e. articulation, interferes with postural control and that the reduction in sway reflects increased musculoskeletal stiffening as a result of arousal associated with the mental task. Fear of falling produces a similar stiffening strategy which is more marked in the elderly and is accompanied by a rise in blood pressure; again, this points to increased arousal.[59] As noted earlier, increased stiffness improves balance during quiet standing, but impairs the response to perturbations. Fear, mental distractions or talking would be expected to reduce postural control when walking.

Parkinsonian patients are at particular risk of falling when their balance is threatened if at the same time they are distracted by a cognitive task, especially when off levodopa.[53] The role of attentional strategies is clearly important in the rehabilitation of PD patients. Developing a mental picture of an ideal stride size is as effective as asking patients to walk over lines on the floor in improving gait, and when distracted by cognitive tasks the deterioration in gait is proportional to the complexity of the task.[36]

Effect of surgery on motor function

The motor problems due to PD are thought to be a result of over-activity of the globus pallidus interna (GPi) caused by excessive drive from the subthalamic nucleus (STN). The excessive inhibitory activity of GPi on the thalamus results in rigidity, bradykinesia and tremor. There are, therefore, three potential surgical targets for ablation or deep brain stimulation (DBS), which produces a similar effect by blocking neuronal output:

1. Thalamotomy: this is particularly good for tremor control (90 per cent improvement), but is much less useful for control of rigidity and dyskinesias, and has no effect on bradykinesia.
2. Pallidotomy: this is effective in controlling dyskinesias and improving total motor score in the 'off' state,[60,61] and generally improves contralateral bradykinesia, rigidity and tremor. However, balance, freezing and bulbar problems are not helped.
3. DBS or lesioning of the STN: tremor and bradykinesia are either resolved or improved in all patients. Dyskinesia improves in most, and gait freezing in about one-half. Bilateral stimulation improves instability in all patients. Bilateral lesioning tends to be avoided because of the risk of hemiballismus. The advantage of surgery on the STN is that levodopa dosage can be reduced to a much greater extent than following pallidotomy. Gait laboratory studies on patient who have undergone DBS in either STN or GPi show that DBS improves step initiation, the force of lateral COP shift before a self-initiated step is increased, and the latencies of foot-off are reduced, this improvement being more marked with DBS than with levodopa. DBS also improves the scaling of automatic postural responses following a backwards platform perturbation, and this is not seen with

levodopa. The effects of DBS in STN or in GPi are probably not very different.[62]

Conclusions

Patients usually find that their most significant motor problem is impaired balance control. Falls occurring as a result of this have a major effect on quality of life, and only when patients become chair- or bed-bound is there a reduction in fall risk. L-Dopa (levodopa) appears to have little effect on preventing falls, but physiotherapy can be helpful in teaching patients to use visual cues and attentional strategies. Recent advances in surgery promise considerable improvement for patients with advanced disease and gait and balance impairment. The question of which non-dopaminergic pathways are involved in the control of balance still remains unanswered, and standardized, reliable functional balance tests which can be used in the clinic need to be developed.

References

1. Hely MA, Morris JGL, Reid WGJ, et al. Age at onset: the major determinant of outcome in Parkinson's disease. Acta Neurol. Scand. 1995; 92: 455–63.
2. Bennett DA, Beckett LA, Murray AM, et al. Prevalence of Parkinsonian signs and associated mortality in a community population. N. Engl. J. Med. 1996; 334: 71–6.
3. Klawans HL. Individual manifestations of Parkinson's disease after ten or more years of levodopa. Movement Disord. 1986; 1: 187–92.
4. Winter DA. ABC of Balance during Standing and Walking. Waterloo, Ontario: Waterloo Biomechanics, 1995.
5. Baloh RW, Fife TD, Zwerling L, et al. Comparison of static and dynamic posturography in young and older normal people. J. Am. Geriatr. Soc. 1994; 42: 405–12.
6. Lord SR, Rogers MW, Howland A, Fitzpatrick R. Lateral stability, sensorimotor function and falls in older people. J. Am. Geriatr. Soc. 1999; 47: 1077–81.
7. Horak FB, Nutt JG, Nashner LM. Postural inflexibility in parkinsonian subjects. J. Neurol. Sci. 1992; 111: 46–58.
8. Mitchell SL, Collins JJ, DeLuca CJ, et al. Open-loop and closed-loop postural control mechanism in Parkinson's disease: increased mediolateral activity during quiet standing. Neurosci. Lett. 1995; 197: 133–6.
9. Schieppati M, Hugon M, Grasso M, et al. The limits of equilibrium in young and elderly normal subjects and in parkinsonians. Electroencephalogr. Clin. Neurophysiol. 1994; 93: 286–97.
10. Imms FJ, Edholm OG. Studies of gait and mobility in the elderly. Age Ageing 1981; 10: 147–56.
11. Bloem BR, Haan J, Lagaay AM, et al. Investigation of gait in elderly subjects over 88 years of age. J. Geriatr. Psychiatry Neurol. 1992; 5: 78–84.
12. Winter DA. The Biomechanics and Motor Control of Human Gait. Waterloo, Ontario: Waterloo Biomechanics, 2nd edn, 1991.
13. Waite LM, Broe GA, Creasey H, et al. Neurological signs, aging and the neurodegenerative syndromes. Arch. Neurol. 1996; 53: 498–502.

14. Bloem BR, Gussekloo J, Lagaay AM, et al. Idiopathic senile gait disorders are signs of subclinical disease. *J. Am. Geriatr. Soc.* 2000; **48**: 1098–1101.
15. Nutt JG, Marsden CD, Thompson PD. Human walking and higher-level gait disorders particularly in the elderly. *Neurology* 1993; **43**: 268–79.
16. Trenkwalder C, Paulus W, Krafezyk S, et al. Postural stability differentiate 'lower body' from idiopathic parkinsonism. *Acta Neurol. Scand.* 1995; **91**: 444–52.
17. Yamanouchi H, Nagura H. Neurological signs and frontal white matter lesions in vascular Parkinsonism. *Stroke* 1997; **28**: 965–9.
18. van Zagten M, Lodder J, Kessels F. Gait disorders and Parkinsonian signs in patients with stroke related to small deep infarcts and white matter lesions. *Movement Disord.* 1998; **13**: 89–95.
19. Piccini P, Pavese N, Canapicchi R, et al. White matter hyperintensities in Parkinson's disease. *Arch. Neurol.* 1995; **952**: 191.
20. Kuhtz-Buschbeck JP, Jöhnk K, Mäder S, et al. Analysis of gait in cervical myelopathy. *Gait Posture* 1999; **9**: 184–9.
21. Mitchell SL. Extrapyramidal features in Alzheimer's disease. *Age Ageing* 1999; **28**: 401–9.
22. Martin JP. *The Basal Ganglia and Posture.* London: Pitman Medical, 1967.
23. Burleigh-Jacobs A, Horak FB, Nutt JG, Obeso JA. Step initiation in Parkinson's disease: influence of levodopa and external sensory triggers. *Movement Disord.* 1997; **12**: 206–15.
24. Crenna P, Frigo C, Giovannini P, Piccolo L. The initiation of gait in Parkinson's disease. *Motor Disturbances* 1990; **II**: 161–73.
25. Lee RG, Tonolli I, Viallet F, et al. Preparatory postural adjustments in Parkinsonian patients with postural instability. *Can. J. Neurol. Sci.* 1995; **22**: 126–35.
26. Halliday SE, Winter DA, Frank JS, et al. The initiation of gait in young elderly and Parkinson's disease subjects. *Gait Posture* 1998; **8**: 8–14.
27. Georgiou N, Iansek R, Bradshaw JL, et al. An evaluation of the role of internal cues in the pathogenesis of Parkinsonian hypokinesia. *Brain* 1993; **116**: 1575–87.
28. Quinn NP. Classification of fluctuations in patients with Parkinson's disease. *Neurology* 1998; **51** (Suppl. 2): S25–9.
29. Giladi N, Kuo R, Fahn S. Freezing phenomenon in patients with Parkinsonian syndromes. *Movement Disord.* 1997; **12**: 302–5.
30. Shabtai H, Treves TA, Korczyn AD, et al. Freezing of gait in patients with advanced Parkinson's disease. Poster, International Symposium on Gait Disorders, Prague, 1999.
31. Imai H. Clinicophysiological features of akinesia. *Eur. Neurol.* 1996; **36** (Suppl. 1): 9–12.
32. Sandyk R. Freezing of gait in Parkinson's disease is improved by treatment with weak electromagnetic fields. *Int. J. Neurosci.* 1996; **85**: 111–24.
33. Fabre N, Brefel C, Sabatini U, et al. Normal frontal perfusion in patients with frozen gait. *Movement Disord.* 1998; **13**: 677–83.
34. Hughes AJ, Bishop S, Kleedorfer B, et al. Subcutaneous apomorphine in Parkinson's disease: response to chronic administration for up to five years. *Movement Disord.* 1993; **8**: 165–70.
35. Morris ME, Iansek R, Matyas TA, Summers JJ. The pathogenesis of gait hypokinesia in Parkinson's disease. *Brain* 1994; **117**: 1169–81.
36. Morris ME, Iansek R, Matyas TA, Summers JJ. Stride length regulation in Parkinson's disease. *Brain* 1996; **119**: 551–68.
37. Bowes SG, Clark PK, Leeman AL, et al. Determinants of gait in the elderly Parkinsonian on maintenance levodopa/cardidopa therapy. *Br. J. Clin. Pharmacol.* 1990; **30**: 13–24.

38. Morris M, Iansek R, Matyas T, Summers JJ. Abnormalities in the stride length – cadence relation in Parkinsonian gait. *Movement Disord.* 1998; **13**: 61–9.
39. Steiger MJ, Thompson PD, Marsden CD. Disordered axial movement in Parkinson's disease. *J. Neurol. Neurosurg. Psychiatry* 1996; **61**: 645–8.
40. Duncan G, Wilson JA. Extrapyramidal signs in dementia of Alzheimer type. *Lancet* 1989; **ii**: 1392.
41. Bloem BR, van Vugt JPP, Beckley DJ. Balance and falls in Parkinson's disease. Paper presented at International Symposium on Gait Disorders, Prague, 1999.
42. Koller WC, Glatt S, Vetere-Overfield B, Hassanein R. Falls and Parkinson's disease. *Clin. Neuropharmacol.* 1989; **12**: 98–105.
43. Maki BE, McIlroy WE. Postural control in the older adult. *Clin. Geriatric Med.* 1996; **12**: 635–58.
44. Overstall PW. Falls. *Rev. Clin. Gerontol.* 1992; **2**: 31–8.
45. Colledge N. Falls. *Rev. Clin. Gerontol.* 1997; **7**: 309–15.
46. Dick JPR, Rothwell JC, Berardelli A, *et al.* Associated postural adjustments in Parkinson's disease. *J. Neurol. Neurosurg. Psychiatry* 1986; **49**: 1378–85.
47. Horak FB, Frank J, Nutt J. Effects of dopamine on postural control in Parkinsonian subjects: scaling, set and tone. *J. Neurophysiol.* 1996; **75**: 2380–96.
48. Rogers MW. Disorders of posture, balance and gait in Parkinson's disease. *Clin. Geriatric Med.* 1996; **12**: 825–45.
49. Bloem BR, Beckley DJ, van Dijk JG, *et al.* Influence of dopaminergic medication on automatic postural responses and balance impairment in Parkinson's disease. *Movement Disord.* 1996; **11**: 509–21.
50. McIlroy WE, Maki BE. Controlling change-in-support reactions. *Gait Posture* 1999; **9** (Suppl. 1): S10.
51. Maki BE, McIlroy WE, Perry SD, *et al.* Control of change-in-support reactions to whole body instability. *Gait Posture* 1999; **9** (Suppl. 1): S10.
52. Maki BE, McIlroy WE. Control of foot placement during compensatory stepping. *Gait Posture* 1999; **9** (Suppl. 1): S6.
53. Horak FB, Jones C, Nutt J. Patients with Parkinson's disease perseverate postural adjustments for compensatory stepping. *Gait Posture* 1999; **9** (Suppl. 1): S9.
54. Smithson F, Morris ME, Iansek R. Performance on clinical tests of balance in Parkinson's disease. *Physical Therapy* 1998; **78**: 577–92.
55. Redfern MS, Jennings JR, Furman JM. The influence of attention on postural control during stance. *Gait Posture* 1999; **9** (Suppl. 1): S11.
56. Brauer S, Woollacott M, Shumway-Cook A. Balance impaired elderly: secondary task influences EMG response to perturbation. *Gait Posture* 1999; **9** (Suppl. 1): S33.
57. Yardley L, Bronstein AM, Davies R, Luxon L. Concurrent performance of mental tasks and dynamic control of balance. *Gait Posture* 1999; **9** (Suppl. 1): S11.
58. Dault MC, Frank JS, Allard F. Interference of a visuo-spatial and a verbal working memory task on postural control. Poster, International Symposium on Gait Disorders, Prague, 1999.
59. Carpenter MG, Frank JS, Brawley LR, Adkin AL. Influence of threat on postural control in young and older adults. Poster, International Symposium on Gait Disorders, Prague, 1999.
60. Golbe LI. Pallidotomy for Parkinson's disease: hitting the target? *Lancet* 1998; **351**: 998–9.
61. Quinn N, Bhatia K. Functional neurosurgery for Parkinson's disease. *Br. Med. J.* 1998; **316**: 1259–60.
62. Gross AK, Nutt J, Jones C, *et al.* Deep brain stimulation: the effects of stimulation site on postural control. *Gait Posture* 1999; **9** (Suppl. 1): S49

12 Safe mobility

D. O'Neill

The importance of safe mobility

The irresistible rise of the internal combustion engine has had a profound effect on our society. In a little over 100 years, there has been a revolution in our expectations of safe and accessible transportation. Never in history has personal and public transportation been so widely available. This mobility is important at all ages, and is particularly so in later life. At the White House Conference on Ageing in 1971, transportation was rated as third in importance in older people's lives, after health and finance.[1]

There is also a negative cost to this ease of mobility, in terms of pollution, land use and injuries and deaths due to crashes. Deaths from road crashes are set to rise from ninth to sixth place in the global burden of disability. Society has accepted a certain toll from car crashes, and safety is not the over-riding concern in transportation policies: indeed, if it were, speed limits would be fixed at 20 miles per hour and car engines would be fitted with governors to limit their speed at this level. Convenience, financial efficiency and other factors shape policy with equal force. A consciousness of this unstated, but accepted, level of risk should form the background to any discussion of transportation policies, particularly in the context of neurodegenerative illness.

Medical approaches to illness and safe mobility are relatively under-developed, and in automotive terms are still at the stage of the man with the red flag walking in front of the car. Much of the medical and regulatory literature is couched in terminology which is negative. It seems more concerned with limiting personal mobility than in providing solutions as to how people with disease and disability can participate fully in society. Those sections which deal with fitness to drive concentrate on detecting those who cannot drive rather than on enabling them to drive more safely and with ease.[2]

Enabling or policing?

Although the literature on enabling drivers is embryonic, the underlying philosophy is all-important. Patients attend their physician in the expectation of achieving health and social gain. Safe mobility, increasingly (but not exclusively) by means of driving, is a key function which needs to be safeguarded, just as we attempt to do for continence, mobility and balance. The handful of studies on mobility in Parkinson's disease (PD) have also shown this bias, with an emphasis on risk rather than on mobility.[3-5] Although it is too early to be certain, it is likely that even the perceived risk may be an overstatement of actual risk, representing selected populations and not taking into account restrictions on driving practices and mileage by the patients,[6] their carers and physicians. This can be seen in studies on driving in Alzheimer's disease: in public health terms, there does not appear to be an increased risk for the group, but in clinical terms a proportion of patients will present a dilemma for clinicians.

As PD is an age-related illness, it is important to appreciate the changes in how older people fulfil their mobility needs. In developed countries, this is increasingly by using cars. In the US, less than 3 per cent of trips by older people are made with public transport. While the European experience is somewhat different, in the UK the car accounts for over half of trips less than 100 km made by those aged 65–74 years. Older people are in general safe drivers: an oft-quoted statistic (especially by those seeking research grants) is that older drivers are involved in more crashes per mile travelled than younger people. However, as they drive considerably less miles than their younger peers, the calculation is not relevant to their contribution to morbidity and mortality. Health is a major determinant of older driver ease and eventual cessation. There is some concern that older drivers may quit driving without appropriate assessment and remediation of age-related disease. Older people who stop driving seem to have difficulty with adapting to public transportation: even when provided cost-free, they use it with a lesser intensity than those who have never driven.

Models of driving behaviour

While the geriatrician is aided in the assessment and rehabilitation of problems with balance and gait by an understanding of the underlying mechanisms, driving is a complex task, and there has been a marked lack of progress in developing a comprehensive and clinically relevant model of driving behaviour. At least five main types of model have been explored: psychometric, motivational, hierarchical controls, information processing and error theory.[7]

Due to the relative ease of measuring cognitive function, clinicians may look to psychometric measures as a means of assessing older drivers. A preliminary emphasis on psychometric measures relating to accident-causing behaviour has been faulted for having been conducted without the benefit of a process model of driving, for focusing primarily on accident-causing behaviours and not on everyday driving, and on relying heavily on post hoc explanations.

Motivational models which distinguish between drivers' performance limits and on-road driving offer a different perspective. For example, a pioneering Swedish study showed that when drivers are asked to remember road signs, the accuracy ranged from 17 per cent to 78 per cent, depending on the subjective importance of the sign, i.e. the amount of risk involved in ignoring the sign.[8] Early models assume risk to be a primary motivating factor: second-generation motivational models have given emphasis to motives other than risk, i.e. pleasure in driving, traffic risks, driving time and expense.[9] They also factor in concurrent activity at operational, manoeuvring and strategic levels, and portray the driver as an active decision-maker rather than as a passive responder implicit in early information-processing models. The driver's allocation of attention depends on the immediate driving situation and the driver's motives, which include the level of risk and other motives relating to the purpose of the trip. The main research interest is in identifying factors that influence the driver's allocation of attention among the tasks of the different control levels.

Much of routine driving is done automatically. Automaticity, which is fast, effortless cognitive processing, can occur at all three levels of control, and contrasts with control processing which is demanding of attention and resources. This automaticity can develop as a response to several types of stimuli and underlies much of experienced driving behaviour until knowledge-based problem solving is required. A combined model of a control hierarchy and a automaticity/controlled processing scheme is illustrated in Table 12.1.

Table 12.1 A combined model of a control hierarchy and a automaticity/controlled processing scheme

	Strategic	Tactical/manoeuvring	Operational/Control
Knowledge	Navigating in unfamiliar area	Controlling skid	Novice on first lesson
Rule	Choice between familiar routes	Passing other vehicles	Driving unfamiliar vehicle
Skill	Route used for daily commute	Negotiating familiar intersection	Vehicle handling on curves

A practical, hierarchical approach

One practical scheme has been outlined, with an emphasis on a hierarchy of strategic, tactical and operational factors.[10] Strategic performance includes the planning of choice of route, time of day (avoiding rush hour), or even the decision not to drive and to take public transport. Tactical decisions are those aspects of the driving style which are characteristic of the driver and are consciously or unconsciously adopted for a great range of reasons, e.g. decisions on whether or not to overtake, go through amber lights or signalling in good time before turning. Operational performance is the response to specific traffic situations, such as speed control, braking and signalling. Driving a car requires organisation of action at and between all three levels.

Clinical assessment up to now has tended to dwell on deficiencies on the operational level, i.e. whether an illness affects the subject's appreciation of distracting stimuli or the reaction time to a hazardous situation. This emphasis is misguided: reaction time (a measure which is an integral part of operational tasks) is shortest in the 15- to 25-year age group – the group with the highest accident rate. This places the delayed reaction time noted in PD[11,12] in context. It is very likely that decisions at a strategic and a tactical level are much more important in causing accidents. Older drivers are known to use strategic and tactical measures widely to avoid delay, stress and risk by driving less at night and during bad weather, avoiding rush hours and unfamiliar routes, etc. Drivers with PD also limit their mileage and their speed,[13] both of which are safety-enhancing manoeuvres.

The application of these three levels of function can be of practical help in decision-making. This is illustrated by studies of drivers with acquired brain damage, particularly stroke.[14] Evidence for impairment at all levels may be collected by discussion with patient and relatives, as well as by clinical observation. At a strategic level we would look for evidence of inappropriate planning of trips or lack of selective use of cars. Poor planning, poor judgement, lack of insight and impulsivity affect both strategic and tactical levels. Impulsivity is attributed to disinhibition and/or cognitive impairment. Factors which interfere with the operational level include inadequate visual scanning of the environment, poor visual tracking, slowness in acting and confusion when more complex acts have to be carried out.

Assessment

The methodology for assessment and intervention of mobility is beginning to appear in the geriatric and rehabilitation literature, with chapters on driving assessment in two of the three main textbooks in geriatric medicine. This has paralleled the appearance of papers, which show positive effects for interventions to improve driver ease and safety in illnesses such as cataract and arthritis.

The first step is the recognition of transportation needs as a relevant part of assessment of those with PD. This is not as clearly recognized as it might be: studies of patients with dementia,[15] stroke,[16] syncope[17] and arthritis[18] show a poor appreciation by healthcare providers of the interaction between disease and driving.

PD is of particular interest as there may be multiple influences on driving skills. The illness may involve:

- problems of motor function, including fluctuations, on-off syndrome;
- depression;
- impaired cognitive function; and
- impact of medications (whether through dyskinesia, neuropsychiatric effects or sudden disabling sleepiness[19]).

Rather than stating that PD is dangerous for driving, it is vital to take a phenomenological approach. The depression and the motor function must be treated, psychoactive medications minimized, and cognitive function assessed and managed before any decisions are made about the most appropriate approach to mobility, whether public transport or driving.

Assessment strategy

The schedule for the assessment of a driver with PD is akin to that of geriatric assessment of older people – a process which is marked by the following qualities: medical and functional assessment, detection and prioritization of diseases, interdisciplinary assessment and remediation (Table 12.2). Functional assessments, such as a comprehensive test of visual processing, a falls history, and a review of current medications may be of greater relevance than specific medical aspects in the identification of older at-risk drivers.[20] Early specialist referral may prove beneficial for the primary care physician who does not have access to an interdisciplinary team.

A cascade system for interdisciplinary assessment is probably the most cost-effective way to approach the patient (Fig. 12.1). For example, if the physician detects visual acuity below the standard for the jurisdiction, referral to an ophthalmologist and maximal remediation of vision should occur before returning to the assessment cascade. Similarly, should a patient in the European Union have a homonymous hemianopia (one of the few absolute medical contraindications to driving), then referral to the social worker for developing strategies for alternative transportation is the next step in the cascade.

Table 12.2 The assessment process

History
Patient, family/informant
Driving history
Examination
Functional status
Other illnesses and drugs
Vision
Mental status testing
Diagnostic formulation and prioritization
Disease severity and fluctuations
Remediation
Re-assess
In-depth cognitive/perceptual testing
± On-road assessment
Overall evaluation of hazard
-      Strategic
-      Tactical
-      Operational
Advice to patient/carer ± DVLA (Driver and Vehicle Licensing Authority)
If driving is too hazardous, consider alternative mobility strategies

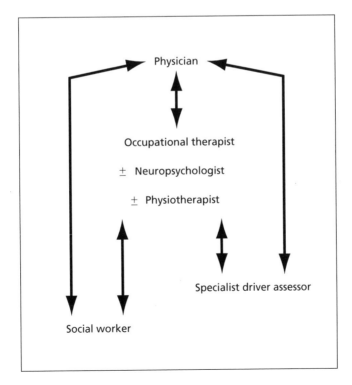

Fig. 12.1 The assessment cascade.

Decision-making

It is worth remembering that many dementia clinics do not use the same neuropsychological batteries. Their high rate of accuracy depends on the care that clinicians take in developing a liaison and familiarity with local occupational therapists and neuropsychologists. This means that results can be taken in context, not only of the patients but also of the training and quirks of the assessors. It is likely that the same approach is critical to good assessment practice in driving competency in PD.

To most clinicians, it is relatively easy to detect those patients who represent a low risk and those who represent a high risk for driving. A caveat to this is one study showed that a single neurologist tended to over-rate the driving performance of drivers with PD.[5] It is those in between who represent the greatest challenge. Using the meagre literature on PD as well as that of the dementias, some interesting information can be gleaned from various components of the assessment and treatment processes outlined above.

Disease severity scales

It is unclear if there is a correlation between disease severity scales and driver performance. Although Dubinsky *et al.* report more crashes in patients with Hoehn and Yahr stage 3 than those with Hoehn and Yahr stage 1 or controls, they concluded that disability scales did not reliably predict ability to drive.[21] On simulator performance, Madely *et al.*[22] found a correlation between the Webster scale in 10 patients, while others found a correlation with the Unified Parkinson's Disease Rating Scale (UPDRS), but not the Webster, with 28 patients![4] A Finnish on-road study showed no correlation with disease severity.[5] It is likely that in estimating safety to drive that disease severity ratings are secondary in importance to cognitive/behavioural changes as measured by occupational therapy/neuropsychology testing: however, they are clearly important as target for remediation, and also as a focus in car choice and adaptation.

Medication review

The potential and actual effect of drugs on driving may be an important factor in the safe mobility of older people.[23] It is a complex area, and very difficult to separate the effects of the disease from those of the medications. Treatment could improve psychomotor performance or impair driving due to side effects such as drowsiness. The use of the synthetic dopamine agonists, ropinirole and pramipexole has been associated with sudden disabling, unheralded attacks of sleepiness, apparently with no warning.[19] Some of these patients were subsequently treated with other agents, with no recurrence of attacks. The drug manufacturers have issued a warning regarding this potential side effect for ropinirole and pramipexole, and advised against driving. If sudden drowsiness occurs during driving, the medication should be modified, or patients should be advised not to drive. The relationship between driving ability and timing and side effects of medication is extremely complex, and must be assessed on an individual basis in discussion with the patient, general practitioner, specialist team, driving assessment centre and the Driver and Vehicle Licensing Authority (DVLA). Some specialist sleep experts doubt the true existence of the phenomenon of very sudden onset of sleep, though we are probably all subject to sleepiness under certain circumstances (e.g. sleep deprivation). The DVLA have stated that the risk of somnolence is low after taking dopamine agonists, and that taking such medication should not lead to automatic cessation of driving.

The effect of other medications for PD is not well quantified. Overt neuropsychological side effects, such as drowsiness or psychotic phenomena, should be indicators for driving cessation until the symptoms have resolved.

Mental status testing

Cognitive impairment or slowing has been found to correlate with an increased crash rate in PD.[3] There are no clear guidelines, although there may be some guidance from studies of dementia and driving. Although a correlation has been established in numerous studies between various cognitive tests and driving skills in dementia – i.e. the Mini Mental State Examination (MMSE)[24–26] – this is not sufficiently well-delineated to provide a useful screening measure. A consensus statement in 1994 could only state that at an MMSE of 17, drivers should have a further evaluation![27] In view of the complex nature of the driving model, it is not likely that this approach offers much above its utility in the generic assessment of cognitive function

Occupational therapy assessment

Although some good reviews on occupational therapy assessment in driving exist,[28,29] there is little yet by way of consensus for tests which are clearly superior in determining those who and are not unfit to drive. It is likely that the opinion of an interested and experienced therapist, backed up by standard test of cognition and perception is the most useful approach. Specific tests aimed at driving have as yet been disappointing.[30]

Neuropsychology tests

No specific battery has yet been established as intrinsically helpful in the assessment of driving skills in PD. A thorough cognitive assessment is important. Heikkila et al.[5] suggest that the test battery should include the following measures: vigilance and concentration, visual perception, choice reaction times and information processing in a complex situation. A battery including these measures correlated with an on-road assessment of driving ability with visual perception being the best predictor.[5] Such test batteries can, however, be criticised for poor construct validity.

On-road tests

Although only a proportion of patients with pleuritic pain undergo a ventilation/perfusion scan, physicians would not be expected to diagnose a pulmonary embolus without access to this diagnostic technology. The on-road driving assessment with a specialist driving assessor is an equally important diagnostic tool. All specialists dealing with PD need to identify a specialist driving assessment centre to which they can refer patients when required. Equally, all patients – except the most severely affected – should have the right of access to a road test. A very large number of 'standardized' road tests have been described, but those developing driver assessment centres or liaising with specialist driving assessors could consider some of those described in the recent past which have been developed with healthcare professionals. Examples include the Washington University Driving test[31] and the Alberta Driving Test.[32] The results from the latter indicated that hazardous errors were the single best indicator of membership in a group of older drivers with early dementia. A regression analysis showed that five classes of driving errors accounted for over 57 per cent of the variance associated with global ratings provided by expert driving instructors. Specialist driving assessors are available at a number of centres throughout North America and the USA. The discipline is achieving academic recognition, with University level courses developing, e.g. Greenwich University in the UK. Addresses of centres for specialist on-road testing are available from the Forum of Driving Centres in the UK (see Appendix 2 for Mobility Advice and Vehicle Information Centre address).

A course of lessons may be prescribed to help the patient to adapt to any deficits uncovered during the assessment. The on-road test may also be invaluable for advising on car adaptation or choice if the patient is changing cars. Large door apertures, high chassis, built-up keys, mirrors and controls as well as power steering and automatic gears may help certain patients. An unresolved issue is the cost of these assessments in some countries: it will be important to stress to healthcare purchasers that retention of safe mobility is a healthcare gain.

Advising the patient

All assessments and advice should be documented in the patient's file. The driver should be advised to consult the documentation from both their insurance companies and driving licensing authorities with regard to disclosure. In the UK, a driver has a legal obligation to disclose to the DVLA any disability that the licence holder knows he or she has. This disclosure must be in writing, and should contain full name, date of birth and details of the nature of the condition. The driver should also inform their insurance company of any change in health-affecting ability to drive, and this includes PD. The patient should be advised to re-attend for review at 6- to 12-month intervals or sooner should they or the carer detect any deterioration in driving habits. Some early data exists suggesting that restrictions to driving locally, by day, may be associated with fewer accidents in drivers with medical impairments.[33] A summary of the advice given by the Parkinson's Disease Society of the United Kingdom and other information leaflets is listed in Table 12.3.

When driving is no longer possible

When driving cessation is indicated, it is important to explore alternatives with the patient. A sympathetic social work intervention may be helpful, and this can operate though the various options available to the patient. Public transport, even if free, is often irrelevant to older, compromised adults . Older drivers who stop driving have been shown to use less public transport than those who have never driven.[34] Family members may be able to provide some driving input. The ideal situation is to provide a system of paratransit: affordable, tailored individual transportation. Various models have been developed (an excellent example is the service in Portland, Maine, USA), but the funding remains problematic.[35]

Dangerous driving: reporting to driver-licensing authorities

The breaking of confidence between physician is not be undertaken lightly. It is likely that there will be wide-ranging differences in the cultural acceptance

Table 12.3   Sleepiness and driving: patient advice

- If anti-PD drugs are causing significant drowsiness, seek advice from a specialist – the dose may need to be adjusted or, rarely, the treatment stopped
- Avoid other medications that cause drowsiness, e.g. antihistamines
- Avoid sleep deprivation – seek advice if your night-time sleep is disturbed
- Be aware of the symptoms of drowsiness – pay attention to these warnings
- Avoid bad times of the day – especially 'off' periods, after meals and evenings, when you are more likely to be sleepy
- Avoid long drives – especially on motorways, or at night or twilight
- If possible, drive with a passenger who is also a driver
- If drowsiness warnings occur, stop, have a break, have a short sleep – and wake up naturally
- Safety is the highest priority – if in doubt about your ability to drive, it is safer NOT to drive

of reporting, and only some indication of the issues can be given. In the United Kingdom and Ireland, standard practice is that confidentiality cannot be broken unless: (i) there is evidence of hazardous driving; (ii) the patient has been informed of the risk but fails to stop driving; and/or (iii) the family has been informed but cannot stop the patient driving. There is concern that reporting over and above this may deter patients from seeking treatment for treatable illnesses if they perceive their physician as an agent for the licensing authority (DVLA in the UK). In Canada, the CMA seems to promote reporting, whether or not it is mandatory in the province. This presupposes a trust in the DVLA assessment procedures, as well as faith that patients with severe impairment will stop driving if their driving licences are withheld. Whatever the case about the former, clinical experience does not necessarily support the latter, and working with the patient and the family may be more ethical and practical.[36,37]

The future

It will be important to develop specialist assessment centres which build on the expertise already developed. To date, geriatricians on both sides of the Atlantic have produced guides for clinicians,[38,39] and an emerging research trend further strengthens the role of the geriatrician in the process. Several epidemiological studies have shown a strong association between falls and crashes;[20,40] it is tempting to speculate that the assessment and intervention strategies for falls (an area of expertise for geriatricians) may be developed to aid in assessing and intervening in compromised driving ability in later life.

Other areas of interest will be the possibility of cognitive training, and studies are underway using the Useful Field of View – a dynamic measure of the functionally useful field of view.[41] Information technology may also be of help, but at present the technology is at a pre-testing phase.

The preservation of safe mobility will also require some adequate substitute for the car for those who can no longer drive. Patterns of usage are developed at an earlier age and in health: this will require careful education of transportation planners. This should focus not only on including those with mental and physical disability in the development of transportation but also on the seamless integration of public and private transport so as to encourage usage of a variety of transport measures at all ages.

References

1. Carp FM, Byerts T, Gertman J, et al. Transportation. Gerontologist 1980; 12: 11–16.
2. White S, O'Neill D. Health and relicensing policies for older drivers in the European Union. Gerontology 2000; 46: 146–52.
3. Dubinsky RM, Gray C, Husted D, et al. Driving in Parkinson's disease. Neurology 1991; 41: 517–20.

4. Lings S, Dupont E. Driving with Parkinson's disease. A controlled laboratory investigation [see comments]. *Acta Neurol. Scand.* 1992; **86**: 33–9.

5. Heikkila VM, Turkka J, Korpelainen J, Kallanranta T, Summala H. Decreased driving ability in people with Parkinson's disease. *J. Neurol. Neurosurg. Psychiatry* 1998; **64**: 325–30.

6. Campbell MK, Bush TL, Hale WE. Medical conditions associated with driving cessation in community- dwelling, ambulatory elders. *J. Gerontol.* 1993; **48**: S230–4.

7. Ranney TA. Models of driving behaviour: a review of their evolution. *Accid. Anal. Prev.* 1994; **26**: 733–50.

8. Johansson G, Backlund F. Drivers and road signs. *Ergonomics* 1970; **13**: 749–59.

9. Rothengatter T, de Bruin R. Risk and the absence of pleasure: a motivational approach to modelling road user behaviour. *Ergonomics* 1988; **31**: 599–607.

10. Michon JA. A critical review of driver behaviour models: what do we know, what should we do? In: Evans L, Schwing RC (eds). *Human Behaviour and Traffic Safety.* New York: Plenum, 1985: 487–525.

11. Bloxham CA, Dick DJ, Moore M. Reaction times and attention in Parkinson's disease. *J. Neurol. Neurosurg. Psychiatry* 1987; **50**: 1178–83.

12. Jahanshani M, Brown RG, Marsden CD. Simple and choice reaction time and use of advance information for motor preparation in Parkinson's disease. *Brain* 1992; **115** (Pt. 2): 539–64.

13. Gimenez-Roldan S, Dobato JL, Mateo D. Vehicle drivers with Parkinson disease: behavior schedules of a patient sample from the Community of Madrid. *Neurologia* 1998; **13**: 13–21.

14. van Zomeren AH, Brouwer WH, Minderhoud JM. Acquired brain damage and driving: a review. *Arch. Phys. Med. Rehabil.* 1987; **68**: 697–705.

15. O'Neill D, Neubauer K, Boyle M, Gerrard J, Surmon D, Wilcock GK. Dementia and driving. *J. R. Soc. Med.* 1992; **85**: 199–202.

16. Fisk GD, Owsley C, Pulley LV. Driving after stroke: driving exposure, advice, and evaluations. *Arch. Phys. Med. Rehabil.* 1997; **78**: 1338–45.

17. MacMahon M, O'Neill D, Kenny RA. Syncope: driving advice is frequently over-looked. *Postgrad. Med. J.* 1996; **72**: 561–3.

18. Thevenon A, Grimbert P, Dudenko P, Heuline A, Delcambre B. Polarthrite rhumatoïde et conduite automobile. *Rev. Rhum. Mal. Osteoartic.* 1989; **56**: 101–3.

19. Frucht S, Rogers JD, Greene PE, Gordon MF, Fahn S. Falling asleep at the wheel: motor vehicle mishaps in persons taking pramipexole and ropinirole. *Neurology* 1999; **52**: 1908–10.

20. Sims RV, Owsley C, Allman RM, Ball K, Smoot TM. A preliminary assessment of the medical and functional factors associated with vehicle crashes by older adults [see comments]. *J. Am. Geriatr. Soc.* 1998; **46**: 556–61.

21. Dubinsky RM, Williamson A, Gray CS, Glatt SL. Driving in Alzheimer's disease [see comments]. *J. Am. Geriatr. Soc.* 1992; **40**: 1112–16.

22. Madeley P, Hulley JL, Wildgust H, Mindham RH. Parkinson's disease and driving ability. *J. Neurol. Neurosurg. Psychiatry* 1990; **53**: 580–2.

23. Alvarez FJ, Del Rio MC. Drugs and driving. *Lancet* 1994; **344**: 282.

24. Fitten LJ, Perryman K, Ganzell S, Williams J, Ganzell D, Bonebakker A. Driving ability and Alzheimer's disease: a prospective field and laboratory study. *Gerontologist* 1991; **31** (special issue II): 88–9.

25. Fox GK, Bowden SC, Bashford GM, Smith DS. Alzheimer's disease and driving: prediction and assessment of driving performance. *J. Am. Geriatr. Soc.* 1997; **45**: 949–53.

26. Odenheimer GL, Beaudet M, Jette AM, Albert MS, Grande L, Minaker KL.

Performance-based driving evaluation of the elderly driver: safety, reliability, and validity. *J. Gerontol.* 1994; **49**: M153–9.

27. Lundberg C, Johansson K, Ball K, *et al.* Dementia and driving – an attempt at consensus. *Alzheimer's Dis. Rel. Disord.* 1997; **11**: 28–37.

28. Quigley FL, DeLisa JA. Assessing the driving potential of cerebral vascular patients. *Am. J. Occup. Ther.* 1983; **37**: 474–8.

29. Taira ED (ed.). *Assessing the Driving Ability of the Elderly* . Binghampton NY: Haworth Press, 1989.

30. Mitchell RK, Castledent CM, Fanthome YC. Driving, Alzheimer's disease and ageing: a potential cognitive screening device for all elderly drivers. *Int. J. Geriatr. Psychiatry* 1995; **10**: 865–9.

31. Hunt LA, Murphy CF, Carr D, Duchek JM, Buckles V, Morris JC. Reliability of the Washington University Road Test. A performance-based assessment for drivers with dementia of the Alzheimer type. *Arch. Neurol.* 1997; **54**: 707–12.

32. Dobbs AR, Heller RB, Schopflocher D. A comparative approach to identify unsafe older drivers. *Accid. Anal. Prev.* 1998; **30**: 363–70.

33. *Evaluating drivers licensed with medical conditions in Utah, 1992–1996.* Washington, DC: Transportation Research Board, 1999.

34. O'Neill D, Bruce I, Lawlor B. Mobility in an older population. *Clin. Gerontol.* (in press).

35. Freund K. The politics of older driver legislation. *Gerontologist* 1991; **31** (special issue II):162.

36. Bahro M, Silber E, Box P, Sunderland T. Giving up driving in Alzheimer's disease – an integrative therapeutic approach. *Int. J. Geriatr. Psychiatry* 1995; **10**: 871–4.

37. Donnelly RE, Karlinsky H. The impact of Alzheimer's disease on driving ability: a review. *J. Geriatr. Psychiatry Neurol.* 1990; **3**: 67–72.

38. Carr DB. Assessing older drivers for physical and cognitive impairment. *Geriatrics* 1993; **48**: 46–8, 51.

39. O'Neill D. The older driver. *Rev. Clin. Gerontol.* 1996; **6**: 295–302.

40. Marottoli RA, Cooney LM, Jr, Wagner R, Doucette J, Tinetti ME. Predictors of automobile crashes and moving violations among elderly drivers [see comments]. *Ann. Intern. Med.* 1994; **121**: 842–6.

41. Ball K, Owsley C. Predicting vehicle crashes in the elderly: who is at risk? In: Johansson K, Lundberg C (eds). *Aging and Driving* . Stockholm: Karolinska Institute, 1994: 1–2.

Part 4: Therapy and management of Parkinson's disease

Organization of services, concepts of management and health economics

D.G. MacMahon

Introduction

Parkinson's disease (PD) has a considerable impact upon the mental, emotional and physical well-being of those affected. Moreover, it may also impinge on the patient's lifestyle, as well as that of their family and other carers. Both patients and carers are likely to require access to a wide range of services throughout the duration of the disease, as direct or indirect consequences of the condition or of its complications. While this may be true at all ages, diagnosis may be particularly difficult in elderly patients, and they have also traditionally been the recipients of services that were unplanned, uncoordinated, poorly managed, and often inaccessible. There is accumulating evidence that properly planned, accessible and integrated multidisciplinary services delivered by skilled, multidisciplinary teams can improve not only the care given to these patients, but also the quality of their lives and that of their carers – in a cost-effective manner. This chapter investigates models of care, and introduces some of the current concepts of disease management applied to PD. It will also explore the context of the economics of providing this care and treatment, and the concept that appropriate team-working and disease management from diagnosis onwards can deliver better care by preventing or solving many of the problems that this disease causes.

Services and structures

In the UK healthcare system, it is necessary to consider primary, secondary and tertiary healthcare, social services, and also the role of self-care, volunteers (and voluntary societies such as the Parkinson's Disease Society) and – most importantly – of carers.

All patients have access to a general practitioner, working in primary care. It has been suggested that with appropriate training and effective teamwork, primary care teams could manage complex chronic illnesses intensively, without losing the benefits of an effective primary care system. However, this is not the usual pattern, and currently most patients are referred to specialists – usually neurologists or geriatricians who are based in hospitals. This is termed secondary care, and is the preferred model in recently published guidelines.[1]

The delivery of care by a coordinated team of individuals has been assumed by many geriatricians to be a good thing, even though objective evidence has not been widely available. Patients are thought to benefit from the deployment of more staff bringing the insights of different bodies of knowledge, and a wider range of skills.

During the past decade, intervention studies have begun to show clear advantages to chronically ill patients of care by a team, within protocols designed to make best use of the particular team roles and functions (Table 13.1). These have consistently been associated with better outcomes. The involvement of – or even leadership by – appropriately trained nurses or other staff who complement the doctor in critical care functions (such as assessment, treatment, management, self-management support and follow-up) has been demonstrated to improve professionals' adherence to guidelines. This can free the doctor to attend to those areas that only they have the training to complete, for example diagnosis and medical treatment. The other elements – best performed by skilled nurses – include population management, protocol-based regulation of medication, support for self-management, and intensive follow-up (face-to-face, or by telephone). The participation of medical specialists in consultative and educational roles outside conventional

Table 13.1 The essential components of effective management of chronic disease[2]

Treatment plans for each patient	Formal written plans help to organize the work of teams and help patients navigate the complexities of multidisciplinary care. Those that include patients' treatment preferences are more likely to result in satisfied, compliant patients
Evidence-based clinical management	The identification or addition of team members to achieve greater concordance with complex treatment protocols by providers and patients has significantly improved outcomes in several chronic conditions
Self-management support	Educational and supportive interventions directed at helping patients to change behaviour and become better self-managers have been shown to improve outcomes across a range of chronic illnesses. Effective interventions tend to emphasize the acquisition of skills rather than just knowledge, and systematically try to bolster patients' motivation and their confidence in managing their condition rather than encouraging dependency. The advantages of the team having a nurse or other professionals trained in behavioural counselling, has been demonstrated in several studies
More effective consultations	The limitations of a brief consultation with a chronically ill patient, who will have multiple needs, are obvious. Group consultations may provide a particularly efficient vehicle for the complementary functions of team care
Sustained follow-up	Close follow-up ensures early detection of adverse effects, problems in compliance, failure to respond to treatment, and recrudescence of symptoms. It affords opportunities to solve problems and demonstrate the concern of the care team. Randomized trials have shown the effectiveness of telephone follow-up by other staff (including nurses) in chronic care

referrals may also be beneficial. It is therefore apparent that sharing care between primary and secondary care would have significant advantages, and a specialist nurse can be in a pivotal position to facilitate these arrangements.

Self-care

Self-care is increasingly recognized as an important component of the management of all chronic illnesses, and has recently been flagged as a government health priority in England. Patients are known to obtain information from a wide range of sources, although little systematic research has been carried out on the factors which inform healthcare-seeking decisions.

Concepts that have been developed recently such as that of patient empowerment, telephone triage (e.g. NHS Direct), 'Expert Patient' programmes, and the concordance model of doctor–patient interaction may help understanding and implementation of self-care programmes . The apparently insatiable demand of more traditional media (television and tabloid journalism particularly) for stories with medical interest demonstrates that the quality of this information may range between extremes of technical accuracy and nonsensical garbage. Whether the spreading accessibility of the Internet and other electronic media will improve the quality of this information or compound the distribution of inaccurate myths remains to be seen.

It is widely agreed that healthcare professionals need better to understand patients' constructions of symptoms and illnesses, and also their needs and expectations of healthcare – particularly in different cultural contexts. There is also a need to have a better understanding of the best ways of providing information to enable people to deal with their health concerns themselves, and of ways to help them to use services most effectively and efficiently. This must be particularly true for conditions with known cognitive components such as PD.[3]

Drawing on experience in asthma, partnerships with patients are central to effective disease control. Teaching of doctors and other healthcare professionals needs to be aware of this and the methodologies that can facilitate this approach.[4]

Commercial disease management partnerships may not be the most appropriate solution, for a variety of reasons including professional and lay suspicion of commercial motives, and the results seen so far from such partnerships.[5]

Needs assessment

The needs of individuals with PD are frequently overlooked, and several surveys have shown under-recognition of cases in the community. Even once recognized, individuals often have a multiplicity of problems that change as the disease evolves, but are often not recognized by the primary health care team.[6,7] Many problems (such as constipation) are easily dealt with once identified. However, many patients are only seen as result of a crisis occurring when management is rendered much more difficult. Evidence is accruing that well-planned interventions can avoid such crises with their attendant miseries, and can not only improve quality of life but also reduce wastage of health and social care budgets.[8,9]

Additionally, it needs to be emphasized throughout that the impact of this disease falls on a similar number of carers. Carers typically perceive problems at and around the making of the diagnosis, and also later in the complex and palliative phases when they perceive themselves no longer able to cope. Referrals for residential and nursing home care (with attendant cost implications) may be necessary, initially for respite care, and ultimately for long-term placement.

Services need to be designed to address each population group, recognizing cultural, ethnic, and social issues as well as those related to the differing needs and wishes of patients at different stages of the disease. Information technology should be capable of informing and supporting disease management packages. In addition to electronic communication, the value of a database – which could act as a disease register – has obvious potential. There remain issues of confidentiality, ownership of information (especially between different agencies) and also of commercial confidence. However, it is hoped that none of these is insurmountable. To make comprehensive plans for the whole of this population in one group is exceedingly difficult. This chapter will examine the issues involved in planning and delivering these services, and offer some solutions to the challenges raised. Because of the complexity and scale of the problem, the chapter has been structured around the four-stage clinical scale developed to simplify the management of this disease (Fig. 13.1).[10] The average duration of each stage for patients with typical and atypical PD is given in Table 13.2

Table 13.2 Audit of 'Pathways paradigm': duration of stages (n = 59 idiopathic PD, 14 atypical)[12]

Stage	Years (idiopathic PD)	Years (atypical)
Diagnosis	1.6 ± 1.5	1.8 ± 2.9
Maintenance therapy	5.9 ± 4.8	3.0 ± 2.0
Complex	4.9 ± 4.4	3.5 ± 3.5
Palliative care	2.2 ± 2.2	1.5 ± 1.2
Total	14.6	9.8

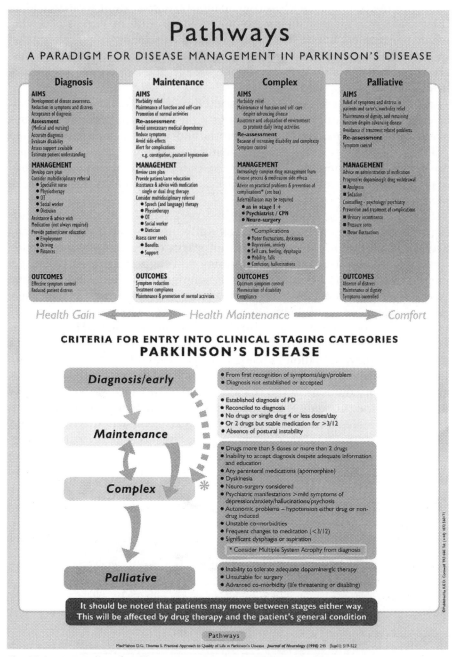

Fig. 13.1 A paradigm for disease management in Parkinson's disease

Diagnosis

Idiopathic PD is a common, age-related, disabling neurodegenerative disorder. Parkinsonism is a term used to describe movement disorders characterized by similar symptoms to those of idiopathic PD. It represents the cause of approximately three-quarters of cases of parkinsonism, the others being either similar neurodegenerative diseases with other features (Parkinson's-plus syndromes such as multisystem atrophy and progressive supranuclear palsy), cerebrovascular disease, and drug or toxic cases. In this chapter, the principles discussed refer to all causes of parkinsonism, since these patients' problems are often similar to those with PD, and they will often present with that diagnosis although their prognosis and response to treatment differs. Some units are organized to manage all movement disorders, of which PD is by far the most common.

To plan a service, it is sensible to quantify the number of cases that may need to access it. It is known that PD can occur at any age, but becomes very much more common in older age groups, with peak incidence in the seventh decade, and a prevalence of at least 2 per cent in the ninth decade.

Other chapters will emphasize the fact that the diagnosis of PD can often be difficult, as each case is different and in some patients it may be quite difficult to distinguish PD from normal ageing, or a number of similar conditions (parkinsonism) which have different, often worse prognoses. For this reason, referral to a specialist with an interest in this condition is recommended in all recently published guidelines.[1] Although most cases can be diagnosed sufficiently well on clinical grounds, computed tomography (CT) or magnetic resonance imaging (MRI) scans are useful in atypical cases, while the definitive imaging is derived from positron emission tomography (PET) scans, with single photon emission computed tomography (SPECT) scans a cheaper alternative. Similarly, most cases will not require many haematological or biochemical tests, although in younger patients Wilson's disease should be excluded. On occasion, there is also a need to perform serological tests for syphilis.

For some patients, the time of diagnosis can be quite traumatic, and this distress needs to be handled carefully by an experienced multidisciplinary team.[11] Depression can frequently coexist with anxiety at this time, and has a major impact on the patient's quality of life.

While the majority of patients will be able to cope at home for many years with the illness, older patients are more likely to suffer cognitive problems, and carry a higher risk of admission to residential or nursing home care as a result of both physical and mental morbidity. PD carries a high mortality in such institutions, and evidence suggests that few patients admitted because of PD survive more than one year from admission.[13] While PD is a common cause of admission to institutional care,[14,15] it should be remembered that the condition can also develop in nursing home residents.

Incidence

In a recent 3-year prospective study the average incidence of PD was estimated at 13 new cases per 100 000 population per annum. The mean age at onset is typically in the seventh decade, but in 1 in 7 cases the onset is below the age of 60 years, while 1 in 50 cases occurs below the age of 40 years.

Prevalence

Since PD is a chronic disease, it is not simply the incidence but also the prevalence that is an important factor in commissioning and providing services. World-wide age-adjusted prevalence ratios vary between 30 and 180 per 100 000, with a commonly accepted estimate in Western populations of 160, depending on demographic factors, especially weighting for age.[16] The prevalence rises to 2 per cent of the population over the age of 80 years.[17] The prevalence of features of parkinsonism in the normal population is even higher (Table 13.3).[18]

The finding of parkinsonism is certainly not benign, the mortality due to parkinsonism having increased over a 10-year period from 49 per cent to 78 per cent. When adjusted for age and sex, this was double that of the control population (95 per cent confidence interval, 1.6 to 2.6).[18] This difference was strongly related to the presence of gait disorders, and suggests that falls prevention strategies should be targeted on this group. There are also clear public health implications in this respect.

Thus, a typical Primary Care Group in the UK commissioning and providing care for 100 000 patients would require services for ~160 patients (and their families), while perhaps 13 new cases each year will need to be distinguished from considerably more who will have features of parkinsonism. Pro rata, a health authority with responsibilities for a population of 500 000 can expect to have 800 adults with PD, and another 65 who will develop it each year.

Table 13.3 Prevalence of parkinsonism

Age group (years)	Prevalence (%)
65–74	14.9
75–84	29.5
85+	52.4

Medical care

Most patients will have an established professional relationship with their general (primary care) practitioner. On suspicion of a problem, this is usually the first person to be consulted, and hence starts the process of identification, diagnosis, and referral. Most GPs would concur with the UK guidelines and wish to refer a suspected case for confirmation of their diagnosis, and for the establishment of a plan for the patient's future treatment and care. Medical referral differs around the country, with younger patients almost universally being referred to a neurologist, while many older patients (and those with complex needs) are referred to geriatricians, the varied referral patterns depending on local expertise and resources. The UK differs from many other countries by having a fewer number of neurologists, and a relatively well-established geriatric service. Since the majority of patients with disease are relatively elderly, geriatricians care for most. As most departments have established multidisciplinary teams, this has the advantage of facilitating access to therapy staff, particularly for more advanced cases.

While most cases will be cared for in primary and secondary care facilities, a few patients will need to access tertiary care centres, either because they have atypical features or because of difficulties with their treatment. The former category would include juveniles or PD appearing in relatively youthful persons, or suspected variants such as multi-system atrophy. These cases may require complex investigations (e.g. PET scans and/or chromosomal analysis)

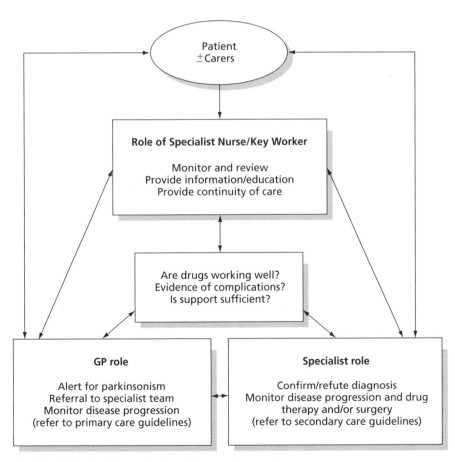

Fig. 13.2 Relationships and roles: primary and secondary care.

that are not normally required in the more typical, older cases. In the latter situation, neurosurgery is dealt with elsewhere. In many other countries, neurologists take full medical responsibility for patients, irrespective of their age or circumstances. Whether 'managed care' or 'shared care' can improve the medical care arrangements remains to be seen.

The role of the PD nurse specialist

The value of the PD nurse specialist is being increasingly recognized. In the medical literature, most successful interventions in chronic diseases have utilized a nurse who has additional experience or training in the treatment of such conditions. The nurses may be nurse practitioners, advanced practice nurses or nurses with additional experience and credentials in a particular chronic disease. The nurses personally 'manage' patients by using local protocols, and adding clinical and self-management skills as well as a greater intensity of care than would be considered standard. In the UK, the PD nurse specialist is now well-established, and well-validated research has demonstrated their value.[9] These nurses work in a variety of settings at the interface of primary and secondary care, including geriatric and neurology units, and also in the community alongside general practice.

The role of these nurse specialists is specifically around disease management and education of patients, carers and other professionals. Patient education is an important part of their role, and this in turn can ensure an improved quality of life for the PD patient and the prevention of complications, together with support and identification. The breakdown of care in the community may be precipitated by ignorance of self-management strategies.

Lay health workers

The importance of lay health workers has often been underestimated by healthcare professionals. Community health workers have been shown to have important roles in bridging language and cultural gaps, especially between middle class health professionals and culturally or ethnically different patient populations. Lay volunteers who have experience of certain illnesses have also been used to support and coach patients facing similar challenges. The effectiveness of self-management programmes led by lay workers has been shown for patients with arthritis and for chronic illness in general. There is no evidence of the specific use of lay workers in the management of PD, but this is an area worthy of further study, and perhaps should be included in the 'Expert Patient' programme.

Treatment

Treatment for PD has advanced in spectacular fashion since 1969, when *Brain's Diseases of the Nervous System*[19] gave standard therapy advice as: 'The sufferer should be encouraged to lead an active life as long as possible, but should avoid fatigue. A 'zip' fastener on the trousers is a convenience'. As an afterthought, the subeditor (presumably) inserted 'L-dopa in doses up to 5 grams looks promising', heralding the new therapeutic age for PD.

Treatment strategies now include the following components:

- Information and education
- Health maintenance/promotion
- Diet, exercise, and activity
- Neurorehabilitative education and training strategies (occupational therapist and physiotherapist)
- Drugs
- Surgery

It is generally agreed that there is no single way to treat and manage PD; controversies exist concerning initial treatment, and also the supplementary regimens required when initial treatment proves insufficient. To some extent therapy algorithms can provide graphical aids to assist decision making, and also suggest options. However, ultimately decisions are individual, pragmatic, and require negotiation between the patient and their doctor, often assisted and informed by carers and other health professionals such as specialist nurses.

Early treatment: maintenance stage

The disabling effects of the disease can be reduced or limited with drug therapy, but when this should be initiated – and with which drug – remain individual decisions. Most specialists advocate that drug treatment be reserved until symptoms cause significant problems, or if there is difficulty in maintaining independence, employment or social activities. Essentially, the choice of initial treatment lies between levodopa preparations and other drugs (such as direct agonists, and in younger patients anticholinergics), but this will be discussed elsewhere in this volume. To encourage the provision of some uniformity of care, algorithms have been published, and the first UK specific guidelines on the management of Parkinson's have been produced.[1] A further awareness document[7] expands on the care options for primary care.

Maintenance therapy

The aims in this phase are for morbidity relief, prevention of complications, and the promotion and maintenance of good health. The main primary care team priorities are to be available for patients and their carers, and to watch out for complications. In order to care further for patients in primary care, the relationship and access to secondary care needs to be explicit, and the primary care team may need to consider whether further referrals (or re-referrals) are indicated.

Many patients in this stage will access their hospital consultant occasionally (e.g. 6- or 12-monthly), but the availability of telephone contact has been shown to be highly beneficial in general terms, and specifically so in PD. As far as possible, patients should be encouraged to stay away from hospitals, and to develop coping strategies that minimize the impact of the disease. At this stage, specialist nurses and lay workers might provide valuable inputs, but tertiary care should have no role.

Education, education, education

Most patients are often hungry for information in the early stages, though others may be frightened or in a state of denial. This requires an individual assessment to be made that involves often both the doctor (usually a specialist) and specialist nurse.

In addition, the potential of a highly effective clinical service may not be realized in practice because of a lack of appropriate education and knowledge among other health and social care professionals. This is clearly a matter for those responsible for the design of undergraduate and postgraduate [continuing medical education (CME), continuing professional development (CPD), vocational training scheme (VTS)] and other educational programmes for the full range of healthcare professionals, including those who commission services or education.

Complex care

In this phase, increasingly complex arrays of potentially toxic drugs will be deployed to counteract the advancing effects not only of the disease, but also of its complications – many of which, are at least in part, iatrogenic. Ultimately, surgical options may be required, usually delivered from tertiary care (specialist neurosurgical units – typically in regional centres). In addition, throughout the care phase, a range of ancillary therapies will be required that includes physiotherapy, occupational therapy, speech and language therapy, dietetics, chiropody, and also social care, advocacy and advice.

Surgical treatment of PD

Surgical treatment of PD can be broadly categorized as follows:

- Lesioning
  - Thalamotomy
  - Pallidotomy
  - Subthalamotomy

- Deep brain stimulation
  - Functional stimulators – Activa™
- Grafting
  - Foetal
  - Cultured dopaminergic cells ± neurotrophic factors

Palliative care

The main aims in this phase are to relieve symptoms and distress for both patient and carers; retention of dignity is also paramount. The needs of patients in the final, palliative care stage are often underestimated. At the time when their needs are at a maximal level, it may be difficult for them to visit a hospital (or even a community-based) specialist because of immobility, and it may also be difficult to assess their needs in a typical out-patient environment. For these reasons, day hospital attendance may be easier, or domiciliary-based services – in which the specialists visit the home – might be beneficial. This has the additional advantage of not only facilitating a better assessment of the domestic circumstances and current problems, but also providing a platform to allow the diffusion of practical advice and guidance. This is especially true where the patient is in institutional care. To achieve these aims, often there is a need progressively to reduce and eventually even to withdraw dopaminergic drugs. There may be needs for other palliative measures such as analgesia, sedation, and other therapies such as physiotherapy. However, the delivery of these modalities of care will usually be a function of residence – that is, the patient's own home, residential, or nursing home and, for a few, long-term hospitalization. The services may be from primary and/or secondary care, depending on circumstances.

Dementia is the major concern, and some longitudinal studies make concerning reading. The cumulative proportion of patients with PD who developed dementia in one longitudinal series exceeded 50 per cent at 10 years.[20] An earlier paper published on this cohort (up to 5 years) suggested that age of onset, duration of PD and disability all correlated with the development of dementia. In addition, those who became demented had minor intellectual changes at inclusion, suggesting that even slight reduction in a generic mental test score (in this case a Folstein mini-mental test score of 25–29) may be significantly associated with the later development of dementia.[21]

The prevalence of PD in nursing homes has been variously estimated as between 5 per cent and 10 per cent of residents. While some may have developed PD since entering care, we know from American figures[13] that PD is a common cause of admission, and predictors of admission include hallucinations and the combination of both mental and physical disability. Those PD patients admitted to nursing homes showed a mean survival of less than 1 year, and all had died within 2 years.[14]

Health economics: costs and 'burden'

Parkinson's disease has a major socioeconomic impact on society that has not been extensively quantified, partly because of difficulties in estimating the prevalence, and partly also in identifying and measuring costs.

It is the sum total of these factors that contribute to the 'economic burden' of this disease. The direct health costs reflect expenditure on drugs, primary and secondary care services, and are matched by direct social costs of domiciliary support, and residential or nursing home care. Indirect costs are comprised of lost earnings both of the individual patient with PD, and also of any carer. In addition, if an economic value were to be placed on time spent by carers in the processes of caring (including lost work and costing domestic and caring inputs at an economic rate), the sum total economic burden is vast.

In 1992, the annual direct health and social costs were estimated in the UK at £383 million.[22] More recently, the direct medical costs of PD were estimated in Germany in 1995[23] at DM 3.0 billion (approximately £1 billion). In this study, hospitalization was the largest component, while drug treatment accounted for the next highest expense. The cost of treatment for patients with motor fluctuations (i.e. complex stage) was more than double that of those without. The average daily expenditure for drug treatment in the German study was DM 10.70 (£3.50) per patient (including patients on subcutaneous apomorphine), whereas in the earlier UK estimate, the sum of £26 900 000 per annum was used for drugs. This equates to £0.66 per day, and may well have been an underestimate of the true cost, perhaps by a factor of 6. The pharmaceutical industry estimated the cost of PD drugs in 1999 as £46 m. In addition, there has been an increasing range of drug and other therapeutic measures, including high-technology electrical functional stimulation and stereotactic surgery. UK estimates are typically lower than others for a variety of reasons, reflecting local practice. If the German costs were extrapolated to the UK scenario, this would increase the total cost of drugs to £140.5m. Therapy and nursing costs are typically low, largely because of low referral rates in direct contrast to both professional and lay opinion.[24] Considerable sums are also expended on other issues, including the treatment of constipation, incontinence, or of erectile dysfunction (and the costs of sildenafil, Viagra) which increase the hidden costs of this disease.

In terms of the 'burden of disease' the costs are even greater, when the impact on the individual, the family and Society are considered. One American study estimated the mean cost at $6000 (£4000) per annum, but also recognized that the costs of care giving meant that the direct costs represent only a small proportion of the total burden.[25] This is reflected in the impact upon families in which such a disease may affect several generations, not only financially, but also emotionally and physically. The impact on health status is estimated to be even greater.[26] Another American study has shown a strong relationship between declining health-related quality of life and use of resources, except for the cost of physicians.[27]

Recent work investigating the value of nurse interventions by Professor Sir

Brian Jarman has shown specialist nurses not only to be well received by patients and their carers, but also to be both effective (reduced mortality and fewer falls and fractures) and cost saving (approximately £300 per patient per annum).[9]

Haycock's UK estimated annual costs for patients are listed in Table 13.4. The figures understate the actual burden of disease, since the cost of treating related disorders such as falls and fractures are excluded from the costing. The costs to informal carers, as well as indirect costs (e.g. loss of earnings, benefits), are not included.[22]

A recent British study was conducted to evaluate a sample of patients with PD to calculate the true economic impact (direct and indirect costs) of PD. The mean direct annual costs per patient were found to increase from around £4000 at age <65 years to £9400 at 85+ years, and over £19 000 in the highest-cost cases in nursing care. Total costs increased both with age and with advancing disease stage. In younger patients, the greatest single costs were drugs (11 per cent) and lost earnings. In older patients, long-term institutional care was the greatest cost. An interesting phenomenon was that drug cost was inversely proportional to age, with drugs accounting for only 6 per cent of total costs in older patients. Secondary health services account for an increasing proportion of costs with advancing disease (27 per cent in Hoehn and Yahr stages 0–1, 62 per cent in Hoehn and Yahr stage 5). The direct costs of patents cared for at home were found to be only 22 per cent of those in long-term institutional care. A move to long-term care implies a net annual increase of almost £12 000 per annum, much of which is a cost falling upon individuals and their families in the present funding systems. These figures confirmed Haycock's earlier predictions that PD is an expensive disease, but quantified a much

Table 13.4 Estimated total annual cost of treatments, UK 1992 (£ 000)[21]

Out-patient management	
Hospital doctors	7 696
General practitioners	3 388
Physiotherapists	1 492
Speech and language	169
Occupational therapists	45
Social workers	284
Health visitors	6 073
Home care management	
Meals-on-Wheels	4 852
Day centres	20 904
Home helps	82 159
Residential care	179 358
Hospital in-patients	49 386
Drugs	26 900
TOTAL	382 706

Out-patient costs are based on average hours of consultation for each profession.

higher expenditure than the earlier study, with costs falling on patients, their carers, and both health and social care agencies.[28]

Estimated direct costs of PD were:[29]

- £3500 to £10 000 per patient
- £7000 to £20 000 per GP
- £560 000 to £1.6 m per Primary Care Group (PCG)

Commissioning services in the new NHS

Chronic illness is increasingly recognized as the dominant feature of health-care expenditure. Its impact on health services will grow with increased focus on disability, the move towards managed healthcare, lay expectations about the benefits from healthcare, and the anticipated growth of the elderly population in all societies. As a relatively common chronic disabling disease, PD has a widespread impact upon patients, carers, social services, primary and secondary health services, and is a common cause of admissions to institutional care. However, there is evidence that these services currently are often poorly structured and uncoordinated. In a number of studies, and even more anecdotes, it has been demonstrated that the health and well-being of patients with chronic progressive neurological diseases can be significantly improved through a well-developed service.

There is mounting evidence that a properly planned and commissioned service would better deliver these services; in addition, there are also data to suggest that this approach would deliver more effective care more cost effectively.

Changes in the specification and configuration of services will, in future, be commissioned by Primary Care Groups (Trusts) in conjunction with District Health Authorities and Social Services according to a Health Improvement Programme (HIMP) and Joint Investment Plan (JIP).

Demands for the service

Evidence about consumers' perspectives on PD services is growing. International interest has also been focused on the neurodegenerative diseases, and in 1997 the World Health Organization made PD a public health priority. With an increasingly ageing population and greater public awareness, demands for comprehensive PD services are predicted further to increase during the next few decades.

Sustained improvements in managing chronic diseases require better practice systems, improvement in doctors' skills, and more effective use of non-physician providers. Practice system changes that have shown the greatest promise of success integrate self-management support programmes, guideline-based treatment plans, nurse case management, more intensive follow-up, and registries that provide reminders and feedback.[30]

In summary, planned services are required because:

- PD is a devastating disease.
- PD is costly, to all health and social agencies, as well as to individuals.
- Early detection is important to prevent falls and other costly morbidity, to avoid complications, and delay the onset of the complex care stage.
- Treatment has advanced remarkably during the 30 years since the advent of levodopa, but remains palliative (directed at overcoming functional difficulties, symptoms and signs) rather than curative.
- Each GP will have experience of a few (typically two or three) patients, but insufficient experience to handle them alone through a disease which can span several decades.
- Ongoing support for this chronic disease is required intermittently and at irregular intervals for some years. This requires good liaison between primary and secondary care providers.
- Coordination and integration of services is necessary to reflect the interplay between medical, social, and functional issues.

There been a lack of effective liaison for individuals with neurodisability across hospital, community and social services. Services are often fragmented, and links between specialist consultant-led facilities and primary care may be uncoordinated. Increasingly, the management of PD is based on a multidisciplinary coordinated service in which the PD nurse specialist will play a pivotal role.[31-33]

To plan services, commissioners will need to engage in a complicated set of activities to produce a template. This template could then be used as an exemplar for other neurological diseases. Stages include:

- Assessment of need (single, or adjoining PCGs)
- Appraisal of the options available to meet that need
- Review of existing or planned 'Care Pathways'
- Evaluation of the effectiveness of interventions
- Prioritization of the competing needs for development or change of services

Extrapolations from prevalence figures should enable a calculation of the likely total population with PD. This will need to be adjusted if there are any local population demographic factors differing from national norms (e.g. a disproportionately high proportion of elderly people). It cannot be assumed that all these people would want to use the service, even if it were made easily accessible. Within the overall need of the local population, commissioners should consider how best to spend scarce resources to enable individuals and their carers to enjoy a reasonable quality of life. Although the perception is that PD is a disease of older persons, one in seven is diagnosed before their sixtieth birthday, and one in 50 before their fortieth. Communication and cultural differences may impinge in ethnic groups, and special consideration is required in planning for those in nursing homes, where PD may account for up to 10 per cent of residents.[15]

Reviewing current services

Current provision is often very patchy; involving a number of providers and contracts usually based upon local interests and residual facilities available as a historical legacy. It will span a wide variety of services, professional personnel, and locations. It is important to include all aspects in a comprehensive review to ascertain the current situation. The current service may include any or all of the elements in Table 13.5.

A wide variety of other services and organizations also have an interest in this service, and their views should be considered when planning services.

In some cases, it is difficult to obtain an overview if local services are fragmented, and involve many elements and different budgets. It can be very difficult to determine how much is being spent, and what level of service is being provided. It is clear that any review of services must be multidisciplinary and include a broader scope of primary, secondary and tertiary care. It should be noted that the key to an effective service is that services are properly coordinated, and that the clinicians involved have special training in the care of people with PD.

One approach that can be used in the collation of such information is the preparation of a matrix in which the services available in each community are plotted. This may necessitate several PCGs working together, perhaps those

Table 13.5 Service involvement for patients with PD

- Medical specialists, neurologists, geriatricians, rehabilitationists, psychiatrists
- Nurse specialists (PDNSs)
- Generalist and specialist nursing services, e.g. district nursing services, continence nurse specialists
- Acute hospitals for medical and rehabilitation services
- Specialist PD clinics either secondary- or primary care-based
- Day hospitals
- Physiotherapy
- Speech and language therapy
- Occupational therapy
- Dietetics
- Services for people with cognitive impairments [neuropsychiatry and Elderly Mental Infirm (EMI) services]
- Services to long-term care, respite care, residential and nursing homes
- Psychology
- Chiropody
- Voluntary sector services may provide complementary facilities
- Tertiary centre for neurological advice and neurosurgical treatment

There should also be consultation with:
- Community and hospital nursing services through Primary Care Groups/Trusts, including General practitioners and primary healthcare teams
- Social services departments
- Community health councils
- Local Parkinson's Disease Society branch(es); user groups and other voluntary organizations, e.g. Age Concern, Carer's National Association
- Disabled Living Centres

utilizing a local hospital service. In each location, a starting point is whether there is an identifiable person/service, and this can thereafter be quantified in terms of hours/sessions/staffing levels.

While most services are provided locally, tertiary neuroscience services are mainly provided on a regional or supra-regional basis serving a population of >1 million. These will include highly specialist neurology, imaging and neurosurgery.

A population of 100 000 (i.e. a typical PCG size) may be the best level at which to commission this PD Nurse Service, with primary care strongly linked to secondary care, as the correct focus for a disease which is relatively rare but largely managed in the community.

In order to satisfy the requirements of clinical governance, PCGs should adopt a formal quality assurance system. Comprehensive evaluations of service provision will benefit greatly from the framework that an established system would provide. In recent years, a wide range of approaches to quality systems has been developed, although almost all are based on self-assessment against a specific model. Any system is only as good as the way it is used, and the culture of each PCG will be unique and the systems should match the culture. To retain ownership of any changes or improvements (and to be cost-effective), service users and staff should be actively involved in the implementation of any quality system. Providing a quality service should not necessarily imply higher costs as the more efficient use of resources may reduce the overall cost.

Health outcome measures

Outcomes from PD are more diffuse and difficult to measure compared with the 'harder' indicators from, for example, coronary heart disease. Measures of well-being are individual, subjective and variable, and very much perceived. Management of PD has naturally focused on treating symptoms of the disease, but quality of life is also a primary concern. A Global Parkinson's Disease Survey[11] suggests that maintaining and improving quality of life is the desired outcome of any therapeutic intervention. It may therefore be more pertinent to measure the standards of service in terms of clinical governance and outcomes in terms of quality of life rather than the strict performance indicators of disease severity, which may have little bearing on the perceptions of the parkinsonian patient. A survey has shown that personal control and teaching people with PD how to improve their quality of life increases their satisfaction with the service received by up to a factor of four.[34]

Audit

An on-going or rolling audit review should be in place to satisfy clinical governance criteria. This could be undertaken using performance indicators for each for each of the four stages of PD, i.e. at the diagnostic, maintenance, complex, and palliative care stages. All audits should include the views of users and carers.

Additionally, any audits should ensure that PCGs, GPs and primary care staff are able to attend study days in order to review results and update their skills.

Some purchasers have found it useful to set up a multidisciplinary, inter-agency working group to review current services and plan for future needs. Such a group may meet for a short period only, or may continue to meet to monitor the contract for the PD services.

Addressing the needs of carers

Carers play a vital role in looking after people with PD, and have a right to expect that the NHS and social services help them to fulfil this role. The National Priorities Guidance for health and social services in England issued in 1998 asks GPs, primary care team members and social services to identify carers by April 2000. Their health and ability to undertake tasks which require physical strength or stamina need to be particularly considered. The carers' willingness to act as a carer may reveal emotional or mental health needs and vary with the progression of the disease, and their reaction to life events.

Developing a comprehensive service

A comprehensive service for people with PD should include professional and public education, comprehensive assessment and investigation facilities, a range of multidisciplinary treatment options, and a support and management service for people.

Consideration needs to be given to the following:

- A defined method of referral by GPs, nurses, hospital staff and patients themselves.
- Means of access to appropriate specialist facilities and agreed time scales (as per Table 13.5).
- Attention to the wishes of patients and carers.
- A policy concerning the purchasing and supply of equipment in the community, residential and nursing homes and in hospitals.
- Well-defined audit and quality assurance systems.

The structure required to achieve these aims might include a designated manager, an expert advisory panel, and a budget to provide staff with training and support services.

A neurologist or consultant with a special interest in PD may lead this service. Commissioners must consider whether there will be a single unified service to serve all areas within their remit, or whether they will purchase a separate service from each provider. Careful consideration should be given to whether the service is to be hospital- or community-based, or both. Whichever is chosen, seamless liaison across trust and community boundaries will be needed, and this can be facilitated by a PD nurse specialist.

Teamwork

A major problem in planning is that individuals can present in any healthcare setting. No one professional group has clear overall responsibility for PD. Indeed, it spans both health and social care. It is recognized that different commissioners will have different policies on involvement of providers in planning and consultation. There is potential for a conflict of interest if providers write strategies for services for which they may tender subsequently. This conflict is often outweighed by the providers local knowledge, and desire to enhance local services.

Steering group

Trying to coordinate and liaise between all these different specialities presents a considerable challenge, and should be the responsibility of a key worker designated for each individual practice. It is recommended that a small steering group be appointed for the service with representatives from commissioners, purchasers, providers and service users. This group could meet several times per year to monitor progress and review problems that arise

Care management

Following implementation of the 1990 Community Care Act, the concept of care management for people with long-term disability has gained widespread acceptance. Care management provides an excellent forum for the inclusion of specific objectives aimed to promote independence for individuals with a long-term disability. The cost of caring can be reduced through the inclusion of a comprehensive health promotion strategy using the care management approach. Social service departments should be encouraged specifically to consider PD services when drawing up community care plans.

Example of how a service for PD could be commissioned (reproduced from *Moving and Shaping*,[28] with the publisher's permission)

1. The PCG suggests that PD should become a local priority condition as a disabling degenerative neurological disorder.
2. The PCG identifies a local lead on PD. A multidisciplinary Task Group is

established to examine services. This task group should include medical specialists, e.g. neurologist, geriatrician, a local GP with an interest, a nurse, a physiotherapist, an occupational therapist, a speech and language therapist, and a social worker. The involvement of the clinical governance lead would be appropriate at this stage.

An assessment of the local situation, including information on existing services, is carried out with liaison and help from the public health medicine department, the individual GP practices and representatives of users and carers, Social Services, and the local Parkinson's Disease Society branch.

- Information on nationally developed guidelines for care is obtained, and a specialist reference group consulted on local arrangements.
- The Health Improvement Programme (HImP) may have already acknowledged the problems of chronic disabling neurological diseases, and should assist the task group in identifying deficits in service provision
- Topics that the Task Group will need to examine include primary and secondary care, acute care, continuity of care, rehabilitation, carers support and respite and necessary action regarding community developments
- A comprehensive plan of action for potential commissioning is agreed by the Task Group and put to the PCG board, who may share their findings with neighbouring PCGs.
- The PCG Executive integrates the plan into services within an agreed timetable.
- An audit plan is developed with feedback arranged to the Task Group for reappraisal.

Conclusions

Many of the problems experienced by patients with PD, and by their carers, can be overcome by the application of modern treatments and therapies, and by understanding the organization and management of health, social and voluntary services. A PD team in which the PD Nurse Specialist has a pivotal role in areas of clinical management, liaison, and education can facilitate the coordination of these providers. These services need to be commissioned according to local circumstances, respecting geographical, cultural and logistical features unique to the locality. However, the principles stated in this chapter should help guide this process and allow the development of properly managed cost-effective and evidence-based services.

References

1. Bhatia K, Brooks DJ, Burn DJ, *et al*. Guidelines for the management of Parkinson's disease. The Parkinson's Disease Consensus Working Group. *Hosp. Med.* 1998; **59**: 469–80.

2. Wagner EH. The role of patient care teams in chronic disease management. *Br. Med. J.* 2000; **320**: 569–72.
3. Jones R. Self care. *Br. Med. J.* 2000; **320**: 596.
4. Clark NM, Gong M. Management of chronic disease by practitioners and patients: are we teaching the wrong things? *Br. Med. J.* 2000; **320**: 572–5.
5. Greenhalgh T, Herxheimer A, Isaacs AJ, *et al.* Commercial partnerships in chronic disease management: proceeding with caution. *Br. Med. J.* 2000; **320**: 566–8.
6. Koplas PA, Gans HB, Wisely MP, *et al.* Quality of life and Parkinson's disease. *J. Gerontol. Biol. Sci. Med. Sci.* 1999; **54**: M197–202.
7. The Parkinson's Disease Task Force. *Parkinson's Aware in Primary Care.* London: Parkinson's Disease Society, 1999.
8. Hurwitz B, Bajekal M, Jarman B. Evaluating community-based Parkinson's disease nurse specialists: rationale, methodology, and representativeness of patient sample in a large randomised controlled trial project. *Adv. Neurol.* 1999; **80**: 431–8.
9. Jarman B. The Community Nurse Specialist Project. Conference presentation. British Geriatrics Society Special Interest Group Meeting, 1998.
10. MacMahon DG, Thomas S. Practical approach to quality of life in Parkinson's disease *J. Neurol.* 1998; **245** (Suppl. 1): S19–22.
11. Findley L. Global Parkinson's Disease Survey (GPDS). Conference presentation, Vancouver 1999.
12. MacMahon DG, Thomas S, Campbell S. Validation of the pathways paradigm for the management of Parkinson's disease. *Parkinsonism Rel. Disord.* 1999; **5**: S53.
13. Goetz CG, Stebbins G. Risk factors for nursing home placement in advanced Parkinson's disease. *Neurology* 1993; **43**: 2227–9.
14. Goetz CG, Stebbins G. Mortality and hallucinations in nursing home patients with advanced Parkinson's disease. *Neurology* 1995; **45**: 669–71.
15. Larsen JP. Parkinson's disease as community health problem: study in Norwegian nursing homes. The Norwegian Study Group of Parkinson's Disease in the elderly. *Br. Med. J.* 1991; **303**: 741–3.
16. de Rijk MC, Tzourio C, Breteler MM, *et al.* Prevalence of parkinsonism and Parkinson's disease in Europe: the EUROPARKINSON Collaborative Study. European Community Concerted Action on the Epidemiology of Parkinson's disease. *J. Neurol. Neurosurg. Psychiatry* 1997; **62**: 10–15.
17. Mutch WJ, Dingwall-Fordyce I, Downie AW, Paterson JG, Roy SK. Parkinson's disease in a Scottish City. *Br. Med. J.* 1986; **292**: 534–6.
18. Bennett DA, Beckett LA, Murray AM, *et al.* Prevalence of parkinsonian signs and associated mortality in a community population of older people. *N. Engl. J. Med.* 1996; **334**: 71–6.
19. *Brain's Diseases of the Nervous System.* 7th edn. Lord Brain, Walton J (eds). London: Oxford University Press, 1969.
20. Hughes TA, Ross HF, Musa S, Bhattacherjee S, Nathan RN, Mindham RH, Spokes EG. A 10-year study of the incidence of and factors predicting dementia in Parkinson's disease. *Neurology* 2000: **54**: 1509–602.
21. Biggins CA, Boyd JL, Harrap FM, *et al.* Prognostic features for the development of dementia in PD. *J. Neurol. Neurosurg. Psychiatry* 1992; **55**: 566–71.
22. Haycock J. In: *Meeting a Need.* Parkinson's Disease Society, London, 1994.
23. Dodel RC, Eggert KM, Singer MS, Eichhorn TE, Pogarell O, Oertel WH. Costs of drug treatment in Parkinson's disease. *Movement Disord.* 1998; **13**: 249–54.
24. Oxtoby M. *Parkinson's Disease Patients and their Social Needs.* London: Parkinson's Disease Society, 1982.
25. Whetten-Goldstein K, Sloan F, Kulas E, Cutson T, Schenkman M. The burden of

Parkinson's disease on society, family, and the individual. *J. Am. Geriatr. Soc.* 1997; **45**: 844–9.

26. Rubenstein LM, Chrischilles EA, Voelker MD. The impact of Parkinson's disease on health status, health expenditures, and productivity. *Pharmacoeconomics* 1997; **12**: 486–98.
27. Chrischilles EA, Rubenstein LM, Voelker MD, Wallace RB, Rodnitzky RL. The health burdens of Parkinson's disease. *Movement Disord.* 1998; **13**: 406–13.
28. MacMahon DG, Findley L, J Holmes, K Pugner. The True Economic Impact of Parkinson's disease: A Research Survey in the UK. Movement Disorder Society 6th International Congress of Parkinson's disease and Movement Disorders, Barcelona, June 2000.
29. Thomas S, MacMahon DG, Henry S. *Moving and Shaping*. London: Parkinson's Disease Society, 1999.
30. Wagner EH. Chronic disease management: what will it take to improve care for chronic illness? *Effect. Clin. Pract.* 1998; **1**: 2–4.
31. MacMahon DG. The Parkinson's disease clinic: a focal point for multi-disciplinary care. *Care of the Elderly* 1990: **2**: 406–11.
32. MacMahon DG. Parkinson's disease nurse specialists – an important role in disease management. *Neurology* 1999; **52** (Suppl. 3): S21–5.
33. Royal College of Nursing. *The Developing Role of the Parkinson's Disease Nurse Specialist*. London, 1999.
34. Fujii C, Aoshima T, Sato S. Quality of life for patients with intractable diseases: subjective satisfaction of patients with Parkinson's disease. *Kango Kenkyu* 1997; **30**: 11–21.

Parkinson's disease and the general practitioner

14

C.M. Hindle and J.V. Hindle

Introduction

The general practitioner (GP) plays a unique pivotal role in the diagnosis and management of Parkinson's disease (PD). James Parkinson himself was in general practice in Shoreditch, following in his father's footsteps. It was the broad and eclectic interests of James Parkinson, working in the family practice, which enabled him to be aware of the cases of this syndrome. To this day, the majority of the day-to-day care of people with PD occurs in primary care.

The role of the primary healthcare team

The basic unit of care in the community is the general practice based primary healthcare team. The Royal College of General Practitioners has identified core primary healthcare team membership as consisting of general practitioners, practice nurses, community nurses, health visitors, midwives, practice managers and administrative staff. The exact composition of any primary healthcare team may depend on the particular circumstances, and patients may require the services of a varying number of members of this team. The GP provides the common link with the team, and therefore often assumes leadership. GPs have adapted their medical roles to incorporate management and business skills, including the employment of some of the staff within the team. The roles of such a team relevant to conditions such as PD include the following:

- The diagnosis and management of acute and chronic conditions, when necessary in the patients' homes.
- Prevention of disease and disability.
- Follow-up and continuing care of chronic and recurring disease.
- Rehabilitation after illness.
- Care during terminal illness.
- The coordination of services for those at risk, including the mentally ill, the bereaved and elderly
- Helping patients and their relatives to make appropriate use of other agencies for care and support, including hospital-based specialists.[1]

The general practitioner's role

The GP provides the first point of contact with health services. This is at the request or demand of the patient, and can be for any problem deemed medical by the patient. The GP's role is to evaluate the patients' presenting complaint to identify symptoms and signs of illness. The GP has a vital 'gatekeeper' function which helps to prevent the over-investigation of the worried but well, while ensuring that further assessment and treatment are obtained by those who require it. The GP has the only fully integrated medical record containing information from primary care and specialist advice. GPs usually have knowledge of the patient and the family prior to the onset of the illness. They have an awareness of premorbid factors that may affect the outcome of illness and disability. They can assess the wider effects of chronic disease. GPs are able to review events in relation to a span of time rather than as individual episodes, and this role continues throughout the disease. The GP is part of the wider community of which the patient is a member, and may be aware of other factors that might help or hinder the patient in their disease. GPs do not normally have special expertise in the management of PD, although some have set up community PD clinics.

Parkinson's disease carries a considerable health burden, which increases with advancing stages of the disease, irrespective of age.[2] GPs are able to intervene in PD through looking holistically at the patient. When treating symptoms, practitioners need to be aware of the high level of pain, fatigue and depression associated with this condition, even in the early stages. Family relationships are affected early in the disease, indicating the importance of providing prompt referral to services such as home care, social work, therapy, counselling and PD support groups.[3] Practitioners must also be aware that caring for a spouse with PD produces considerable social, psychological and physical effects,[4] and contributes to depression in carers.[5] The GP is in an ideal position to evaluate the many effects on the sufferer and wider family. The main tool the general practitioner has at his/her disposal is the primary healthcare team.

Primary care nursing

There may appear to be a confusing variety of nursing posts within primary care teams. The local hospital or community trust usually employs community nurses who specialize in physical care (historically called district nurses). These nurses work outside the practice setting, often in the patients' own home, and provide vital support for patients with advanced PD. Health visitors have a role in working with families and individuals in preventive medicine and health promotion, which is not confined only to children under the age of 5 years. From January 2001, nurses with health visitor or district nursing qualifications will be able to prescribe for their patients from a limited list of drugs and dressings. In some areas, community mental health nurses are also integrated into the primary care team. Primary care trusts and some Primary Care Groups have increased the integration of team working by the direct purchasing of community nursing services.

Practice nurses are employed by the GP partnership. Their roles and duties vary between practices and may include immunization, counselling, family planning, cervical cytology screening and the management of common chronic diseases. Some practices have enhanced this to a nurse practitioner role, which requires a higher level of education and training. This role can include a limited degree of diagnosis and management, and may set a precedent for the employment of PD nurse specialist within the primary healthcare group.

The document *Parkinson's Aware and Primary Care*, developed by the primary care task force of the Parkinson's Disease Society for the United Kingdom (see Chapter 13), outlines the priorities and referral requirements in the diagnostic, maintenance, complex and palliative stages of PD. This document is a useful aid to the management of patients with PD in primary care, in close liaison with specialist clinics. It envisages a key role for the PD nurse specialist.[6]

The general practitioner consultation

The doctor–patient relationship is central to general medical practice. It is an important predictor of quality of life for patients with PD,[7] and can be enhanced – but not replaced – by team working.[1] Consultation is the main process through which this relationship is established. In 1992–93, in the UK, over 70 per cent of patient contacts were face-to-face consultations in the surgery, 12 per cent were telephone contacts, and 12 per cent were home visits. People aged 75–84 years accounted for 25 per cent of the home visits. Patients attend the GP, on average, five times per year (women six, men four), but patients aged over 75 years attend (on average) seven times (women = men). Each surgery consultation averaged 9.36 min, and each home visit took over 25 min. Almost one-third of consultations were for respiratory conditions, while 17 per cent were for nervous and sensory system conditions, the majority of which were due to depression and anxiety or non-specific symptoms.[8]

The frequency and intensity with which patients with PD utilize the services of the GP varies tremendously. In a survey of GPs to ascertain the frequency of consultation with PD patients, nearly half (42 per cent) reported seeing the patients three to four times a year, with 22 per cent seeing patients once or twice a year, and 20 per cent only when problems arise. Few GPs saw patients more than four times per year.[9] The frequency of consultation depends upon many factors, including comorbidity, attendance at specialist clinics, severity of disease and domicile.

Perspectives on PD in practice

After stroke, Parkinson's disease is the second most common cause of chronic neurological disability. The prevalence of PD in the general population is 2 per 1000. In the elderly, this increases to 2 per 100, and in nursing home residents it may be as high as 1 in 10. Although, in terms of formal neurological disease, PD is relatively common, in relation to the spectrum of neurological symptoms seen by the GP in daily practice, it is relatively rare. This was confirmed by a survey conducted through the National Hospital for Nervous Diseases in two GP surgeries over a period of one year. The incident neurological disorders were described and extrapolated to populations of 100 000 people. The relative incidence per 100 000 population of these disorders is summarized in Table 14.1.[10] The incidence of PD was estimated to be 26 cases per 100 000 per year. This same group of workers in London found, in a GP survey, that the age-adjusted prevalence of parkinsonism is 254 and of PD is 168 per 100 000 population,[11] which is similar to that found in other studies.

It can be seen the vast majority of the GP's time in relation to neurological symptomatology is taken up with non-specific illness, headaches and back syndromes. It may be easy for a GP to fail to recognize early symptoms of PD, thereby remaining unaware of the implications of the diagnosis and the requirement for multidisciplinary assessment.

The accuracy of diagnosis by GPs has been well studied through a community register in North Wales. Computerized prescribing records in general practice were used to create a community-based disease register, and subjects were examined to establish the likely diagnosis using recommended clinical

Table 14.1   The incidence of neurological syndromes in GP surgeries[10]

Condition	Frequency per 100 000 population
Headache	210
Back syndrome	313
Cerebrovascular disease	128
Non-specific neurological symptoms	514
Migraine	64
Parkinson's disease	26
Epilepsy	23

diagnostic criteria. Parkinsonism was confirmed in 74 per cent of cases, and clinically probable PD in 53 per cent. The most common misdiagnoses were essential tremor, Alzheimer's disease and vascular pseudo-parkinsonism. It was concluded that diagnosing parkinsonism and PD in elderly subjects is difficult, and that GPs should refer patients for specialist assessment.[12] Using this community register, the services received by patients attending a specialist PD clinic were compared with those received by patients being cared for by the GP.[13] In total, 172 patients were interviewed, of whom 102 attended a specialist clinic. Those attending the specialist clinic had significantly more contacts with therapists, social workers ($P < 0.05$) and, interestingly, with GPs ($P < 0.05$). The utilization of other community services was similar for both groups.[13] Attendance at specialist clinics may have stimulated an increased frequency of review by the GP, or alternatively the patients may have had more severe disease requiring more medical input. The results suggest that there remains the need for an increased awareness within primary care of the importance of the diagnosis and multidisciplinary management of PD.

Practice survey of PD patients

In a survey of a general practice in North Wales, 33 patients suffering from parkinsonism were identified from a computerized practice list of ~12 000 patients (26 clinically probable or definite PD).[14] The case notes and correspondence were analysed by a GP and hospital PD specialist to ascertain predictors of GP consultation over a period of one year. There were 10 men and 23 women with a median age of 77 years.

The result of the consultation survey is presented in Table 14.2, and the significant correlation results are shown in Table 14.3. The average attendance of seven per year was identical to the national average for the whole population in this age group. Although PD was the largest single cause of consultation, most of consultations were taken up with co-morbid problems unrelated to PD, and on average only one consultation per patient was directly related to PD. Higher doses of levodopa correlated with advanced disease. Frequent attendance at a movement disorder clinic was associated with higher doses of levodopa and more use of direct-acting dopamine agonists. Increasing age was associated with increasing institutionalization (residential or nursing home placement). Elderly and institutionalized patients were less likely to attend the movement disorder clinic, and elderly patients were less likely to be on a direct-acting dopamine agonist. The best predictor of GP consultations was the number of co-morbid conditions, with no relationship to the severity of PD (Fig. 14.1). The overall number of GP consultations was less in institutionalized patients (particularly in nursing homes), but these consultations were more likely to be home visits. Home visits were more likely with increasing age and co-morbidity. Although there was not a significant correlation between GP consultations and overall stage of PD, there was a tendency for patients in the late stages of PD to be seen less often (Fig. 14.2).

The results of this survey confirm the importance of the GP in the care of patients suffering from chronic disease. Co-morbidity and institutionalization had much more effect on the frequency of consultation than any factors related to PD.

Table 14.2 GP consultations over one year in 33 cases of parkinsonism

Consultations	Total	Range	Median	Mean
GP	241	2–17	7	7.3
Home visits	116	0–13	2	3.5
All out-patient visits	109	0–11	3	3.3
PD clinic visits	77	0–11	2	2.3
In-patient weeks	64.5	0–20	0	1.9
GP PD- related consultation	52	0–6	1	1.5

Table 14.3 Significant correlation in GP practice Parkinson's disease survey

Factor	Age	Stage PD	GP total consultation	GP visit	PD clinic
Age	NA			+ve	−ve*
Agonist use	−ve**				+ve**
Levodopa dose		+ve			+ve**
Institutionalization	+ve**		−ve	+ve**	−ve**
Co-morbidity			+ve**	+ve	

($n = 33$; Spearman's rho. SPSS package calculated significance $P < 0.05$, *$P < 0.01$, **$P < 0.005$.)
NA = not applicable.

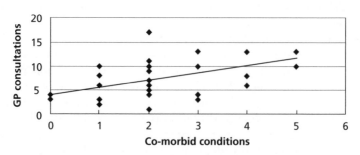

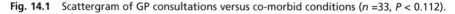

Fig. 14.1 Scattergram of GP consultations versus co-morbid conditions ($n = 33$, $P < 0.112$).

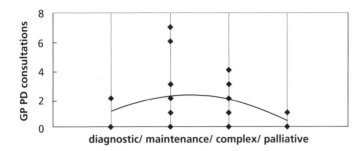

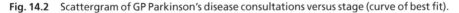

Fig. 14.2   Scattergram of GP Parkinson's disease consultations versus stage (curve of best fit).

The specialist PD team and nurse specialists are only one component in the wider medical and social care of elderly PD patients managed through the primary healthcare team. Guidelines and disease management strategies used in commissioning services for patients with PD must take account of the burden of comorbidity and the utilization of primary care resources.

Disease management

The role of the primary healthcare team in the care of a patient with PD has been well described in the Parkinson's Aware in Primary Care document and in Chapter 13. Although it is widely accepted that GPs should refer all cases of possible PD and related disorders to a specialist team,[15] it is important to emphasize that the role of the GP continues through the whole of the patient's disease process, complementing the activities of the more specialized team (see Fig. 14.3).[16] The level of involvement of the GP in the day-to-day management of patients may vary. Some clinics will assess patients, confirm diagnosis and then refer back to the GP pending any change in the condition. Other clinics tend to review patients on a regular basis.

Shared care

In recent years there has been increasing emphasis on the concept of integrated care pathways, in which one or more members of the primary healthcare team work with other specialist groups in the shared care of patients. This sharing enables patient care to be integrated across organizational boundaries. Examples of shared care in general practice have included asthma and diabetes, terminal care, maternity care and health promotion. The Parkinson's Aware in Primary Care project promotes the shared care of patients with PD (see Fig. 14.3).

Prescribing

Decisions regarding the prescription of medication, or a change in the medication regime, can lead to disagreement and confusion between specialist

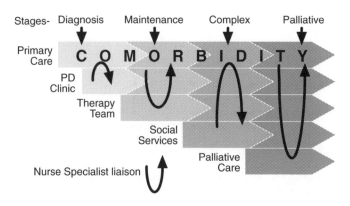

Fig. 14.3 Interdisciplinary disease management. (Adapted from *Parkinson's Disease Aware in Primary Care.*[6])

services and general practice. In the majority of cases, medication is prescribed by the GP following specialist advice although, in some areas, drugs such as apomorphine may be part of a restricted list of medications that can only be prescribed by a specialist. It is important always to remember that the responsibility for medication rests with the prescriber, so GPs must have confidence in the proposed arrangements. Many GPs prefer the clarity of hospital prescription of drugs such as apomorphine, but the practicalities of this may lead to substantial difficulties in the community. Agreement and discussion with the GP prior to the commencement of new or expensive medications may clarify the issues and avert difficulties. Whatever the local regulations, local agreement and clear guidelines for the prescription of such drugs across the boundary between specialists and primary care are needed. There must be clear arrangements for the prescription and continuation of medication, for adjustments in medication within a spectrum of doses, and for access to advice should side effects or problems occur. This is particularly important with patients on apomorphine, who may develop local skin reactions and difficulty with infusion pumps or obtaining the medication. In many areas, easy access to advice and support for the prescription of complex medication regimes is obtained by the provision of a PD nurse specialist. The nurse may adjust medications within stated limits, to avoid unnecessary visits or discussions with the specialist, according to guidelines agreed between primary and secondary care. This is not nurse prescribing, since the prescription of the drugs still lies with the GP or specialist. Nurse prescribing is being developed in the UK, but is limited to items such as laxatives, disinfectants, dressings and skin preparations taken from the Nurse Prescribers' Formulary.[17] Discussion about drug treatments can be informed by the development of a joint formulary between Trusts and primary care, and through regular meetings or a prescribing forum, which could include a community pharmacist.

Patient-held record

The potential for good quality care is enhanced when patients are in partnership with the practitioners involved in their care. Patient education is important, and patients and carers must be involved in the decision-making process. Confidence can be increased by the provision of a cooperation card, which could be held by the patient as a patient-held record. There are some commercially available cards or patient-held records, which have been adapted by many clinics. Information which should be recorded on such cards includes the name, address and contact number of the clinic, the key worker and the GP, the diagnosis and a medical alert to avoid unnecessary cessation of medication during hospitalization. The name, dose, frequency and limit of dose adjustment of medication for PD must be included with any special instructions, particularly relating to subcutaneous apomorphine. A record of unwanted side effects or occurrence of fluctuations or dyskinesia is useful. A space for the recording of comments by the hospital or GP, and the date of the next clinic should be included. Such a card could be produced through utilization of a PD register, or databases in the clinic or GPs surgery, which would enable regular updating and communication with the GP.

Commissioning

With the development of Primary Care Groups (local health groups in Wales), GPs have an increasing awareness of benefits and cost of community services. This has occurred through increased liaison with (or in Wales, involvement of) local government officers (e.g. directors of social services) and representatives of the voluntary sector in these groups, and through increased awareness within these groups of the impact of social care services on the health of vulnerable people. Each Primary Care Group, servicing a population of about 100 000 people, will have around 200 patients suffering from PD, costing social and healthcare over £1 million per year.[18] The magnitude of these costs has increased interest in reducing the burden of PD. There is evidence that a PD nurse specialist can reduce the cost of social care, and improve care in moderate disease,[19,20] and this may provide the incentive for Primary Care Groups to promote the appointment of PD nurse specialists either through Trusts or employed directly through the Primary Care Group.[18]

At present, the development of health improvement programmes and national service frameworks drives the commissioning of services. These programmes and frameworks are concentrating initially on diseases with a high mortality, which affect large numbers of people and which have a good evidence base for treatment and intervention, such as cardiovascular disease and diabetes. Diseases which cause premature death tend to have a higher political and media profile and to receive priority in commissioning, particularly those which involve large potential numbers of years of life lost in younger people. Chronic diseases, such as PD, will inevitably be given a lower priority.

PD is predominantly a condition of the elderly, and the effects of the disease lead to loss of function and a poorer quality of life rather than to large numbers years of life lost. Decisions on commissioning of services should also be based on the potential quality of life, since mitigating the effects of chronic disease can have health and socioeconomic benefits for both the sufferer and the community. Through the work of the Parkinson's Disease Society and the awareness programme in primary care, the true extent of the effects of PD are being realized in general practice. The potential for avoiding unnecessary nursing home admissions, avoiding unnecessary social care costs, and improving the quality of life of both patients and carers will drive the commissioning of better services for patients with PD.

Conclusions

Neurological symptoms are commonly seen in general practice, and the GP must be aware of the symptoms and signs of PD. The GP consultation is the cornerstone of the management of PD patients through the primary healthcare team. The frequency of consultation with the GP may be affected more by the presence of co-morbidity than by factors related directly to PD. It is important that specialist services and the GP work together as key components of the interdisciplinary team in the care of patients with PD. The development of shared care protocols and the commissioning of specialist interdisciplinary services should improve the quality of care that we are able to offer PD patients in primary care.

References

1. The Primary Health Care Team. *The Royal College of General Practitioners Information sheet. No. 21, January 1998.* London: Royal College of General Practitioners.
2. Chrischilles EA, Rubenstein LM, Voelker MD, Wallace RB, Rodnitzky RL. The health burdens of Parkinson's disease. *Movement Disord.* 1998; 13: 406–13.
3. Whetten-Goldstein K, Sloan F, Kulas E, Cutson T, Schenkman M. The burden of Parkinson's disease on society, family and the individuals. *J. Am. Geriatr. Soc.* 1997; 45: 844–9.
4. O'Reilly F, Finnan F, Allwright S, Daveysmith G, Ben-Shlomo Y. The effects of caring for a spouse with Parkinson's disease on social psychological and physical wellbeing. *J. R. Coll. Gen. Pract.* 1996; 46: 513–19.
5. Meara J, Mitchelmore E, Hobson P. Use of the GDS-15 Geriatric Depression Scale as a screening instrument for depressive symptomatology in patients with Parkinson's disease and their carers in the community. *Age Ageing* 1999; 28: 35–8.
6. Parkinson's Aware in Primary Care. A guide for primary care teams developed by the primary care task force of the Parkinson's Disease Society United Kingdom. London: Parkinson's Disease Society, 1999.
7. Pinder R. *The Management of Chronic Illness – Patient and Doctor Perspectives on Parkinson's Disease.* London: MacMillan, 1991.

REFERENCES 249

. *General Practitioner Workload. RCGP Information sheet No 3. August 1999*. London: Royal College of General Practitioners, 1999.
. Grace J. Parkinson's disease- your views. *Geriatr. Med.* 1995; June: 28–31.
. Cockerell OC, Goodridge DM, Brodie D, Sander JW, Shorvon SD. Neurological disease in the defined population: the results of a pilot study in two general practices. *Neuro-Epidemiology* 1996; 15: 73–82.
11. Schrag A, Ben-Schlomo Y, Quinn NP. Cross sectional prevalence survey of Parkinson's disease and parkinsonism in London. *Br. Med. J.* 2000; 321: 21–2.
12. Meara J, Bhowmick BK, Hobson P. Accuracy of diagnosis in patients with presumed Parkinson's disease. *Age Ageing* 1999; 28: 99–102.
13. Meara J, Hobson P. Levels of service provision for people with Parkinson's disease – a survey of community registered patients perceptions. *J. Br. Assoc. Service to the Elderly* 1997; 64: 3–10.
14. Hindle CM, Hindle JV. Hobson P. The General Practitioner consultation in Parkinson's disease (manuscript submitted).
15. Bhatia K, Brooks DJ, Burn DJ, et al. Guidelines for the management of Parkinson's disease. *Hosp. Med.* 1998; 59: 469–79.
16. Hindle JV. Interdisciplinary care of the older P.D. patient. *Prog. Neurol. Psychiatry* 1999; 3: 16–21.
17. *The report of the Advisory Group on Nurse Prescribing*. Crown Report. London: Department of Health, 1989.
18. Henry S. Wanted: 240 Parkinson's disease nurse specialists. *Geriatr. Med.* 2000; April: 19–20.
19. Jarman B. The Imperial College School of Medicine Parkinson's Disease Nurse Specialist Project. Presented at 'The Science and Practice of Multidisciplinary Care in Parkinson's Disease'. The Royal College of Physicians, London, June, 1998.
20. Jarman B, Hurwitz B, Cook A. Parkinson's disease specialist nurses in primary care, a randomised controlled trial. *Movement Disord.* 2000; 15 (Suppl. 3): 860.

15 # Rehabilitation and the interdisciplinary team

D. Robertson, A. Aragon, G. Moore and
L. Whelan

Introduction

The increasing social and financial burden of chronic disease has focused attention on the neglected area of chronic disability,[1–4] renewing interest in the concept of care management to avoid crisis management.[5,6] In Parkinson's disease (PD), studies show that under-reporting of problems is common and the evolving needs of patients and carers are often overlooked within primary care.[7] The emphasis has very much been on developing new drugs as the means of improving the outlook for patients. Whilst important, the evidence suggests that, as in stroke,[8] attention to perhaps more mundane issues such as the organization and delivery of care pays dividends.

Much lip service is paid to the concept of multidisciplinary rehabilitation in PD, but unfortunately there is a considerable gap between the rhetoric and the reality. A survey of the PD Society Membership by Marie Oxtoby in 1979[9] found that only 20 per cent of patients had ever seen a physiotherapist, 13 per cent an occupational therapist (OT), and 3 per cent a speech therapist. In 1997, the Parkinson's Disease Society commissioned the Policy Studies Institute to repeat the membership survey[10] and, with the exception of speech therapy (20 per cent) found little change in the proportion reporting physiotherapy (27 per cent) and occupational therapy (17 per cent). Clearly, access to therapists remains far from being the norm, even among Parkinson's Disease Society members. It should be emphasized that questions regarding therapy input were couched in terms of 'have you ever' seen a physiotherapist. etc. When a shortened version of the Oxtoby Questionnaire was sent to our local Parkinson's Disease Society membership in Bath prior to establishing a PD day hospital, it was clear from the returns that people tended to have either seen a physiotherapist *and* an OT, or neither. Comments in the margin such as 'Yes – when I broke my hip' indicated that the therapy input had often been in response to a crisis.

Patients with PD experience a wide variety of symptoms and functional problems despite their drug therapy. Dependency is particularly high for elderly patients.[11] The 1997 Parkinson's Disease Society membership survey[10] gives some insight into the size of the problem. Although most patients managed the majority of their personal care unaided, 75 per cent admitted to difficulty with at least six common activities of daily living, and 20 per cent with sixteen such activities. The commonest reported problems, occurring in more than half the respondents were: writing, doing up buttons and zips, turning over in bed, getting in and out of a chair, opening bottles, jars and tins, and controlling the flow of saliva. These figures underestimate the situation, since patients aged over 70 years are under-represented in the sample. A community-based study in Aberdeen found a similar pattern of multiple functional problems.[12] It is clear that the traditional out-patient clinic, with its focus on pathology and drugs rather than function, has limited relevance to patients with PD who need access to a wide variety of health professionals and Social Services.

The past few years has seen the introduction of around 80 PD specialist nurses initiated through the Parkinson's Disease Society and supported by the pharmaceutical industry. As outlined by Noble,[13] these nurses play a key role in facilitating multidisciplinary input, supervising medication and coordinating care in their locality. Preliminary results from an evaluation by Jarman[14] indicate patient and carer satisfaction, as well as cost effectiveness with reduced mortality, fewer falls and fractures and cost savings of around £300 per patient per annum, despite increased drug costs. Unfortunately, only a minority of patients in the UK have access to this resource at present.

Rehabilitation

Rehabilitation involves a complex and poorly understood interaction between patients, carers, health professionals and Social Services. The literature contains numerous definitions, as it is difficult to encapsulate the concept and philosophy in a single sentence.[15–17] A recent King's Fund report defines it as 'a process aiming to restore personal autonomy in those aspects of daily living considered most relevant by patients or service users, and their family and carers'.[18]

The essence is the focus on function (of the person as a whole) rather than pathology, with the aim of reducing the impact of the disease on the individual's quality of life. It follows that patients and carers must be at the centre of the process since their perception is the only truly valid outcome measure.

Although provision is patchy, the concept of multidisciplinary management is generally accepted in PD due to the wide variety of problems that can occur. Good practice guidelines advocate a team approach,[19,20] but it is important to emphasize the difference between multidisciplinary input and true interdisciplinary team working.[21,22] In the former, parallel or sequential referrals occur, with each discipline evaluating the situation and providing their expertise and developing goals independently. One person – usually the doctor – makes the overall treatment decisions based on information from the various disciplines. Although superior to input from a single individual, this approach in complex situations can result in duplication of effort and conflicting advice. Problems also arise when the involvement of one discipline depends on referral from another who may not appreciate what they could contribute. In contrast, interdisciplinary working entails professionals simultaneously and cooperatively evaluating the problems and developing a joint action plan with input from the patient and carer.

Terminology and concepts in rehabilitation

In 1980, the World Health Organization[23] categorized the experience of illness into three different levels, namely impairment, disability, and handicap. In the context of PD, the underlying pathology is the degeneration of neurones and consequent deficiency of dopamine within the basal ganglia, whereas *impairment* relates to the resulting damage or dysfunction. Examples of impairment in PD include gait disturbance, bradykinesia, rigidity, poor balance and tremor. *Disability* refers to the functional consequences of the impairment such as difficulty turning in bed or dressing. The term *handicap*, defined as 'the disadvantage suffered by the individual as a result of ill-health compared with what is normal for someone of the same age, sex and background', tries to capture the impact of impairment and disability in the context of the patients social functioning. For example, tremor and bradykinesia may cause problems feeding, but the handicap is the loss of confidence to eat out.

Whilst disability, impairment and handicap are related concepts, the relationship is neither linear nor predictable. Reduced facial expression in PD is clearly an insignificant impairment in terms of disability, but the handicap via effects on social isolation and self-esteem can be considerable, for example when children avoid 'unfriendly' Grandpa. Even health professionals are more likely to judge a person with PD as hostile, unhappy, introverted, passive and dull compared with controls matched for similar levels of disability.[24] The character of Mr Omer in Charles Dickens's novel *David Copperfield* nicely illustrates the distinction between disability and handicap. He describes his new wheelchair to David as 'an ingenious thing, ain't it? . . . and I tell you what – it's an uncommon thing to smoke a pipe in. . . . I see more of the world I can assure you in this chair than I ever see out of it. You'd be surprised at the number of people who looks in of a day for a chat. You really would! There's twice as much newspaper since I've taken to this chair as there used to be'.

This original International Classification of Impairment, Disability and Handicap (ICIDH) was an important first step in moving away from a purely biomedical approach to illness, and provided a conceptual framework and common language for research, service planning and rehabilitation.[25] Its weakness lies in the emphasis on disability and handicap as a consequence of medical problems within the patient. In contrast, social models of disability emphasize the influence of political, financial and environmental factors such as building design, services and social attitudes on the experience of illness.[26] A revised version (ICIDH-2) is now being field-tested to encapsulate this social dimension of disability.[27] Although the acronym ICIDH is preserved for historical reasons, the terminology has changed. Impairments are subdivided into body function and body structure, while disability and handicap are replaced by the terms 'activity limitation' and 'participation restriction'. The interaction with 'contextual factors' is rightly emphasized and subdivided into the social and physical environment and the personal factors that make up the individual such as past experience, education, lifestyle, habits, coping style, etc. A useful departure from the previous classification is the recognition of positive factors at all levels, i.e. functional and structural integrity, preserved activities and participation as well as the contextual factors that act as facilitators (see Table 15.1).

An additional facet described by Wade[28] is that of 'well-being', which equates broadly with quality of life and satisfaction with life. Well-being, he suggests can be reduced in two ways. Some impairments such as chronic pain

Table 15.1 Revised terminology employed by the World Health Organization in the International Classification of Functioning and Disability – ICIDH-2[27]

	Impairments at body level	Activities at person level	Participation at social level	Contextual personal and environmental
	Body function and structure	Person's daily activities	Involvement in the situation	Features of the physical, social and attitudinal world
Positive aspects	Functional and structural integrity	Activity	Participation	Facilitators
Negative aspects	Impairment	Activity limitation	Participation restriction	Barriers

and anxiety will directly reduce well-being, even in the presence of good social role function. Well-being is also affected by discrepancy between the patient's expectations and their actual situation.

The scope for inter-individual variation increases with each level. The variation at the level of 'activity' and 'participation' is immense as multiple factors relating to the physical and social environment and psychological aspects come into play. It is this variation which provides the challenge for rehabilitation staff working predominantly at the 'activity' and 'participation' end of the spectrum. Whilst the same principles underlie the approach to all patients there are no 'off the peg' text-book solutions to bringing out the 'Mr Omer' in our patients.

Rehabilitation services

The concepts contained in the ICIDH-2[27] provide a framework for examining rehabilitation strategies, and the document *Moving and Shaping – the Future. Commissioning Services for People with Parkinson's Disease* is a helpful starting point for discussing local service provision with Primary Care Groups (PCGs).[29] The following principles should underpin the organization of care for elderly patients with PD.

The need for regular review

Patient and carer needs evolve due to the degenerative nature of the problem and the age group primarily affected. Although some patients can be relied upon to report if they are running into problems, all too often people quietly accept the fact that, for example, it is getting more difficult to turn over in bed or they are starting to stumble. To avoid crisis management, which merely reacts to problems when they have developed there needs to be a mechanism for regular review within an agreed care plan.

The need for a specialist team

Every patient is different! While this applies to patients in general, it is particularly the case in PD, in which the clinical picture can vary enormously both at presentation and in terms of the rate and nature of progression. In addition, many patients exhibit wide fluctuations in disability and symptoms throughout the day as part of the 'on–off' syndrome. This complicates both assessment and the delivery of care – it is much easier to plan for a fixed disability. To be effective, health professionals need to be seeing enough patients to understand the vagaries of this condition, and develop and maintain their skills. In practice, this requires a specialist service in partnership with primary care.

Old age doesn't come alone

Since two-thirds of PD patients are over the age of 70 years, other health-related problems are to be expected. Treatment must take place in the context of their general medical background and include regular review of all medications. Cognitive problems, depression and drug-induced psychosis are all more common in older patients[30,31] and complicate treatment.

Patient and carer needs are inter-dependent and cannot be considered in isolation. Looking after someone with PD is extremely demanding,[32,33] yet elderly patients often have elderly carers with health problems of their own. Around three-quarters of carers responding to the Parkinson's Disease Society Survey[10] mentioned at least one condition – the most common being arthritis (48 per cent), anxiety (33 per cent) and cardiovascular disease (30 per cent). In addition, 14 percent had difficulty hearing and 12 per cent mentioned visual problems, while 27 per cent were depressed.

A key worker is essential

The greater burden of problems in older patients can result in a bewildering array of people being involved in the care – all with their own assessment forms! It is not surprising that patients and carers can be unclear as to who is dealing with what and who to call. A key worker is essential to ensuring the right care at the right time by the right person, and that the relevant people are kept informed. An example of good practice is the North Tyneside Parkinson's Disease Service (contact person Dr Richard Walker, North Tyneside General Hospital, Reke Lane, North Shields, Tyne and Wear, NE29 8NH, UK). A key worker is allocated to coordinate management, and patients are given an Information and Resource File with contact details for the rehabilitation team, along with an explanation of the Service and individual roles. A 'Use of Service Sheet' is included for the patient or carer to record any contacts or meetings related to their PD, and a patient-held Communication Sheet facilitates communication between health professionals and Social Services and encourages patients to note any questions or comments as they arise.

Interdisciplinary rehabilitation and team working

A central tenet of rehabilitation medicine is the importance of the 'team' as a means of delivering care in partnership with primary care. Unfortunately, applying the label 'team' will not in itself cause individuals to function as a team. Many factors can undermine team working, including managerial barriers, dominance by individuals or professions (usually doctors!), tensions over professional boundaries, devotion to uni-professional notes, resistance to change and poor definition of roles and objectives.[34,35] A common problem is failure to establish (both within the team and with patients and carers) if there is a common understanding of what is wrong, why and what can be achieved within the limitations of the disease process.

Successful teams don't just happen – they must be developed. Sensitive leadership is required, and regular face-to-face contact is essential. Shared documentation and joint educational opportunities also promote the changes in culture and practice that team working requires.

In the context of PD, a specialist interdisciplinary team should ideally contain the following: PD specialist nurse, physiotherapist, occupational therapist, speech and language therapist, social worker, dietician and a consultant with an interest in movement disorders (usually a neurologist or geriatrician). Ready access is also needed to continence advisors, mental health services, neuropsychology, dentistry and chiropody. The actual size of the core team will vary from area to area depending on resource issues, but if gaps exist every effort should be made to establish good channels of communication and involve more peripheral staff in education sessions and service development discussions.

Blurring and overlap of roles characterize an effective team, but the core areas of expertise are summarized below. Different combinations will provide input depending on the situation – not all patients need to see everyone.

The main ingredients for an effective interdisciplinary team in PD are listed in Table 15.2. The role(s) of the team members are outlined in the following section.

Table 15.2 The main ingredients for an effective interdisciplinary team in Parkinson's disease

1. A shared understanding of normal basal ganglia function and what goes wrong in Parkinson's disease.
2. A common approach and language based on (1)
3. Shared goals negotiated with patient and carer and understood by all the team
4. Consistency and re-enforcement of advice by other disciplines
5. Shared understanding and respect for team member roles
6. Equal involvement in decision making
7. Regular face-to-face contact
8. Shared PD oriented notes
9. Enthusiasm fired by opportunities for on-going education and staff development
10. Administration and Information Technology support

PD nurse specialist (PDNS)

The PDNS provides the link between primary and secondary care for patients, carers and the rehabilitation team. His/her roles include:

- assessment of patients' needs and problems in the home or clinic setting using a structured assessment with validated scales;
- counselling and education of patients and carers and liaison with the Parkinson's Disease Society;
- facilitation of access to rehabilitation and encouragement of realistic goal setting;
- ongoing follow-up of care management and education issues;
- serving as a point of contact for patients, carers and the primary healthcare team should new problems occur;
- provision of regular follow-up to highlight new difficulties before they become established problems affecting quality of life;
- management of urinary problems;
- advice regarding medication and supervision of drug changes; and
- education resource for other health professionals.

Physiotherapist

The role(s) of the physiotherapist include:

- the assessment and measurement of impairments and functional problems;
- providing proactive advice to maintain/improve general fitness and avoid secondary problems;
- the promotion of a home exercise regimen;
- the education of patients and carers in the use of visual, auditory and cognitive cues to enhance movement;
- analysis and management of balance problems to reduce the risk of falls; and
- the promotion of postural awareness and advice regarding walking aids.

Occupational therapist

The role(s) of the occupational therapist include:

- assessment of daily living activities (in the patient's home, when relevant);
- education of patients and carers about the nature of PD and the use of practical techniques to improve or maintain functional abilities;
- advice regarding ways of reducing the impact of PD on interpersonal communication and social and recreational activities;
- the promotion of safety and ergonomics in daily life;
- providing advice on the selection, acquisition and use of assistance aids and equipment to increase personal independence and/or reduce carer stress; and
- liaison with Social Services.

Social worker

The role(s) of the social worker include:
- the assessment of non-medical care needs of patient and carers, including social and financial aspects;
- counselling;
- providing advice regarding services, including voluntary organizations, nursing and home care agencies, day care and respite;
- the coordination of service providers;
- providing advice regarding eligibility for disability benefits; and
- providing support and advice regarding nursing home or residential home placement.

Speech and language therapist

The speech and language therapist is responsible for:

- analysis of communication and swallowing problems;
- education of patients, carers and healthcare professionals regarding strategies to improve/maintain communication; and
- liaison with dieticians and advice on reducing the risk of aspiration and maintaining nutrition; and
- assessment for communication aids.

Dietician

The dietician has responsibilities for:

- assessment of the patient's nutritional status;
- giving practical advice on the maintenance of body weight and nutrition (including calcium), and the avoidance of constipation; and
- liaison with speech and language therapists in the management of patients with swallowing problems.

Consultant

The consultant is responsible for:

- diagnosis of the movement disorder and assessment of the general medical context;
- assessment of impairments including motor, cognitive and autonomic aspects;
- reviewing medication and PD treatment modification; and
- providing advice to the patient, carer and team members regarding medical problems and prognosis.

Rehabilitation strategies: the theory

A shared team understanding of current concepts of basal ganglia function and what goes wrong in PD is essential when dealing with patients – not only in terms of understanding their physical and mental problems, but also as a pathophysiological basis for developing rehabilitation strategies.[36-40]

Cerebral blood flow activation studies indicate that complex movement sequences are particularly dependent on basal ganglia function, especially when they are internally driven rather than externally cued.[41-43] The basal ganglia, along with the supplementary motor area (SMA) act as an 'auto-pilot', allowing well-learned movement sequences such as walking, speech and fastening buttons to run automatically while attention is focused elsewhere. Phasic neuronal activity in the globus pallidus, within the basal ganglia is thought to act as an internal motor cue terminating pre-movement activity in the SMA and allowing sequences of sub-movements to occur.[44,45] The basal ganglia also contribute to cortical motor preparedness for the whole motor sequence or 'motor set'.[46,47]

In PD, degeneration of neurones in the basal ganglia impairs the ability to plan, sequence and 'run' well-learned motor skills with appropriate force generation.[48-50] This manifests clinically in problems with initiation, under-scaling of movements, motor instability as the sequence proceeds and global slowing.[37,51] As predicted, well-learned movement sequences such as talking and walking are particularly affected due to the defective production of internal cues. The dependence on conscious attention is apparent from the deterioration noted with simultaneous tasks.[52,53]

In addition to this motor loop, the basal ganglia are involved in cognition and mood via connections with frontal and limbic areas. Depression is common in PD, and the risk of dementia increases with age.[54] However, even in the absence of dementia some disturbance of cognitive function is common. Information processing is slowed (bradyphrenia) and can be erroneously interpreted as dementia. Mental inflexibility results from problems shifting mental set, and impaired executive function causes difficulties with planning, problem solving and sustaining attention.[55] Memory problems are more marked when asked to recall information without cues or context.[56] Similarly, when learning new tasks patients are more dependent on external cues and correction feedback.[57,58] These changes complicate rehabilitation and underlie many of the subtle changes in behaviour and personality described by carers such as lack of organization and resistance to change.

Recent information from positron emission tomography (PET) scanning in PD reveals selective underactivity in the SMA and dorsal prefrontal cortex, brain regions linked with the basal ganglia and particularly involved in motor preparation and decision making.[59,60] In contrast, lateral premotor and parietal cortical areas are overactive, explaining why actions that are cued are generally easier in PD.[61] It appears that the use of conscious attention and visual and auditory cues facilitates a switch to non-basal ganglia-dependent nerve circuitry.[62-64]

In summary, these concepts form the basis for a coherent approach based on awareness that conscious attention facilitates movement, dual tasks are counter-productive, 'cues' can enhance function and breaking down sequences and information into simpler parts can be helpful. In addition, the team must understand and take account of cognitive and communication difficulties as well as the potential for both symptoms and function to vary with the time of day and environmental factors.

Interdisciplinary rehabilitation: the practice

Assessment

Depending on the patient and the stage of the illness, the initial assessment may involve one or more members of the team, and take place in a variety of settings. However, most information collected will be of relevance to the whole team at some stage and should be available in an integrated record. While this seems obvious and spares patients and carers from endlessly repeating the same information, the culture change required to achieve this should not be underestimated – but is essential for interdisciplinary working. Assessment aims to determine what the problems are, be they medical, psychological or functional and to establish the severity and impact on quality of life at home. The initial interview also starts the process of establishing a therapeutic relationship and informs the management plan. An example of integrated paperwork used in the Rehabilitation Unit in Bath is shown in Fig. 15.1. The form summarizes the individual assessments and notes patient/carer priorities on the initial visit to the unit. The key problem areas, goals and action plan are then agreed jointly by face-to-face discussion at the end of the day.

Certain principles are important when interviewing patients and are relevant to all professions: allow ample time and provide a quiet environment without distractions; establish rapport and gain focused attention; gauge knowledge base and understanding and use language accessible to the individual. It is important to explain the purpose of the interview and to establish what issues the patient and carer wish to discuss. Use short sentences and stress key words, and provide a written summary of the action plan. Avoid introducing too many new ideas in one session and, above all allow plenty of time for responses and listen, even if several sessions are needed to complete the assessment. Staff should also be aware and take account of factors that may confound the picture. In particular, variations which occur as part of 'on–off' fluctuations as well as fatigue at the end of a long session. The context of the assessment is also important, since awareness of being observed increases conscious attention to the task – a source of frustration for carers when the patient performs well in clinic despite major problems at home. The physical layout is relevant, since gait deteriorates in the more cluttered home environment and again a false impression may be gained when observed in the hospital setting.

MULTIDISCIPLINARY ASSESSMENT FORM
Clara Cross Rehabilitation Unit, St Martin's Hospital, Bath

Patient's Name: .... DOB: .... Registration No: ....

Address/Tel: .... Date: ....

Medical assessment summary:
Diagnosis – Idiopathic PD with on/off fluctuations. Diagnosed 15 years ago. pergolide added 2 years ago. Mini mental 28/30, no hallucinations. Has intermittent Speech Therapy review.
Husband frail with poor memory.
Main problems:
1. Erratic drug response and ? compliance problems
2. Variable mobility – tending to freeze when 'off'
3. Falls – exclude postural hypotension
4. High-risk fracture but not on osteoporosis medication
5. Back pain
6. Weight loss

Occupational therapy assessment summary:
1. Problems with bed mobility
2. Difficulty dressing
3. Difficulty with writing
4. Problems with food preparation
5. Needs education regarding PD and coping strategies for 'off' periods
6. Needs home visit to check armchair, bed and bathing – ? rails needed by toilet
7. Safety aspects re falls
8. May need help at home – carer stress

Physiotherapy assessment summary:
1. Flexed posture with R-sided flexion
2. Neck flexion
3. Poor righting reactions and recent falls
4. Poor gait pattern with freezing
5. Back pain
6. Problems with bed mobility

Nursing assessment summary:
1. Difficulty hearing
2. Constipation
3. Urinary frequency and nocyuria
4. Weight loss
5. Poor fluid intake
6. Difficulty eating and drinking due to neck flexion
7. Drug regime complicated – difficulty remembering drug times

Patient/carer priorities: ....

Fig. 15.1 Example of integrated assessment form to facilitate interdisciplinary working in The Key Problem Areas, Key Goals and Action Plan are agreed jointly at the end of the assessment clinic. Speech Therapy and Social Work assessments not included as unfortunately they are not part of the core team at present.

Exercises for posture, ease back pain

Key problem areas:
1. Back pain through posture
2. Poor mobility with poor righting reactions and freezing
3. At risk further falls and high-risk hip fracture
4. Constipation
5. Assessment required to improve functional abilities at home, including bed mobility
6. Nutrition
7. Medication compliance
8. Carer stress

Key goals:	**Dates achieved:**
1. Promote postural correction and optimise analgesia to ease back pain	....
2. Promote safe mobility and teach strategies to reduce freezing	....
3. Reduce risk of fracture	....
4. Promote healthy bowel function	....
5. Facilitate independence in functional activities	....
6. Management plan to maintain/improve nutrition	....
7. Simplify medication and determine how to improve compliance	....
8. Reduce carer concerns and stress	....

Agreed plan:
• physiotherapy and review of analgesia for back pain
• exclude postural hypotension
• exclude other medical causes weight loss and falls, check bloods, commence calcium and viatmin D
• monitor weight and observe feeding problems at meal times
• advice re fluid intake and review laxatives; likely to need dietician
• home visit and consider care package
• education re movement strategies
• medication review and establish plan for compliance

To attend CCRU:

Days: Tuesday afternoons   Proposed length of attendance: 5–6 weeks

Key worker: Lesley Brooker   Review dates: 29/11/99

Not attend CCRU at present:
Reasons why: ....

Referral to other services: ....

Copies to:	GP	DN	Other

Fig. 15.1 Continued.

Interventions and advice

Detailed description of possible interventions by the rehabilitation team is beyond the scope of this chapter. *Parkinson's Disease: A Team Approach*[38] (edited by Meg Morris and Robert Iansek) draws on the wealth of practical experience within the Movement Disorders Programme in Melbourne, Australia. Other useful sources of information include the Physiotherapy, Speech and Language Therapy, Occupational Therapy and Nurse Information packs obtainable from the Parkinson's Disease Society.[65]

MacMahon and Thomas have devised a clinical management scale that provides a useful framework, together with the ICIDH-2 classification for considering rehabilitation within a care management approach.[66] The scale describes four stages – namely diagnosis, maintenance, complex and palliative (see Chapter 13).

During the first phase the emphasis is on confirming the diagnosis medically, education (including correction of misinformation) and helping patients and carers to accept the diagnosis and develop a positive attitude. Medication may or may not be needed yet, and functional problems will vary depending on the delay in diagnosis and any co-morbidity. Education needs at diagnosis are generally not well met in primary care or with the traditional out-patient approach,[10] and the PDSN as key worker is ideally placed to fulfil this role, with help from the Parkinson's Disease Society. In older patients, input from other disciplines is often needed even in this early stage due to functional problems.

The maintenance phase has been described as the 'honeymoon phase', implying a stable situation with improvement due to starting medication. Patients are often referred back to primary care with a 'send her back if she runs into trouble' comment. However, the opportunities and pitfalls of this period should be emphasized. The use of the term 'Maintenance' is perhaps unfortunate as it implies something passive. However, the management scale emphasizes an active approach with follow-up arrangements being defined to provide education and to watch out for complications. Often patients (especially the elderly) expect gradually to get worse – after all they have PD, and don't complain. This may result in unnecessary disability, and once unhelpful ideas, practices and family dynamics are established they are very difficult to change. In contrast, establishing access and relationships with a specialist team allows patients and carers to acquire the understanding and skills they will need to live with this disease and to build on the positive aspects which will facilitate continued 'participation'. During this second phase, points to be communicated and re-enforced by team members include general aspects of maintaining health and fitness and measures to avoid secondary problems. These include encouraging suitable exercise, good dental hygiene and nutrition, as well as the importance of a positive attitude with continuance of household activities and outside interests and hobbies. A variety of simple interventions such as ensuring optimum height of furniture, advice to pace and simplify the domestic routine, and the provision of grab rails or a bed stick can maintain independence. In addition, as functional difficulties increase, the concepts underlying the more specific rehabilitation techniques outlined below can be gradually introduced and practised.

Attention

Concentration is essential. The relevance of concentrating on the task in hand needs to be explained to patients and carers, and re-enforced by the team. Avoid distractions during therapy sessions and avoid chatting to patients when they are performing a task.

Avoiding simultaneous tasks

Doing two things at once should be avoided whenever possible. Again, this concept should be re-enforced by the team. For example, by advising patients to sit while dressing or making a phone call, and to 'walk then talk'.

Cues and triggers

Patients and carers should be taught a variety of techniques to facilitate movement, such as the use of visual and auditory cues, mental rehearsal and internal commentary. Experimentation is needed to find what is most effective, since different methods work in different situations and patients vary in their response.

Visual cues

Increased stride length can be achieved using strips of coloured tape approximately 60 cm (24 inches) in length, stuck to the floor where freezing or deterioration in gait regularly occur (Fig. 15.2). Strips are placed parallel at intervals to match the individuals normal stride length (~45 cm; 18 inches). Where a 90° turn is the problem, strips are placed to fan around the bend. Whether the feet fall on or between the strips is not important, but such strips are only effective if the patient is able (spontaneously or with prompting) to pay attention to them. In the absence of orthopaedic or other problems, stairs rarely cause difficulties for patients with PD, since the edge of the step seems to act as a visual cue.

Visual environment

The environmental layout has a major impact on gait in PD,[67] and simple advice from an occupational therapist on repositioning furniture can be very effective. Central coffee tables should be moved to the side, thus allowing direct access from the armchair to the door or television, and patterns and multiple floor colours should be avoided.

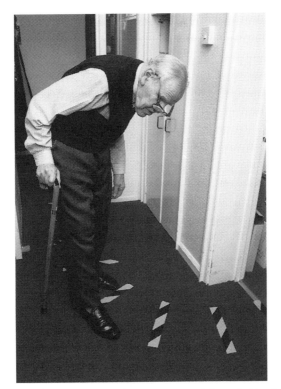

Fig. 15.2 Visual cues for the prevention of 'freezing' and falls. Individually tailored floor markers are applied by the physiotherapist or occupational therapist in areas which provoke shuffling or freezing. A week later their effectiveness and the need for any additional markers is assessed. This patient is prone to 'freezing' with frequent falls. The visual cues significantly improved his gait, with a marked reduction in falls.

Auditory cues

The beneficial effects of music and rhythm on gait in PD are well known, and portable metronomes have been used to facilitate movement.[68,69] However, simple commands such as 'One-Two'; 'Left- Right' or 'Big step' are also very effective. Patients poised and ready to stand may be helped by the firm command '1 ... 2 ... 3 ... Stand'. Similarly, problems with swallowing may respond to the carer saying '1 ... 2 ... 3 ... Swallow' and repeated verbal reminders to 'write big' can improve micrographia.[70]

Mental rehearsal, planning and visualization

In patients able to master the technique and maintain concentration, attentional strategies such as visualizing and then focusing on the desired step length is as effective as strips at improving gait.[37] Freezing can be overcome by stepping over an imaginary log, and negotiating a crowded supermarket will be easier if the route is first planned and visualized from the door. If patients find a particular task difficult, the illustration of sports training in

Table 15.3 Strategy to promote independence and safety in dressing

1. Collect all the clothes you plan to wear, lay them in the correct order for dressing.
2. SIT DOWN on a chair or the bed close to your stack of clothes
3. Concentrate on dressing, avoid distracting thoughts, sounds or conversations
4. Before doing each item, imagine yourself doing it
5. Describe each body movement while you are dressing, e.g. 'put right hand into this sleeve and pull up'
6. Stand to pull up pants/trousers, making sure the body is well balanced.
7. Sit down to do buttons and fastenings
REMEMBER
Do only one task at a time
    Concentrate fully on the task
        Describe each movement to yourself

which athletes visualize the precise movements involved in scoring a goal can be used as an analogy to encourage mental rehearsal prior to movement.

Breaking up the sequence

Long movement sequences such as getting out of bed or standing from a chair flow more easily if they are broken down into smaller parts and attention focused on each sub-movement in turn. For example, when standing from a chair think: shuffle bottom forward, feet well back, 'nose over toes', push forwards and up to stand. Similarly, sentences should be divided into short phrases when speaking. If communication is very difficult, a pacing board can help patients to divide speech into more manageable phrases as they point to each section in turn.

In practice, a mixture of techniques is used. For example, mental rehearsal of the individual steps for standing is combined with a running commentary out loud or internally while performing the task. Similarly, the auditory cue 'big step', combined with the carer placing their foot at right-angles to the patient's toes, provides an auditory and visual cue to prompt stepping when patients 'freeze'. Table 15.3 illustrates a strategy for promoting independence and safety in dressing.

As the disease moves into the 'complex' phase, more intensive input is required to manage and prevent problems. Patients are generally less able to use internal cues such as mental rehearsal and internal commentary, and are more reliant on verbal cues and prompts from carers as well as aids. Since care will involve several disciplines and probably social services, coordination by a key worker and communication with primary care is vital. Psychiatric symptoms and fluctuations in drug response often complicate management, and flexible access to medication advice is essential. In the presence of response fluctuations it is essential for the whole team to have a clear picture of both symptoms and function during the various phases of 'off', 'on' and 'in-between'. Out-patient assessment can be misleading, as patients often manipulate their medication to be 'on' for the doctor. A careful history is essential, and asking the patient or carer to complete a diary prior to clinic can also help. A day hospital is very useful in this situation as it allows the patient to be observed over a longer period, and problems with mobility, eating and toileting observed first hand. Mood swings often accompany the ups and downs of motor performance, and need to be explained to carers. A vital role of the key worker is to ensure that everyone involved appreciates how the patient's physical and emotional needs vary with the 'on' and 'off' state, and adapt their care accordingly. It is particularly important to ensure that care-home staff understand about PD. In this complex phase, the team is often involved in 'brokering' compromise to try and meet the needs of both the patient and carer. For example, when views differ on respite or care provision or when the carer but not the patient wants continence problems to be managed with a catheter.

In the 'Palliative' phase the model emphasizes relief of symptoms and distress, support for carers and maintenance of dignity. Drug side effects may require a gradual reduction in PD medication, and nursing aspects of management become increasingly important.

Examples of interdisciplinary working

To justify itself, an interdisciplinary approach should have more impact than the sum of its parts. The added benefit of a team approach can best be illustrated in the context of the management of falls, and also problems at night. Some of the interventions that may be needed are listed in Tables 15.4 and 15.5, and require close collaboration between the disciplines involved and re-enforcement by the team.

Falls

Falls are a major source of anxiety, morbidity and, indeed, mortality in PD. Assessment and management lends itself to a team approach since numerous factors may be involved (Table 15.4). If 'freezing' is a problem, a careful history may determine if this is an 'on' or 'off' phenomenon, or is unpredictable and provoked by the environmental layout.[67] Turning is a high-risk activity in PD, as due to faulty weight transference the feet may cross, or 'freezing' may occur mid-turn. Other common situations provoking falls include hurrying to the toilet in the dark at night, walking while carrying things, dressing, getting in and out of bed or a chair, walking on uneven ground, and negotiating a crowded or unfamiliar environment. From the medical point of view, postural hypotension and other medical causes should be excluded, the drug therapy

Table 15.4 Interdisciplinary assessment and management of falls in Parkinson's disease

- assessment and treatment of relevant medical factors – remember osteoporosis
- re-enforce movement strategies such as the use of planning, attention and cues and remind to do one thing at a time – don't walk and talk!
- re-enforce techniques for safe turning – don't swivel but use 'clock turn' or wide arc if space allows
- examine footwear
- balance practice in sitting, standing and walking
- reduce clutter at home to maximize floor space
- ensure adequate night lighting
- consider strips on floor in areas provoking freezing
- remove loose mats, check toilet, bed and chair heights and install grab rails at danger spots
- assess possible need for walking aid
- teach techniques for getting up and consider a 'life-line' to summon help
- common-sense advice to reduce unnecessary risk taking
- confidence building to alleviate fear of falling

reviewed and calcium and vitamin D supplementation considered. Precipitating factors can be highlighted by the use of a 'falls diary'[71] to document the time of day, relation to medication times, where the patient was and what they were doing when they fell, as well as any associated symptoms such as dizziness. Specific patterns may emerge such as falls when 'off' or a tendency to fall when turning in the kitchen, or when carrying things, or dressing; such patterns help to target management.

Nocturnal problems

Problems at night are common in PD[72–74] and, if unresolved often lead to nursing home placement. Problems include sleep fragmentation, vivid dreams/hallucinations, restlessness and pain. Depression disrupts sleep, and poor mobility compounds the problem of nocturia, causing incontinence. As with falls, assessment and management lends itself to a team approach, since several inter-related factors may be involved (Table 15.5).

Table 15.5 Interdisciplinary assessment and management of nocturnal problems in Parkinson's disease

- Medical review of medication. Consider depression and analyse why sleep is disturbed. Consider slow-release levodopa or dopamine agonist at bedtime if mobility poor or discomfort; reduce levodopa if hallucinations, restlessness or unpleasant dreams
- Mental health input if significant psychosis/agitation or depression
- Joint medical and nursing assessment of continence problems. Agree plan for management with patient, carer and District Nurse
- Joint physiotherapy and occupational therapist assessment of bed mobility. Review technique and re-enforce strategies including planning, attention and cues. Involve carer
- Occupational therapist advice regarding equipment, e.g. commode, satin draw sheet, bed stick or 'silent riser'
- Nursing advice to avoid pressure sores
- Assess impact on carer
- Advice regarding Attendance Allowance, Care Agencies and Respite Care

Conclusions

The specialist team functions within a wide network of people involved with the patient's care. Strong links are needed with a two-way sharing of knowledge and expertise. Rehabilitation is not something that is done to someone, but rather patients and carers must be central to the process. Regardless of the management stage certain principles apply, namely the need for regular review, ready access to relevant members of a specialist team and a key worker to coordinate care and facilitate communication.

References

1. Beardshaw V. *Last on the List: Community Services for People with Physical Disabilities*. London: King's Fund Institute, 1988.
2. Robinson J, Batstone G. *Rehabilitation a Development Challenge*. London: King's Fund, 1996.
3. Davis RM, Wagner EH, Groves T. Managing chronic disease. *Br. Med. J.* 1999; **318**: 1090–1.
4. Wagner EH. Chronic disease management: what will it take to improve care for chronic illness? *Effect. Clin. Pract.* 1998; **1**: 2–4.
5. Bernabei R, Landi F, Gambassi G, *et al.* Randomised trial of impact of model of integrated care and case management for older people living in the community. *Br. Med. J.* 1998; **316**: 1348–51.
6. Leville SG, Wagner EH, Davis C, Erothous L, Wallace J, LoGerfo M, Kent D. Preventing disability and managing chronic illness in frail older adults: a randomised trial of community-based partnership with primary care. *J. Am. Geriatr. Soc.* 1998; **46**: 1191–8.
7. Koplas PA, Gans HB, Wisely MP, *et al.* Quality of life and Parkinson's disease. *J. Gerontol. A. Biol. Sci. Med. Sci.* 1999; **54**: M197–202.
8. Collaborative systematic review of the randomised trials of organised inpatient care after stroke. Stroke trialists' collaboration. *Br. Med. J.* 1997; **314**: 1151–9.
9. Oxtoby M. *Parkinson's Disease Patients and their Social Needs*. London: Parkinson's Disease Society, 1982.
10. *Policy Studies Institute Survey of Parkinson's Disease Society Membership*. London: Parkinson's Disease Society, 1997.
11. Tison F, Barberger-Gateau P, Dubroca B, Henry P, Dartigues JF. Dependency in Parkinson's disease: a population based survey of non demented elderly subjects. *Movement Disord.* 1997; **12**: 910–15.
12. Mutch WJ, Strudwick A, Roy SK, Downie AW. Parkinson's disease: disability, review and management. *Br. Med. J.* 1986; **293**: 675–7.
13. Noble C. Parkinson's disease and the role of nurse specialists. *Nursing Standard* 1998; **12**: 32–3.
14. Jarman B. The Community Nurse Specialist Project. Conference presentation British Geriatrics Society Special Interest Group Meeting. Royal College of Physicians, London, 1998.
15. Mair A. Report of the sub-committee of the Standing Medical Advisory Committee, Scottish Health Service Council on Medical Rehabilitation. Edinburgh, HMSO, 1972.

16. Nocan A, Baldwin S. Trends in rehabilitation policy. Audit Commission, 1998.
17. Wade DT. *Measurements in Neurological Rehabilitation*. Oxford: Oxford University Press, 1992.
18. Sinclair A., Dickenson E. *Effective Practice in Rehabilitation*. London: King's Fund, 1998.
19. Bhatia K, Brooks DJ, Burn DJ, *et al*. The Parkinson's Disease Consensus Working Group. Guidelines for the management of Parkinson's disease. *Hosp. Med.* 1998; **59**: 469–80.
20. *Managing Parkinson's: Making the Difference*. Health Services Management Unit, University of Manchester, 1997.
21. Melvin JL Interdisciplinary and multidisciplinary activities and ACRM. *Arch. Phys. Med. Rehabil.* 1980; **61**: 379–80.
22. Davis A, Davis S, Moss N. First steps towards an interdisciplinary approach to rehabilitation. *Clin. Rehabil.* 1992; **6**: 237–44.
23. World Health Organization. *International Classification of impairments, disabilities and handicaps. A manual of classification relating to the consequences of disease*. Geneva: WHO, 1980.
24. Pentland B, Pitcairn TK, Gray JM, Riddle WJR. The effects of reduced expression in Parkinson's disease on impression formation by health professionals. *Clin. Rehabil.* 1987; **1**: 307–13.
25. Thuriaux MC. The ICIDH: evolution, status, and prospects. *Disabil. Rehabil.* 1995; **17**: 112–18.
26. Marks D. Models of disability. *Disabil. Rehabil.* 1997; **19**: 85–91.
27. World Health Organization. *ICIDH-2: International classification of impairments, activities and participation. A manual of dimensions of disablement and functioning. Beta-1 draft for field testing*. Geneva: WHO, 1997. http://www.who.int/icidh
28. Wade DT A framework for considering rehabilitation interventions. *Clin. Rehabil.* 1998; **12**: 363–8.
29. Thomas S, MacMahon D, Henry S. *Moving and Shaping – the Future. Commissioning Services for People with Parkinson's Disease*. London: The Parkinson's Disease Society UK; Primary Care Task Force, 1999.
30. Goetz CG, Stebbings GT. Mortality and hallucinations in nursing home patients with advanced Parkinson's disease. *Neurology* 1995; **45**: 669–71.
31. Tom T, Cummings JL. Depression in Parkinson's disease. Pharmacological characteristics and treatment. *Drugs Ageing* 1998; **12**: 55–74.
32. O'Reilly F, Finnan F, Allwright S, Smith GD, Ben-Schlomo Y. The effects of caring for a spouse with Parkinson's disease on social, psychological and physical well-being. *Br. J. Gen. Pract.* 1996; **46**: 507–12.
33. Carter JH. Parkinson's Disease Study Group. Living with a person who has Parkinson's disease: the spouse's perspective by stage of disease. *Movement Disord.* 1998; **3**: 20–8.
34. Evers HK. Multidisciplinary teams in geriatric wards: myth or reality? *J. Adv. Nurs.* 1981; **6**: 205–14.
35. Strasser DC, Falconer JA, Martino-Saltzmann D. The rehabilitation team: staff perceptions of the hospital environment, the multidisciplinary team environment and interprofessional relations. *Arch. Phys. Med. Rehabil.* 1994; **75**: 177–82.
36. Homberg V. Motor training in the therapy of Parkinson's disease. *Neurology* 1993; **43** (suppl. 6): S45–6.
37. Morris ME, Iansek R, Matyas TA, Summers J. Stride length regulation in Parkinson's disease. Normalisation strategies and underlying mechanisms. *Brain* 1996; **119**: 551–68.

38. Morris M, Iansek R. Parkinson's disease: a team approach. 1997. Order forms from Kingston Centre, Movement Disorder Clinic, Warrigal Rd, Cheltenham 3192, Australia.

39. Iansek R, Bradshaw J, Phillips J, Cunnington R, Morris ME. Interaction of the basal ganglia and the supplementary motor area in the elaboration of movement. In: Glencross D, Pieck J (eds). *Motor Control and Sensorimotor Integration.* Amsterdam: Elsevier, 1995: 49–60.

40. Iansek R. Interdisciplinary rehabilitation in Parkinson's disease. *Adv. Neurol.* 1999; **80**: 555–9.

41. Deiber MP, Passingham RE, Colebatch JG, Friston KJ, Nixon PD, Frackowiak RSJ. Cortical areas and the selection of movement: a study with positron emission tomography. *Exp. Brain Res.* 1991; **84**: 393–402.

42. Seitz RJ, Roland PE. Learning of sequential finger movements in man: a combined kinematic and positron emission tomography (PET) study. *Eur. J. Neurosci.* 1992; **4**: 154–65.

43. Brooks DJ. The role of the basal ganglia in motor control: contributions from PET. (review). *J. Neurol. Sci.* 1995; **128**: 1–13.

44. Brotchie P, Iansek R, Horne MK. Motor function of the monkey pallidus: 1. Neuronal discharge and parameters of movement. *Brain* 1991; **114**: 1667–83.

45. Brotchie P, Iansek R, Horne MK. Motor function of the monkey globus pallidus: 2. Cognitive aspects of movement and phasic neuronal activity. *Brain* 1991; **114**: 1685–702.

46. Robertson C, Flowers KA. Motor set in Parkinson's disease. *J. Neurol. Neurosurg. Psychiatry* 1991; **53**: 583–92.

47. Phillips JG, Bradshaw JL, Iansek R, Chiu E. Motor functions of the basal ganglia. *Psychol. Res.* 1993; **55**: 175–81.

48. Hallet M, Khoshbin S. A physiological mechanism of bradykinesia. *Brain* 1980; **103**: 301–14.

49. Benecke R, Rothwell JC, Dick JPR, Day BL, Marsden CD. Disturbance of sequential movements in patients with Parkinson's disease. *Brain* 1987; **110**: 361–79.

50. Harrington DJ, Haaland KY. Sequencing in Parkinson's disease. *Brain* 1991; **114**: 99–115.

51. Morris ME, Iansek R, Matyas TA, Summers JJ. The pathogenesis of gait hypokinesia in PD. *Brain* 1994; **117**: 1169–81.

52. Talland GA, Schwab RS. Performance with multiple sets in Parkinson's disease. *Neuropsychologia* 1964; **2**: 45–53.

53. Benecke R, Rothwell JC, Dick JPR, Day BL, Marsden CD. Performance of simultaneous movements in patients with Parkinson's disease. *Brain* 1986; **109**: 739–57.

54. Reid WGJ, Broe GA, Hely MA, *et al.* The neuropsychology of de novo patients with idiopathic Parkinson's disease: the effects of age of onset. *Int. J. Neurosci.* 1989; **48**: 205–17.

55. Albert ML, Feldman RG, Willis AL. The subcortical dementia of progressive supranuclear palsy. *J. Neurol. Neurosurg. Psychiatry* 1974; **37**: 121–30.

56. Dubois B, Pillon B. Cognitive deficits in Parkinson's disease. *J. Neurol.* 1997; **224**: 2–8.

57. Vriezen ER, Moscovitch M. Memory for temporal order and associative learning in patients with Parkinson's disease. *Neuropsychologia* 1990; **28**: 1283–93.

58. Dominey PF, Jeannerod M. Contribution of frontostriatal function to sequence learning in Parkinson's disease: evidence for dissociable systems. *Neuroreport* 1997; **8**: iii–ix.

59. Brooks DJ. Motor disturbance and brain functional imaging in Parkinson's disease. *Eur. Neurol.* 1997; **38** (Suppl. 2): 26–32.
60. Brooks DJ. Functional imaging of Parkinson's disease: is it possible to detect brain areas for specific symptoms? *J. Neural Transm. Suppl.* 1999; **56**: 139–53.
61. Martin JP. *The Basal Ganglia and Posture.* London: Pitman Medical, 1967.
62. Samuel M, Ceballos-Baumann AO, Blin J, Uema T, Boecker H, Passingham RE, Brooks DJ. Evidence for lateral premotor and parietal overactivity in Parkinson's disease during sequential and bimanual movements. A PET study. *Brain* 1997; **120**: 963–76.
63. Praamstra P, Stegeman DF, Cools AR, Meyer AS, Horstink MW. Evidence for lateral premotor and parietal overactivity in Parkinson's disease during sequential and bimanual movements. A PET study. *Brain* 1998; **121**: 769–72.
64. Cunnington R, Iansek R, Bradshaw JL. Movement related potentials in Parkinson's disease: external cues and attentional strategies. *Movement Disord.* 1999; **14**: 63–8.
65. Physiotherapy, Occupational Therapy, Nurse and Speech and Language Therapy Packs. Parkinson's Disease Society, 215 Vauxhall Bridge Rd, London, SW1V 1EJ.
66. MacMahon DG, Thomas S. Practical approach to quality of life in Parkinson's disease. *J. Neurol.* 1998; **245** (suppl. 1): S19–22.
67. Giladi N, McMahon D, Przedborski S, Flaster E, Guillory S, Kostic V, Fahn A. Motor blocks in Parkinson's disease. *Neurology* 1992; **42**: 333–9.
68. Thaut MH, McIntosh GC, Rice RR, Miller RA, Rathbun J, Brault J. Rhythmic auditory stimulation in gait training for Parkinson's disease. *Movement Disord.* 1996; **11**: 193–200.
69. McIntosh GC, Brown SH, Rice RR, Thaut MH. Rhythmic auditory-motor facilitation of gait patients in patients with Parkinson's disease. *J. Neurol. Neurosurg. Psychiatry* 1997; **62**: 22–6.
70. Oliviera RO, Gurd JM, Nixon P, Marshall JC, Passingham RE. Micrographia in Parkinson's disease: the effect of providing external cues. *J. Neurol. Neurosurg. Psychiatry* 1997; **63**: 429–33.
71. Yekutiel MP. Patients falls records as an aid in designing and assessing therapy in Parkinson's disease. *Disabil. Rehabil.* 1993; **15**: 189–93.
72. Lees AJ. A sustained-release formulation of L-dopa (Madopar HBS) in the treatment of nocturnal and early-morning disabilities in Parkinson's disease. *Eur. Neurol.* 1987; **27** (suppl. 1): 126–34.
73. Tandberg E, Larsen JP, Karlsen K. A community based study of sleep disorders in patients with Parkinson's disease. *Movement Disord.* 1998; **13**: 895–9.
74. Pal PK. Calne S, Samii A, Fleming JAE. A review of normal sleep and its disturbance in Parkinson's disease. *Parkinsonism Related Disord.* 1999; **5**: 1–17.

The Parkinson's disease nurse specialist

16

E. Morgan and M. Moran

Introduction

The first Parkinson's disease nurse specialist (PDNS) was appointed in 1989. Since then, the role has developed greatly, and it is the intention of the Parkinson's Disease Society of the United Kingdom to have one nurse in each Health Authority throughout the UK. The ability of PDNSs to assess patients in a variety of settings, i.e. hospital, home and workplace, makes them important in the overall management of patients with Parkinson's disease (PD). Other authors have also commented on the vital function that PDNSs fulfil in the clinic, ward area, in education and telephone support.[1] Indeed, the flexibility of their approach to patients and carers, and their ability to communicate effectively across wide educational and social barriers that exist among these patients makes them popular with patients and carers alike. The PDNSs have, in conjunction with Royal College of Nurses and the Parkinson's Disease Society, looked at developing standards of care. These include standards on health education, assessment of functional mobility, assessment of nutritional status, assessment of bladder and bowel function and communication and psychological status.[2] These should be valuable tools to assist when auditing practice.

The healthcare environment is changing rapidly in response to economic factors, demographic changes and the need to provide cost-effective healthcare. These factors – when combined with the rising costs of hospital care and the need to reduce hospital waiting lists – puts extreme pressure on all community-based services. PDNSs are ideally placed to take on the challenges of these changing times, and have been clearly identified as playing a major role in the coordination of services and organizational aspects of patient management in both primary and secondary care teams.[3,4]

The Jarman project looked at the cost effectiveness and healthcare outcomes of the community-based PDNS. Specialist nurses were placed in Health Authorities in England and were randomly based; the patients in these areas were then randomly divided into two groups. One group involved actual contact with a PDNS, while the other group had no PDNS support and was used as a control. Although the report findings are still awaited, interim accounts appear to show that the PDNS is cost-effective, as shown by the reduction in long-term institutional care costs. The results also showed that each PDNS saved her/his own salary and running costs, and produced an additional saving that was sufficient to fund another consultant neurologist (5).

Qualifications for the post of PDNS have been identified by the Parkinson's Disease Society as having to meet the following criteria:[6]

1. Minimum 3 years post registered RGN, and currently registered to practice with United Kingdom Central Council (UKCC).
2. Skilled through training in the treatment and management of PD and other allied conditions.
3. Expertise will be maintained through clinical practice and education obtained in secondary and primary care. This will be facilitated through reflective practice seminars, conferences and related courses, and will be in line with UKCC preparation requirements.
4. Designated to have specialist clinical responsibility for the care and management of patients with PD.
5. The PDNS is central to the effective functioning of the medical and multidisciplinary team, and must aim to coordinate and implement the overall strategy for PD in his/her area.

An English National Board A43 course has been established in several universities, and the number of courses is expected to rise. Recently, Swansea established the first module of Meeting the Specific Needs of People with Parkinson's Disease and Their Carers BSc (Hons) Nursing Degree, which is the equivalent of the English National Board A43 course. Employers are encouraged to support PDNS attendance at this and other relevant educational courses and meetings.

The role of the PDNS

The role of the PDNS has been described as being fundamental in coordination of case management, acting as a resource for information, providing access for advice, and as a catalyst for improved public awareness (Table 16.1).[7]

The role is diverse and challenging and ranges from assessment to carer's support. The important aspects of the role are outlined in the following text.

Table 16.1 The needs of patients and the contribution of nurse specialists[7]

Need of patients and carer	Contribution of nurse specialist	Intended outcome
Counselling following diagnosis	Early identification of diagnosis	Acceptance of diagnosis
		Informed choice
Timely/appropriate Information	Provision of advice	Empowerment
	Continuity of care	Positive attitude
Time and attention		Control
	Coordination, oversight of care	Improved care support and quality of life
Multidisciplinary support		
Regular re-assessment	Supervision, coordination	Long-term planning
Carer support information regarding respite care	Carer contact	Symptom relief
		Reduction in complications

Assessment and evaluation

Direct patient and carer contact is essential at all four stages of the disease process – diagnostic, maintenance, complex, and palliative.[8] The aim is to advise and guide towards maintaining independence for as long as possible, through minimizing disabilities and maximizing abilities. Advice can be offered within the primary or secondary care sector.

Once problems have been identified, a care plan is established by mutual agreement between nurse and patient, providing individual holistic care. The philosophy of a well-informed patient or carer is that they will feel empowered if they are actively involved in the management of care.

Counselling

Helping to facilitate acceptance of diagnosis or addressing issues such as coping with long-term chronic illness are important features of the role. The PDNS will not only focus on the affect of the physical aspects of the disease, but also the psychological, social and spiritual implications that this unpredictable disease may manifest. It has also previously been highlighted how chronic illness can impact all members of the family, with patients sometimes resenting the intrusion and loss of privacy when their home is disrupted by frequent visits from health and social service workers.[9]

The specific counselling and communication skills that PDNSs can provide are used for the purpose of helping either one person, a group or a family live in a more satisfying and resourceful way. Studies have shown that a high proportion of patients felt that the opportunity to talk about their PD was the most important aspect of their contact with a nurse practitioner.[10] It has also been suggested that patients find discussing issues such as sexual dysfunction easier with nurse specialists.[11]

Previous surveys have looked at sexual function in patients with PD, and have shown that factors such as age, carer strain, depression and anxiety had an impact on sexual function and that such problems could not only be attributed to physical symptoms of the disease. The knowledgeable and empathetic approach of the PDNS would appear to be important when dealing with such sensitive issues.[12]

Drug management

Parkinson's disease differs in many respects from other neurological conditions in that the disability that people experience can fluctuate unpredictably over the course of a day, or even an hour. It therefore becomes essential that professional advice on drug management is tailored to individual needs, thereby improving quality of life.

An important aspect of the PDNS role is to advise and offer guidance/information on titration, potential side effects and dietary implications (Table 16.2). A greater understanding of when and how to administer medication should result in the PD patient gaining optimum benefits from prescribed treatment. Drug compliance can be dramatically improved once a patient has been educated about the nature of his/her disease and its treatment.[13]

This advice is extended to all forms of medication, including apomorphine – a powerful dopamine agonist that is currently only available as subcutaneous injection. It has been documented that the success of an apomorphine programme depends very much on the continuing advice and encouragement from the PDNS.[14]

Table 16.2 Drug management points to consider

- Drugs currently available do not offer a cure for Parkinson's disease.
- Drugs improve quality of life.
- Education and understanding of the effect of drugs and their side effects enables patients to manage the condition better in the long term.
- Small changes in dosage or frequency often bring about major improvements in the patient's condition.
- Choice of drugs should depend upon individual patient's needs and symptoms.
- A long-term treatment strategy is of paramount importance in Parkinson's disease and such a strategy should be agreed and shared by the physician, nurse and the patient.

Education

The role includes increasing awareness through education and training. Many PDNSs, although identifying patient care as their key role, also see education as an integral part of that role, providing evidence-based learning to patients and their families as well as junior doctors, nurses, general practitioners and other members of the multidisciplinary team. This is particularly important where healthcare professionals have little experience of PD, or equally where there is a high turnover of staff. The information should be given in a non-threatening manner in an effort to reduce any feelings of de-skilling these members of the healthcare team.

With regard to education, the PDNS:

- is a catalyst to increase public awareness and reduce the incidence of mis-information;
- provides ongoing education of PD to patients and carers;
- is involved with other members of the team in the planning, delivery and evaluation of initial education to patients, their families and carers. The PDNS is a main resource for educating medical and other healthcare professionals on up-to-date issues and effective clinical practices; and
- provides organization of educational study days for health professionals.

The PDNS is committed to ongoing education, and exploring new knowledge and medical advances in treatment strategies.

Audit, quality and clinical effectiveness

Quality of life is of paramount importance, and is gaining prominence with the advent of Clinical Governance. Clinical studies and clinical trials are now routinely using quality of life indicators.[15] Studies involving nurse practitioners have shown previously that easy access to them makes patients more knowledgeable about their condition and its treatment, and also improves the patient's psychological status.[16] All these are important quality outcomes.

Two new approaches to quality improvement in the National Health Service are the National Institute for Clinical Excellence (NICE) and the concept of Clinical Governance:

- NICE has been established with the responsibility for assessing the clinical and cost-effectiveness of new and existing health technologies and providing guidance to the National Health Service on their adoption. NICE is also responsible for directing clinical audit in all specialities.[17] PDNSs need to be aware of these new organizations, and may be useful in assisting with audit at all levels of practice.
- Clinical Governance places a statutory duty of quality on National Health Service Boards as it places a legal duty on National Health Boards to ensure good quality healthcare provision.

Clinical Supervision

One of the strategies for the successful implementation of Clinical Governance is through clinical supervision. Actively participating in this is a clear demonstration of individuals exercising their responsibility under Clinical Governance. PDNSs should take every opportunity to implement clinical supervision in their working area, either locally or nationally.

The multidisciplinary team

Along with the PDNS and patient, this may consist of a neurologist or geriatrician, physiotherapist, occupational therapist, speech and language therapist, dietician and social worker. All should have a specialist interest and expertise in the field of PD. It is also important that the main carer is identified as part of the multidisciplinary team. It has been suggested that the role of the PDNS is the key element in coordinating care management, and that they should be responsible for liasing with the primary care team regarding coordination of activities. It has been indicated that PDNSs should be based and managed in specialist departments.[3]

Patients require a continuum of care, which is best provided by a multidisciplinary team approach.[18]

Contact with other healthcare professionals

This may be within primary or secondary healthcare settings and involve nurses, doctors and the multidisciplinary team giving educational support and advice as necessary. This also incorporates involvement in discharge planning, liasing with community nurses and GPs and facilitating continuity of care.

Links with the pharmaceutical industry

The pharmaceutical industry is committed to improving patient education, and PDNSs are pro-active in creating educational packages, audio visual aids and information sheets for both patients and carers. At the 1999 Pharmaceutical Marketing Awards Ceremony, the Parkinson's Disease Society won the Best Pharmaceutical Alliance Award for establishing a network for PDNSs. The criterion for the award is the productive relationship between patient associations, the NHS and the pharmaceutical industry. The panel agreed that PDNSs have achieved a successful outcome, demonstrating cost savings for the NHS and providing real benefits for the patients.[19]

Links with professional and voluntary organizations

The PDNS works in close contact with many agencies, including the Parkinson's Disease Society and the local PD support branches. Currently, there are 250 support branches within the UK which are run by volunteers, and this creates an ideal arena for the nurse specialist to disseminate up-to-date information to the patient and carers in an informal setting. There is also a national group specifically for young-onset patients YAPP&RS (Young Alert Parkinsonian Partners and Relatives).

Benefits of the role of the PDNS

The benefits of the contributions made by PDNSs to PD patients may be summarized as:

* an enhanced quality of life for both the patient and the carer;
* an empowerment of patients/carers who are satisfied with their care;
* greater compliance among patients;
* improved continuity of care;
* reduced hospital admissions;
* the introduction of PDNS-led clinics;
* reduced lengths of hospital stay;
* reduced numbers of GP visits; and
* the prevention of inappropriate clinic attendance.

Carers

The impact on carers should not be underestimated. It has been well documented that 'Looking after a person with Parkinson's disease can be stressful and may lead to social isolation as well as physical and mental health problems'.[20] A study on carer spouses with PD who were shown to have worse social, psychological and physical profiles, also showed that carers providing extensive care likewise experienced worse health. These results also have implications for targeting appropriate intervention, and identifying the needs of carers should be seen as a priority for PDNSs.[21]

It is generally accepted that carers experience more stress as a consequence of the psychiatric manifestations of PD that occur in patients than the purely physical symptoms.[22]

Hallucinations by patients are predictive of nursing home admission, and re-assessment of the patient would seem to be needed at this stage of mental deterioration.[23]

Again, the role of the PDNS in coordinating care and providing increased support to carers should not be understated (Table 16.3). This is of even greater importance nowadays considering the decreasing number of potential female carers. For example, during the 1920s, a couple in their 80s would

Table 16.3   Action points for carers' support/counselling

- As potential carers are usually female daughters/wives, they may already have extra stress of employment, and growing families and may feel ill-equipped to take on a caring role
- Women may be reluctant to seek out help, as society has a greater expectation on women to be carers than it does on men
- Role reversal may be an issue, particularly when the affected partner has been the breadwinner in the home
- Men may find it easier to take on the role of caring due to their previous delegation in the workplace
- Underlying feelings of guilt when a partner is placed in care can produce strong emotional reactions

potentially have had 42 female relatives in a position to be carers, and 14 of these would not have been employed outside the home. Today, people aged over 75 have an average of 11 female relatives, and only three of these do not work outside the home.[24]

Conclusions

Specialization in nursing is a dynamic and ever-changing phenomenon, and it is important for nurses to be sensitive, flexible and responsive to these changes.[25] The PDNS is pivotal in providing a service in healthcare, bridging a gap where the previous provision was lacking.

The move towards an advanced nursing practitioner level is currently being debated in the UK.[26] Studies on nurse attitudes to the expansion of their clinical role have found that extending the nurses' role could be beneficial as it improves continuity of care. Proliferation of the roles may be due to doctors unloading what they consider to be 'mundane' tasks. There has been long-standing concern that extended roles lead to nurses being used to cut costs in the work force.[27] PDNSs may find it more acceptable to continue to demonstrate their autonomy and develop within the parameters and boundaries of nursing practice through gradual expansion of their role.

Providing effective healthcare, improving quality, evaluation and research, leading and developing practice, innovation, self-development and cross-boundary working are all essential for the implementation of higher level nursing practice.[28] Future purchasers of healthcare from Health Authorities through to Primary Care Groups (local health groups in Wales) will be looking for cost-effectiveness in the future, and nurse specialists must continue to demonstrate clinical effectiveness and aim to meet the above criteria when looking for continued sponsorship.

It is clear that the PDNS has an extremely important role in the holistic management of the PD patient and his/her family. This has evolved steadily over the past decade, and the logical progression to nurse practitioner is inevitable, presenting new and exciting challenges for the PDNS who has chosen to work in the rapidly expanding field of Parkinson's disease.

References

1. MacMahon D. A paradigm for geriatric medicine. *Care of the Elderly* 1994; **April**: 51–8.
2. *The Developing Role of the Parkinson's Disease Nurse Specialist.* London: Royal College of Nursing, 1998, 1999.
3. Marsden D. *Managing Parkinson's – Making the Difference.* Manchester: Health Services Management, University of Manchester, 1997.
4. Bhatia D, Brooks DJ, Burn DJ, *et al.* Guidelines for the management of Parkinson's disease. *Hosp. Med.* 1998; **59**: 467–79.
5. Clarke CE. Managing early Parkinson's disease. *Practitioner* 1994; **243**: 39–47.
6. *The Development of the Parkinson's Disease Nurse Specialist.* London: Parkinson's Disease Society, 1998.
7. Noble C. Parkinson's disease and the role of nurse specialists. *Nursing Standard* 1998; Vol. 12, No. 22, Feb 18th.
8. MacMahon D, Thomas S. Practical approach to quality of life in Parkinson's disease. The nurses role. *J. Neurol.* 1998; **245**: 19–22.
9. Peace G. Living under the shadow of illness. *Nursing Times* 1996; **92**: 46–8.
10. Whitehouse C. A new source of support. The nurse practitioner role in Parkinson's disease and dystonia. *Professional Nurse* 1994; **April**, pp. 448–51.
11. Calne S. Nursing care of patients with idiopathic Parkinson's. *Nursing Times* 1994; **90**: 38–9.
12. Brown RG, Jahanshahi M, Quinn N, Marsden D. Sexual function in patients with Parkinson's disease and their partners. *J. Neurol. Neurosurg. Psychiatry* 1990; **53(6)**: 480–6.
13. Nyatanga B. Psychosocial theories of patient non-compliance. *Professional Nurse* 1997; **12**: 331.
14. Colzi A, Turner K, Lees AJ. Continuous subcutaneous waking day aporphmorphine in the long term treatment of levodopa induced interdose dyskinesias in Parkinson's disease. *J. Neurol. Neurosurg. Psychiatry* 1998; **64**: 573–6.
15. Findley L. Global Parkinson's disease survey. Quality of life. Presented at the 13th International Congress on Parkinson's Disease, Vancouver, July, 1999.
16. Hill J. A nurse practitioner rheumatology nursing clinic. *Nursing Standard* 1992; **7(11)**: 35–7.
17. Brocklehurst N. Quality and the New National Health Service. *Nursing Standard* 1999; **13**: 46–53.
18. Quinn N. Drug treatment of Parkinson's disease. *Br. Med. J.* 1995; **310**: 575–9.
19. Parkinson's Disease Society. News Release. PDS wins award for development of PDNSs. Parkinson's Disease Society News Release, July, 1999.
20. Maguire R. Parkinson's disease. *Professional Nurse* 1997; **13**: 33–7.
21. O'Reilly F. The effect of caring for a spouse with Parkinson's disease on social, psychological and physical well being. *Br. J. Gen. Pract.* 1996; **46**: 507–12.

22. Miller E. Caring for someone with Parkinson's disease: factors that contribute to distress. *Int. J. Geriatr. Psychiatry* 1996; **11**: 263–8.
23. Goetz C. Risk factors for nursing home placements in advanced Parkinson's disease. *Neurology* 1993; **43**: 2227–9.
24. Roy S, Redfern L. Cited by Parkinson's disease. *Nursing Standard* 1998; **12**: 49–55.
25. Castledine X. Editor in Chief. *Br. J. Nursing* 1995.
26. Magennis C, Slevin E, Cunningham J. Nurses attitudes to the extension and expansion of their clinical roles. *Nursing Standard* 1999; **13**: 46–53.
27. Higgins M. Developing and supporting expansion of the nurses role. *Nursing Standard* 1997; **11**: 41–4.
28. Skyte S. Rigorous but not elitist. *Nursing Standard* 1999; **13**: 21–3.

Drug therapy

17

J.R. Playfer

Introduction

Drug therapy is the central pillar around which management plans in Parkinson's disease (PD) are built. Only in cases where there is insignificant disability or the diagnosis in doubt are drugs withheld. At all other stages of the disease, the challenge is to get the best out of the available drugs for the individual patient. Superficially, this should be a relatively simple task. The current *British National Formulary* lists only 18 drugs with which to treat PD, and these have just two general modes of action: (i) drugs which enhance dopaminergic transmission either singly or in combination; and (ii) anti-muscarinic drugs which reduce central cholinergic activity.[1] Such apparent simplicity soon breaks down when the drugs are classified more clearly.

The senior drug is undoubtedly levodopa, which has been the mainstay of treatment for 30 years. Although available in pure form, it is usually used as either Co-beneldopa or Co-careldopa when it is combined with a peripheral decarboxylase inhibitor. Levodopa is an amino acid precursor of dopamine that is absorbed by the large neutral amino acid transport system and able to cross the blood–brain barrier. The precursor loading enables the depleted striatal dopamine to be replenished. Correctly diagnosed PD patients respond in the early stages of the disease, particularly with improvement in bradykinesia and rigidity. In longer-term use, the emergence of tachyphylaxis and abnormal involuntary movements has led to the search for alternative therapies of which the most important are the dopamine agonists.[2] There are six orally acting dopamine agonists, four of which are ergot derivatives: bromocriptine, pergolide, cabergoline and lisuride; and two non-ergot derivatives, ropinirole and pramipexole. These combine directly to stimulate the postsynaptic dopamine receptor. Each of these drugs has a very distinctive pharmacological profile. Initially developed to be adjunct therapy for levodopa, increasingly a case has been made for single use, although not all have a licence for such use. Apomorphine is the most potent dopamine agonist, but can only be used by subcutaneous injection. Levodopa has a notoriously short half-life, and this has led to the development of drugs which block the metabolic pathways by which dopamine is deactivated. Selegiline (a mono amine oxidase B inhibitor) and entacapone [a catechol-O-methyl transferase, (COMT) inhibitor] both work in such a manner. Tolcapone, another COMT inhibitor, was also employed in this respect, but the licence for its use has been suspended because of serious hepatotoxicity.

Amantadine enhances dopaminergic activity, although its actions are as complex as its effects are relatively modest. It acts by releasing dopamine stores and also by modulating the presynaptic autoregulator. It also has actions on N-methyl-D-aspartate (NMDA) receptors and possibly some anticholinergic effects.

Anti-cholinergic drugs having anti-muscarinic actions are the oldest drugs used in PD. The number of these drugs available has decreased markedly, there now only being five available: benzhexol hydrochloride, benztropine mesylate, biperiden, orphenadrine hydrochloride and procyclidine hydrochloride.

Parkinson's disease has very clear age-related distribution, becoming more common with increasing age. General considerations for prescribing to the elderly clearly apply in PD. The patients are more likely to have other illnesses and therefore take other prescribed drugs, leading to problems of polypharmacy, with associated increased adverse reaction(s).[3] Compliance of medication may be difficult and require altered formulations of drugs to be available.[4] Ageing of the nervous system makes the patient more vulnerable to neurotoxicity; this is very evident in the high prevalence of drug-induced parkinsonism. In elderly people, prochlorperazine (which is commonly prescribed for giddiness) given in prolonged use is likely to produce drug-induced parkinsonism, along with postural hypotension and confusion.[5] If a patient is already parkinsonian, this will antagonize the effects of their anti-parkinsonian drugs. Such an increase in sensitivity and susceptibility to side effects must always be borne in mind.

The pharmacokinetics of many of the drugs used in PD is complex, and this relates to their side effects. Pharmacokinetics can be changed by inter-current illness, especially sudden changes in renal function. An unexpected variation in response to drugs may be due to pharmacokinetic factors such as the timing of levodopa dosage relative to meals, when a neutral amino acid may compete with the drug for absorption.

There is a wide range of views on how to best use drugs in PD, the order in which drugs may be introduced, and timing of the treatments. It has become apparent that even with an increasing evidence base in the current literature, many questions remain unanswered. This has led to the growth of a number of algorithms and guideline documents in order to assist clinicians in making the most appropriate clinical decisions.[6–10] None of the available guidelines has been specific to elderly PD patients; hence an attempt will be made in this chapter to appraise the information available on PD drugs, and to conclude which treatment algorithms are most appropriate for this patient group. One of the major difficulties for geriatricians in this field is that the drugs have been assessed almost solely on their effects on motor symptoms. Most physicians in this field would recognize that parkinsonism is not only a motor disease but also a more general neurodegenerative condition with neuropsychiatric aspects. This point is clearly illustrated in many other chapters in this book, and highlighted in Chapter 8.

Dopaminergic drugs in PD

Levodopa

The rationale for levodopa in the treatment of PD centres around the notion that the symptoms of the disease result from a deficiency of the neurotransmitter dopamine in the striatum; this occurs as a result of progressive degeneration of the pigment-containing cells of the pars compacta of the substantia nigra. Levodopa is a precursor of dopamine, and when made available is avidly taken up by depleted dopaminergic neurones where it undergoes decarboxylation in the presynaptic terminal to dopamine, which is then incorporated into the presynaptic vesicle. This helps to replace the endogenous neurotransmitters lost because of progressive pathology in the pars compacta.

EFFICACY

The effectiveness of levodopa was shown in clinical studies during the late 1960s,[11] PD being the first neurodegenerative disease to be treated by neurotransmitter replacement. To date, no other drug has been shown to be more effective than levodopa at relieving the symptoms of PD. Levodopa is used almost universally in combination with a decarboxylase inhibitor, either carbidopa or benserazide. These compounds prevent the conversion of levodopa to dopamine outside the central nervous system, and thus reduce the nausea and vomiting and postural hypotension that are associated with levodopa monotherapy. They also increase the availability of levodopa to the brain.[12] The introduction of decarboxylase inhibitors during the early 1970s was a major step forward in controlling the early complications of levodopa. In the early stages of PD, virtually all patients will show an initial clinical improvement, and failure to do so raises a question mark about the diagnosis.[13] The drug has greatest benefit in akinesia and rigidity, although there is some effect on tremor, but this is often disappointing.[14] Heightened response in initial therapy is due to suprasensitivity from long-term denervation. At the early stages of the disease there is preserved capacity for the presynaptic nerve terminals to store dopamine. The clinical benefit therefore of each levodopa dose lasts for several hours – significantly longer than would be expected from the very short half-life that plasma levodopa levels demonstrate ($t_{1/2}$ = 1.5 h). As the disease progresses, the population of functional nigrostriatal neurones is reduced, and with it the capacity to store dopamine. Some of the initial suprasensitivity to dopamine is also lost. The theoretical disadvantages of levodopa, which are not evident initially, become more evident.[15] Levodopa has poor bioavailability, and in particular its gastric absorption is irregular and can be affected by competition by other large neutral amino acids. The plasma half-life is shorter than would be desirable. Consequently, the first detrimental symptom to emerge is usually end-of-dose deterioration of response, or the wearing-off phenomenon.[16] Patients with a good response to drugs can usually pin-point precisely when the drug begins to work, and also when it wears off. Once this occurs the patient usually notices the symptoms becoming worse over time, and eventually goes on to more unpredictable phenomena such as motor fluctuations, dyskinesia and 'on/off' syndrome. The kinetics of levodopa change in individual patients over time. Reducing striatal storage capacity for dopamine with compensatory changes in modulation of synaptic and postsynaptic mechanisms[17] decreases the area under the curve of plasma concentrations. Chronic levodopa syndrome also involves pharmacodynamic changes involving regulation of dopamine receptors.[18] The fluctuations in the response to the drug are not purely motor, but patients often complain of other phenomenon such as autonomic effects, sweating, a sense of anxiety and psychiatric symptoms.[19]

DYSKINESIA

Dyskinesia begins to appear with levodopa between 3 and 5 years of treatment. For the elderly population, dyskinesias appear to be less common than for patients with early onset of the disease. The widely quoted figure of 50 per cent of patients developing dyskinesia after 5 years was true of earlier high levels of levodopa. Subsequent studies have shown that with low overall levels of levodopa, the rate of dyskinesia can be contained to more manageable levels of under 10 per cent.[20] The most common form of dyskinesia is peak-dose dyskinesia, when plasma levels of levodopa are high.[21] Biphasic dyskinesia occurs secondary to a rapid change of plasma level as patients switch 'on' and 'off'.[22] To complicate matters, dystonic phenomena often occur when plasma levels are low, and are particularly likely to occur in the early morning, when patients complain of painful curling dystonic movements of the foot.[23] Once fluctuations in clinical response with dyskinesia and dystonia emerge with levodopa, the main focus is to try and reduce these unpleasant side effects. Strategies such as fragmenting doses into smaller, more frequent doses, the use of controlled-release preparations of levodopa, supplementing adjunctive therapy with a dopamine agonist (e.g. selegiline or COMT inhibitors) are among strategies which need to be considered.

SIDE EFFECTS

The psychiatric side effects of levodopa are another important consideration in the elderly patient,[24] ranging from mild cognitive impairment to acute confusional states, hallucinosis and frank psychotic states. The symptoms are very likely to arise from the escalation of doses in order to control problems such as freezing and prolonged 'off' periods. Although much attention is drawn to the drawbacks of levodopa, it remains the 'gold standard' in the treatment of PD. How one can sustain the benefit of the drug while reducing the long-term complications has been much debated in the management of PD over the past 10 years or more. Dopamine is a neuromodulatory transmitter, and in most circumstances its release in the striatum is tonic. Experiments using intravenous administration of levodopa or duodenal infusions to maintain constant levels of the drug in the plasma have been shown to abolish fluctuations.[25] This has strongly fuelled efforts to modify the formulation of the drug, with the development of controlled-release preparations. It has also fuelled the debate about the timing of the initiation of levodopa, whether early in the disease or reserved until later. There has been a long-running debate as to whether levodopa itself may be toxic to dopaminergic neurones.[26] There is a theoretical risk that levodopa may increase oxidative stress and thereby accelerate nigral cell death, and this thought has encouraged the use of much lower doses of levodopa than were usual 10–15 years ago. Although there is no evidence in human patients that levodopa is toxic to nigrostriatal neurones, one advantage of lower dosage has been a lower emergence of motor fluctuations. Indeed, quite a strong consensus seems to be developing that the total daily dose of levodopa should be constrained to 600 mg, or less.

FORMULATIONS

There are two sustained-release formulations of levodopa: one is based on Madopar and uses an osmotic principle; the other is based on Sinemet and uses an erodable monolithic matrix.[27] The matrix system appears to give more consistent stable plasma levels over a wide range of dosage. The CR first study group undertook a 5-year multicentre study comparing immediate-release and controlled-release carbidopa/levodopa in PD.[28] This study was unusual in finding a very low prevalence of motor complications, which made it difficult to distinguish statistically between the two preparations. It did have the merit of demonstrating that lower-dose treatment of PD will reduce motor complications. A subanalysis of the study results showed benefits of the controlled-release preparation in quality of life and reduced adverse reactions,[29] and also an improvement in nocturnal symptoms.[30] Open studies have shown consistently an increase in 'on' time on controlled-release preparations. It was thus surprising that this was not confirmed in the controlled trial. Controlled-release forms of levodopa are more expensive, and reduce the bioavailability and peak-dose plasma levels. The pharmacokinetic profile shows a slower rise to a peak level, with an increased area under the curve. Patients used to an immediate effect from conventional-release levodopa often miss the kick-start that this produces, and may need to be supplemented by conventional doses.

DRUG INTERACTIONS

The interaction with levodopa and dietary protein has been the subject of a number of studies.[31] Administering levodopa on an empty stomach, at least 30 min before a meal, reduces competition between the drug and dietary amino acids, both at the level of the gut and transfer through the blood–brain barrier. Although there are claims that this improves the response to levodopa, it can also result in an increase in dyskinesia. Protein restriction is not a good idea in elderly patients, since one of the symptoms of progression of the disease is often weight loss and dietary problems.

Swallowing disorders have been shown to be common in PD, and in response to this liquid forms of levodopa have been developed, notably a dispersible version of Madopar which is available in the UK. This drug has a very quick onset of action and maybe useful in supplementing other forms of levodopa. However, no major study has indicated that 'on' time is increased by the use of such preparations, and swallowing of fluid forms can be just as difficult as solid forms of levodopa in PD patients.[32]

Drugs augmenting levodopa action

COMT inhibitors

The advent of COMT inhibitors has added a new class of drug to the management of PD. Several enzymes control the metabolism of levodopa and dopamine (Fig. 17.1), with levodopa being converted to dopamine by the enzyme dopa decarboxylase. Dopamine itself is metabolized by methylation, transamination or oxidation. Once peripheral decarboxylation is inhibited, COMT accounts for most of the extracerebral metabolism of levodopa, resulting in increased levels of a metabolite, 3-O-methyldopa. This metabolite can potentially compete with levodopa for absorption and transport into the central nervous system, where it may compete at dopamine receptors. COMT is a widely distributed enzyme, most of its activity being concentrated in the splanchnic area, particularly in the liver. The effect of inhibiting the enzyme is to produce sustained and stable plasma levels of levodopa and reduced production of 3-O-methyldopa.[33] Two COMT inhibitors – tolcapone and entacapone – have reached the stage of being licensed for use in the UK. However, the licence for tolcapone was suspended in 1998 because of problems with hepatotoxicity, leaving entacapone the only currently available COMT inhibitor. Studies in animals confirmed that entacapone increased both plasma and brain levels of levodopa when combined with a levodopa decarboxylase inhibitor preparation, while reducing levels of 3-O-mythyldopa.[34] Positron emission tomography (PET) studies demonstrated increased striatal uptake of the levodopa analogue, fluridopa, in a monkey model when the animals were treated with entacapone.[35] In contrast to tolcapone, animal studies with entacapone showed no evidence of hepatotoxicity.[36] Phase I and phase II clinical studies showed that the pharmacokinetics of entacapone and levodopa were similar, and this led to the co-administration of both drugs.[37] Neither age nor renal function changed the pharmacokinetic profile.[38] Patients with severe hepatic impairment showed enhanced drug levels, with no evidence of exacerbation of already existing liver damage.[39] In addition (at least in theory), a lower dose of the drug could be used patients with hepatic failure. At present, the drug is only available in one preparation, which is not scored (and therefore cannot be broken); thus, as dose reduction in these circumstances is difficult, the drug is contraindicated.

Clinical studies on a dosage of 200 mg of entacapone, combined with standard doses of levodopa/decarboxylase inhibitors, have shown that the plasma level of levodopa is sustained without changes to the peak levodopa concentration (C_{max}).[40] The time–concentration curve is flattened, and the area under the curve is increased, such that less dose-to-dose variation is produced. In theory, avoidance of the rapid cycling of plasma levels should reduce the motor complication of dyskinesia. Two major randomized, placebo-controlled trials have been undertaken with entacapone as adjunct therapy in patients with complicated late-stage PD: the 'Nomicomt' study in Scandinavia, and the 'See Saw' Study of North America.[41,42] These studies have provided highly consistent results, with on average an increase of

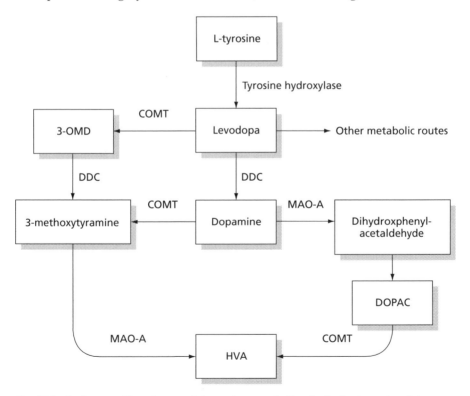

Fig. 17.1 Pathways of levodopa and dopamine metabolism in the brain and periphery. COMT = catechol-O-methyltransferase; DDC = dopa decarboxylase; DOPAC = dihydroxyphenylacetic acid; HVA = homovanillic acid; MAO-A = mono amine oxidase type A; 3-OMD = 3-O-methyldopa.

20 per cent 'on' time in patients treated with entacapone, and with good tolerability. Measurable effects both on motor function and activities of daily living were demonstrable. The use of a COMT inhibitor allowed a reduction of levodopa dosage, on average by 100 mg per day.

Most clinicians have shown considerable caution towards COMT inhibitors following sudden suspension of the tolcapone licence in Europe. Although having a similar target enzyme, there are significant differences between tolcapone and entacapone. Both are nitrocatechols, but tolcapone is more lipophilic due to its hydrocarbon side chain, and this results in increased penetration into the brain and mitochondria. Tolcapone had its action predominantly within the central nervous system, whereas entacapone predominantly affects the splanchnic distribution of COMT. In high concentration, tolcapone has been shown to have actions on oxidative phosphorylation in mitochondria, uncoupling the electron transport chain from ATP production – an essential component on the detoxification of drugs. The reason for the rare idiosyncratic hepatic liver failure with tolcapone may be a combination of an unusual genotype in a patient who is unable to detoxify the drug.[43] Due to this reason, tolcapone's licence in Europe has been suspended. Entacapone has been shown to have no adverse effects on hepatic function, and monitoring of hepatic function is unnecessary. The side effects of entacapone are remarkably benign, with only two side effects standing out in comparison with placebo. The first is an increase in dyskinesia, which is a reflection of increased dopaminergic activity; the second is a slight increase in diarrhoea. Unlike the diarrhoea seen with tolcapone, this is usually not severe and is tolerated by most patients and easily controlled with codeine. Entacapone has the unusual property of chelating iron, and is therefore contraindicated in patients taking oral iron preparations.

Entacapone is licensed for adjunctive use with levodopa, and is a useful tool in managing potential adverse effects of levodopa. The strongest indication for its use is end of dose wearing off (diminution of the effect of levodopa before the next dose is due). COMT inhibition may potentiate dopaminergic side effects, and it is therefore desirable to reduce the levodopa dosage by about 100 mg per day on introduction.

COMT inhibitors can be prescribed safely with other anti-parkinsonian drugs. It must be noted that COMT is involved in the metabolism of apomorphine, methyldopa, antidepressants, dopamine and dobutamine, adrenaline, noradrenaline and isoprenaline, and may theoretically enhance the effects of these drugs.[44] Caution is advised in prescribing COMT inhibitors with some antidepressants, particularly non-selective mono-amino oxidase inhibitors such as phenelzine and meclopamide, and with any of the noradrenaline uptake inhibitors such as venlafaxine. However, no significant clinical interaction has been reported to date.

COMT inhibitors are a welcome addition to the treatment of PD, and promise to be especially helpful in the management of elderly patients.

Selegiline

Selegiline is a selective, irreversible inhibitor of mono amine oxidase type B, the principal enzyme responsible for dopamine metabolism within the central nervous system.[45] The reason for giving selegiline in PD is to slow the breakdown of dopamine, and hence prolong its activity centrally. However, other possible pharmacological properties of selegiline have led to its widespread use. For example, selegiline penetrates the brain extensively, and is also able to target areas of the brain with a high mono amine oxidase type B enzyme content. A mild antidepressive effect is described, although this is less than is achieved with mono-amine oxidase A inhibitors. This mood enhancement may be partly due to mild amphetamine-like effects of the metabolites of selegiline, which include D-methyl selegiline, L-methyl amphetamine and L-amphetamine. Crucial to the argument for the use of selegiline was the hope that it would be one of the first neuroprotective drugs available. The pathogenesis of PD may be due to oxidative stress, leading to the generation of free radicals that damage macromolecules in the mitochondrial complex I, leading to the death of dopaminergic cells. This theory is based largely on the 2-methyl-4-phenyl-1,2,3,6-tetra-hydro-pyridine (MPTP) model of PD. MPTP causes toxicity in animals and man when metabolized by mono amine oxidase B to the free radical metabolite MPP^+; this is taken up selectively by the dopamine transport system and targets mitochondrial complex I. Inhibiting mono-amine oxidase B was shown to render MPTP non-toxic, and selegiline inhibits cell death and has neurotrophic effects.[46] A major study into the value of selegiline and vitamin E as anti-oxidants was undertaken in the United States – the DATATOP trial.[47] The use of selegiline was shown to delay the necessity of introducing levodopa. This was initially thought to be a neuroprotective effect, but it was soon realized that selegiline had its own symptomatic effects on PD. Despite the results of the Sindepar study of 1995 being consistent with a neuroprotective effect,[48] it is now largely discounted that selegiline has any neuroprotective effect. A long follow-up of the DATATOP cohort showed that the initial advantages of selegiline treatment were not sustained.[49,50] The United Kingdom Parkinson's Disease Research Group Trial (UK PDRG) followed over 700 PD patients in a randomized, open study of either levodopa alone, levodopa + selegiline, or bromocriptine alone. Although selegiline was shown to have a levodopa-sparing effect, the combination did not produce the expected benefit in long-term complications, and was associated with a significant (60 per cent) increase in mortality.[51] Not surprisingly, this result has fuelled an on-going debate as to the value of selegiline, as the findings of this study were incompatible with results of other studies with selegiline which did not show an increase, but rather a possible reduction, in mortality.[52-55] The UK PDRG trial was a pragmatic trial, and included many patients who would not normally be included in major trials. Moreover, there has been considerable controversy over the statistical analysis and the design of the trial,[56] a retrospective examination not having provided a clear mechanism or explanation of the excess deaths, though it was noted that a history of falls or dementia would be more likely to be associated with sudden death. The clinical experience with selegiline is extensive, and evidence from controlled trials confirms that adding the drug to levodopa can reduce disability scores and fluctuations in advanced disease. The use of selegiline allows a dose reduction of levodopa of around 30 per cent.[57] Selegiline has a relatively long half-life, and is recommended as a once-daily dose of 10 mg, although in many elderly patients 5 mg is sufficient. Giving the drug later in the day is especially liable to cause sleep disturbance, and is particularly liable to worsen hallucinations or vivid dreams, probably due to the production of amphetamine metabolites.[58] As with any drug that enhances dopaminergic action, dyskinesia may be worsened by the introduction of selegiline. Potentially, the drug may interact with antidepressants, selective serotonin re-uptake inhibitors and non-selective mono-amine oxidase inhibitors. A serotonergic syndrome with episodes of hypotension has also been described. Selegiline potentially can also cause disturbance of autonomic function.[59] Abrupt withdrawal of selegiline is not to be recommended, as in about 50 per cent of patients it leads to an exacerbation of parkinsonian symptoms, while in extreme cases it can be associated with depression and weight loss.

A new sublingual formulation of selegiline – Zelapar 1.25 mg daily – is now available, and this gives much more predictable and constant plasma levels than conventional selegiline, and much reduced levels of amphetamine metabolites.[60] Zelapar is awaiting full appraisal in double-blind, controlled trials. Its major advantage is in patients who are beginning to get hallucinations or cognitive impairment when taking selegiline, but who find it difficult to withdraw from the drug. A quite marked improvement can be made by transferring to Zelapar.

Anti-muscarinic drugs

Muscarinic receptor blockers are the first class of drugs to show any effect on parkinsonian symptoms, and were introduced by Charcot in the nineteenth century in the form of belladonna. Dopamine deficiency in PD leads to failure to inhibit excitatory cholinergic stimulation. Excess cholinergic stimulation is thought to be particularly important in the genesis of tremor, and anti-muscarinic drugs have been shown to have significant anti-tremor effects.[61] These drugs have very little effect on the core disabling signs of rigidity and bradykinesia, however. Anti-muscarinic drugs have been shown to have significant adverse effects on cognitive function. Although these effects are more evident in older patients, they are not limited solely to the elderly, and one study showed that 70 per cent of patients prospectively placed on anti-cholinergics developed worsening of cognitive function. Drugs which have incidental anti-muscarinic effects (e.g. oxybutinin, used to control hyper-reflexia of the bladder) have also been shown to worsen the cognitive and psychiatric symptoms in PD patients.[62] It has been shown that this class of drugs could impair memory even in young, healthy volunteers.[63] Because of this high side-effect profile that included other autonomic effects such as dry mouth, difficulty in swallowing and constipation, these drugs are certainly not to be recommended in older patients, and should largely be of historical interest. It is a common misconception that they are effective in the prevention of parkinsonian signs and tardive dyskinesia in patients on neuroleptic drugs, whereas in fact they may worsen both of these conditions. Procyclidine and benztropine, when given parentally, have been shown to be effective as emergency treatment for acute drug-induced dystonic reactions, and this is probably now their main indication for use.[64]

Amantadine

Amantadine is an unusual drug in that its anti-parkinsonian effect was discovered when it was used as an anti-viral agent; only by chance was amantadine found to improve parkinsonism. The drug has been available for over 30 years, despite which the evidence base of its actions is incomplete.[65,66] Pharmacologically, amantadine is much more complex than was once thought, since although it resembles anti-cholinergic drugs in some respects, its main anti-Parkinson effects appear to be by modulating dopamine re-uptake and releasing dopamine stores. More recently, amantadine has been shown to have anti-NMDA receptor activity, blocking the action of glutamate within the basal ganglia circuitry. There are reports that it may be beneficial in reducing levodopa-induced dyskinesia.[67] The recommended dose for amantadine is 100 mg daily, increased after 1 week to 100 mg twice daily, to a maximum dose of 400 mg. The drug must be used with caution in the elderly, and a daily dose of 200 mg rarely needs to be exceeded. Amantadine is best used as adjunct therapy, and it is useful to give a short-term boost to anti-parkinsonian treatment for a specific event such as a wedding or outing. There are many cautions and potential interactions with this drug. In particular, it should be avoided in patients with hepatic or renal impairment as it may cause significant fluid retention and can cause significant vasculitis.[68] In longer-term use it is difficult to withdraw, and side effects such as weight loss, cognitive impairment and hallucinations become more evident.

Dopamine agonists

Dopamine agonists have been available to treat PD for over 20 years. These drugs have the theoretical advantage that they act directly on the postsynaptic receptors and, unlike levodopa, are not dependent on the degenerating presynaptic nigrostriatal neurones. Like many other neurotransmitters, dopamine does not simply fulfil one function in the brain. This heterogeneity of action and tissue distribution is reflected by the different classes and subtypes of dopamine receptor (D1–D5), which results in as many as 10 recognisably different dopamine receptors. The dopamine receptors are classified into two major classes: D1-like receptors (D1 and D5); and D2 microceptors (D2, D3 and D4). The caudate nucleus and putamen contain a high density of

D1 and D2 receptors which are concerned with motor function, the D1 receptor being involved in the direct motor loop and the D2 receptor in the indirect motor loop. Receptors in the neostriatum are concerned almost exclusively with movement. D3 receptors are localized in the limbic areas, and have effects on behaviour, mood and emotion. D3, D4 and D5 receptors are also expressed in other areas of the brain, but their function is less clearly understood than that of D1 and D2 receptors.[69] The ideal dopamine agonist would target simply motor function. Unfortunately, most of the dopamine agonists available do have non-motor side effects, particularly effects on cognitive function and a tendency to produce hallucinosis. Nevertheless, the potential for selective dopamine receptor activation is an important consideration in choosing drugs to treat PD.[70,71]

Because dopamine agonists reduce the turnover of endogenous dopamine they (theoretically) have a mechanism for producing neuroprotection by producing oxidative stress generated by the metabolism of dopamine. Evidence points towards the possibility of neuroprotection for a variety of dopamine agonists, but the case remains unproven.[72] Dopamine agonists appear to have a longer striatal half-life compared with levodopa – a useful advantage in the management of PD patients.[73]

In most trials of dopamine agonists the withdrawal rate is higher than that for levodopa. In the first major study of a dopamine agonist, 70 per cent of patients were withdrawn from bromocriptine treatment, reporting nausea and vomiting as major problems.[74] The nausea can be helped by using domperidone for a short period only, since there is evidence that long-term domperidone has adverse effects including anorexia and weight loss, especially in older people.

More significantly, neuropsychiatric effects are described with all dopamine agonists, including sleep disturbance and somnolence.[75] Frucht and his colleagues have described a series of eight PD patients involved in car accidents attributable to falling asleep at the wheel.[76] These patients were treated with non-ergot-derived dopamine agonists (either pramipexole or ropinirole). Since this report, patients on these drugs have been advised to be cautious while driving or using machinery. A number of disturbances of sleep have been described in patients on oral anti-parkinsonian medication, including insomnia, fragmented sleep, parasomnias (abnormal behaviour or movement during sleep – most commonly restless legs) and disorders involving excessive daytime sleepiness.[77] Although dopamine is linked with arousal mechanisms, dopaminergic drugs in general can induce daytime somnolence. Patients given dopamine agonists need to be warned about these effects. Particular attention has to be paid to the contribution of other drugs; for example, cimetidine can interfere with dopamine agonist metabolism, while alcohol which can exaggerate the somnolence.[78]

Elderly patients frequently have postural hypotension, and this can be exacerbated by any dopaminergic drug. In all trials so far reported dopamine agonists have caused a higher incidence of dizziness and falls than levodopa, particularly in elderly patients. Most comparative trials show that the complaints of fatigue and tiredness are greater with dopamine agonists. Like all dopaminergic drugs, dopamine agonists may worsen dyskinesia when combined with levodopa, but overall dyskinesia appears to be less severe with this class of drug.[79] A rare side effect of dopamine agonists can be pulmonary fibrosis or retroperitoneal fibrosis, which has been described with ergot-derived agonists.

Dopamine agonists can be used to delay the introduction of levodopa and also to its dosage, holding out the prospect of reducing long-term levodopa syndrome.[80] The sustained receptor stimulation by long-acting dopamine agonists is likely, on theoretical grounds, to lessen the incidence of dyskinesia.[81] Evidence in cultured dopamine neurones of an increase in neurotrophic growth factors, free radical scavenging and reducing dopamine turnover is encouraging to the theory of neuroprotection.[82] Dopamine agonists are more likely to be neuroprotective than levodopa.

There is a balance of arguments about the appropriate use of dopamine agonists, and increasingly attention is being paid to the advantage of starting patients on monotherapy. It is very difficult to evaluate this argument when it is applied to elderly patients. Levodopa provides better symptomatic relief and fewer side effects, and is also considerably cheaper and easier to use; in contrast, dopamine agonists hold out the possibility of causing fewer long-term motor complications. As with many arguments in medicine, the evidence is still incomplete, and the decision whether to use levodopa or a dopamine agonist is very much based on the consideration of what is best for the individual patient.

Bromocriptine

Bromocriptine, an ergot derivative, was introduced in 1974 and is the oldest dopamine agonist used to treat PD. The long-term efficacy of bromocriptine is very much in question. Most published studies show that less than one-third of patients can be maintained on this drug, with most patients stopping treatment in the longer term because of gastric or neuropsychiatric side effects. Bromocriptine has a longer half-life than levodopa, its action lasting between 2 and 6 h. The starting dose is 1.25 mg at night, increasing to an average dose of ~10 mg per day to control motor symptoms, but some advanced patients may require much larger doses (up to 40 mg per day) to produce significant benefit.[83-92]

Lisuride

Lisuride is a highly water-soluble, short-acting dopamine agonist which acts on both D1 and D2 receptors.[93] A starting dose of 0.5 mg can be increased to a maximum of 3 mg. Lisuride was introduced because it could be administered either orally, intravenously or subcutaneously, and was useful to support PD patients through gastric surgery.[94] Lisuride has a reputation for producing more neuropsychiatric side effects than other dopamine agonists, and for this reason is little used in the UK.

Pergolide

Pergolide is the most widely used dopamine agonist in the UK. It has a balanced action of D1 and D2 receptor stimulation, being particularly potent at the important D2 receptor. There is evidence that there is an interrelationship between D1 and D2 stimulation, and this balanced agonist activity is thought by many to be the ideal profile for a dopamine agonist. Pergolide is an extremely well-referenced drug from many clinical studies. It is effective at reversing motor deficits and increasing motor activity, and can reduce dyskinetic movements.[94-96] Pergolide is licensed as an adjunctive therapy to levodopa. It has a relatively low propensity to induce nausea, vomiting and psychosis, but these effects are still seen. Uniquely, it has a beneficial effect on bladder function in PD. Pergolide has an intermediate half-life, its action lasting for up to 6 h. Pergolide requires careful titration on introduction, from low doses to high doses. The starting dose is 50 μg daily for two days, increasing by increments of 100 μg, and 150 μg every third day, titrating up to a dose of 1 mg three times per day. A starter pack is available for titration, and has been validated for use in older people.[97,98] Pergolide has been shown clinically in an open study to be effective in selected elderly patients.[99] Comparative studies with bromocriptine show pergolide in a favourable light.

Cabergoline

Cabergoline is an ergot derivative, which has the longest half-life of any orally acting dopamine agonist (63–68 h), and a high affinity for the D2 receptor.[100] Cabergoline has the advantage of a once-daily dosage, and although its licence is now only for adjunctive use, it has great potential as a monotherapy.[101] Cabergoline has an extremely 'clean' pharmacological profile, with no adverse effects on serotonin or noradrenaline metabolism.[102] The rationale for its use is that it allows continuous dopaminergic stimulation. Controlled clinical studies have demonstrated that cabergoline administered once daily at an average dose of 4 mg is effective in decreasing daily fluctuations in motor performance,[103] while substantially reducing the levodopa/carbidopa dose.[104]

Due to its long half-life, titration of cabergoline in elderly people must be carried out with caution, starting with doses as low as 1 mg per day. Concurrent levodopa doses need to be reduced.[105] The drug appears to have a low incidence of postural hypotension, although careful monitoring in the first few days of treatment is required because of reports of hypotensive reactions.[106] Cabergoline is reported to be effective in restless leg syndrome, and is successful in preventing nocturnal disabilities in PD patients.

One major advantage that cabergoline has is increased compliance due to the once-daily dosage;[107] this is a particularly useful aid to reduce the drug burden in patients with multiple drug regimes.[108]

Ropinirole

Ropinirole is a non-ergot dopamine agonist, which has specific D2 receptor selectivity and a high affinity for the D3 receptor. The drug is licensed for monotherapy as well as adjunctive therapy. In July 1999, a 5-year double blind, placebo-controlled trial of ropinirole versus levodopa was reported in Vancouver at an international meeting, although results have not yet been published in peer review form.[109] Of the ropinirole-treated patients who completed the study, 34 per cent of were receiving monotherapy, and these patients had a very low incidence of dyskinesia. Initial treatment with ropinirole was associated with a lower incidence of dyskinesia when compared with levodopa treatment, regardless of whether the patient subsequently required supplementary levodopa or not. The overall dyskinesia rate in patients taking levodopa was 46 per cent, whereas in those starting on ropinirole it was 20 per cent. The study involved 268 patients with early PD treated for 5 years, with clinicians able to titrate the drugs freely to maximum efficacy. Patients in either group could be supplemented with open-labelled levodopa if they required additional anti-parkinsonian effects. Ropinirole appeared to be as effective as levodopa in the early stages in relieving parkinsonian symptoms, but as the disease progressed levodopa was seen to have a slight advantage.[110]

This study showed a lower than expected risk of neuropsychiatric side effects. Synthetic dopamine agonists such as ropinirole have fewer ergot side effects, but do have a tendency to show central effects – particularly on sleep. Recently, it has become necessary to warn patients taking ropinirole about a possible risk of sleepiness when driving. If sleep attacks do occur when driving the dose should be reduced, but rarely stopped. Patients should refrain from driving until this situation is resolved.

Ropinirole is used initially at a daily dose level of 750 μg in three divided doses, and may be increased by increments of 750 μg weekly until a daily dose of 3 mg is reached. Further titration can then be carried out, with an ultimate daily dose ranging between 3 and 9 mg, and a maximum of 24 mg.[111–113]

Pramexipole

Pramipexole is a synthetic non-ergot derivative, which is highly selective for D2 and D3 receptors.[114] Pramipexole, which has a half-life of ~12 h,[115, 116] has been extensively studied in three major double-blind, placebo-controlled multicentre trials in advanced disease, and two studies in early PD.[117–121] Currently, pramexipole is licensed for adjunct use in advanced PD, where it has been shown that the levodopa dose could be reduced by up to 30 per cent and improvement was scored on motor disabilities, motor fluctuations and reduction of dyskinesia. Pramipexole appears to have particular beneficial effects both on mood and tremor.[122] In the treatment of depression, pramipexole has an efficacy comparable with that of fluoxetine; this could be useful in the treatment of elderly patients in whom depression is common.[123] In addition to anecdotal reports, several studies have now confirmed that there is significant improvement of tremor using pramipexole. It has also shown to be effective in restless leg syndrome.

The side effects of pramipexole include daytime somnolence and sleep disturbance at night, and there have been reports of sudden sleep attacks. People taking this drug have been advised not to drive, and this may limit its use in younger people. There is strong in-vitro evidence that pramipexole causes increased dopamine neurotrophic activity. The drug has only recently been introduced into the UK, and to date no specific studies have been conducted in elderly patients. Sudden hypotensive reactions have been reported in the early stages of treatment, and introduction of the drug needs to be closely monitored. The initial dose should be 264 µg daily in three divided doses (each of 88 µg), after which the dose may be doubled every 5–7 days using the 180 µg tablets until a daily dose of 1.08 mg is arrived at (still in three divided doses). Further titration may occur by larger increments of 540 µg daily at weekly intervals, up to a maximum dose of 3.3 mg/day in three divided doses. Following titration, it is necessary to lower levodopa dosage by 25–30 per cent.[124]

Apomorphine

Apomorphine is a unique drug for use in late-stage PD. It is the most effective dopamine agonist, and has clinical efficacy equivalent to levodopa. It is given by the subcutaneous route by intermittent injection using insulin syringes or by Penject injection, the latter being more straightforward but also more expensive. The intermittent injection rescues the patient from the 'off' state within 5–15 min of administration, and the effects last for about 1 h. In more advanced cases where more than about eight rescue injections are needed each day, apomorphine can be given by continuous waking day subcutaneous infusion using an ambulatory syringe driver. The dosage of apomorphine needs to be titrated for individual patients. The dose range is very wide, from a few milligrams per day by intermittent injection up to 150 mg/day by continuous infusion (the current licence recommends up to 100 mg).[125] Continuous infusions are useful in patients in whom dyskinesia may be a limiting side effect of intermittent injections. Continuous infusion over a period of months, together with reduction of other dopaminergic drugs, may significantly reduce dyskinesia.[125] Most patients ultimately progress from intermittent injections to continuous infusion of apomorphine.

Apomorphine is selective for D1, D2 and D3 receptors, and has no opiate or addictive properties. It cannot be used orally because of extensive hepatic first-pass metabolism.[124] Formulations using other routes of administration have been piloted (e.g. rectal or sublingual), but none is currently available commercially.[127–129]

In order to establish apomorphine therapy, an 'apomorphine challenge' is necessary to ascertain whether the patient responds to the drug and to determine the individual threshold dose. In addition, careful monitoring for side effects, such as postural hypotension or neuropsychiatric symptoms, must be undertaken. Before a patient is exposed to apomorphine it is necessary to pre-scribe domperidone 30 mg orally every 8 h for at least 3 days. Domperidone blocks the very strong emetic effects that previously limited the use of apo-morphine. The patient is initially induced into an 'off' state by withdrawing oral medication overnight. In order to avoid a possible hypotensive reaction it is best to perform the test with the patient recumbent. An initial dose of 1.5 mg of apomorphine is given subcutaneously, after which the patient's motor responses are observed for up to 30 min. If there is no response, a subsequent dose of 3 mg is given, followed by 1.5-mg incremental steps until a response is seen. If no response is seen by 7.5 mg, the patient is classified as a non-responder and is unlikely to benefit from apomorphine. The hourly infusion rate for continuous infusion can be established by using the threshold dose from an apomorphine challenge test, or by transferring the intermittent dose directly to an hourly rate. In frail patients in whom there are concerns about performing a challenge test, a low-dose infusion of 1 mg/h can be started after pretreatment with domperidone, but without withdrawal of any other oral therapy. This infusion rate can be gradually increased hourly or even daily, depending upon the patient, until a response or unacceptable side effects are seen. During any assessment of apomorphine treatment, it is useful to assess patients using a motor scale such as the UPDRS, or alternatively to video patients. The sites of injection must be rotated in order to minimize local skin reactions and the formation of subcutaneous nodules. Nodule formation can be reduced by scrupulous technique, and ultrasound of local nodules can help to reduce their size. The needle site for infusions should ideally be changed daily, but some patients prefer to change on alternate days. Apomorphine treatment is quite demanding, and the support of a PD nurse specialist is valuable in instructing the patient or carers in intermittent subcutaneous injection or infusion pump techniques.

The side effects of apomorphine include dyskinesia, confusion, hallucina-tions, postural hypotension and sleepiness. Eosinophilia associated with myalgia, and haemolytic anaemia (usually in conjunction with levodopa treatment) have also been described. It is recommended that a haematological blood count be performed every 6 months in patients receiving apomorphine.[130]

Apomorphine is useful in pre- and postoperative situations such as gastric surgery, where oral medication may be discontinued. It can also be used in other withdrawal symptoms from dopaminergic therapy such as the rare malignant neuroleptic syndrome.[131]

Apomorphine now has a very firm place in the treatment of advanced PD, and is certainly suitable for the older patient – provided that sufficient super-vision and support can be given.

Future development of anti-parkinsonian medication

As it is perceived that the potential world-wide market for anti-parkinsonian drugs is very large, it follows that at any one time a large number of compounds will be under development for the treatment of PD.[132] A greater understanding of the pathophysiology of PD has led to other neurotransmitter systems being targeted. There is particular interest in anti-glutamate (NMDA) receptor drugs, including riluzole and remacemide, both of which are being investigated for the control of dyskinetic movements. Idazoxan, an alpha-adrenergic antagonist, is being studied for its anti-dyskinetic activity, and a number of adenosine antagonists are also under trial. Nerve regeneration using growth factors may be a future adjunct to surgery. Drugs, which may modify free radical generation (e.g. such as spin-trap agents or anti-oxidants) are still under research. Targets within the dopaminergic system are still being explored, including specific D1 stimulators and drugs that affect the dopamine transporter system, such as prasofensin.

Novel methods to deliver these drugs, such as transdermal patches (a possibility for some dopamine agonists), sublingual preparations involving methyl and ethyl esters of levodopa, and newer systems of controlled release are all at the stage of early development.

Management strategies in elderly PD patients

The concept of a treatment algorithm has gained ground over the past few years with the publication of numerous guidelines for the treatment of PD. In 1998, the Parkinson's Disease Consensus Working Group attempted to weigh the evidence for the differing strategies which may be used in managing the individual PD patient. As the evidence is incomplete and requires interpretation, the individual clinician must produce an effective management plan faced with a unique patient. This plan will include many non-pharmacological interventions as described in other chapters of this book. However, the essential decision points in management are four-fold.

Is this idiopathic PD, which will respond to anti-parkinsonian medication?

Many patients are treated with anti-parkinsonian drugs unnecessarily, particularly patients with arteriosclerotic, pseudo-PD or essential tremor. It is hoped that other chapters in this book will clarify the differential diagnosis and reduce mistakes made in this area.

When should we start treatment?

As all present treatment is symptomatic, the severity of the symptoms should dictate when the drug is introduced. Because of the theoretical involvement of levodopa in the process of oxidative stress, there is controversy as to whether the introduction of levodopa should be delayed. An early study of Markham and Diamond showed that a delay in the introduction of levodopa had no effect on late levodopa complications.[12] Most of the evidence indicates that a delay in the introduction of levodopa has very little benefit in the older patient.

Which drug should be used to initiate treatment?

This is the crucial question, since the choice of initial drug dictates the rest of the strategy over many years. There is a lively debate, with experts arguing for and against initiating with levodopa or a dopamine agonist. Levodopa and decarboxylase inhibitor combined preparations are effective at symptom relief, easy to titrate, well tolerated, and inexpensive. Dopamine agonists have the promise of reducing long-term dyskinetic side effects and good efficacy, but are less well tolerated, require more complicated titration to achieve therapeutic dose, and are more expensive. In the younger patient, the probability of long-term levodopa syndrome is high, within life expectancy. In patients aged over 75 years, with low doses, the majority of patients escape long-term levodopa syndrome, and there is therefore a strong argument for using levodopa as first choice treatment in this group. This is particularly so since multiple pathology and mild cognitive impairment are common in older patients and correlate with intolerance of dopamine agonists. Some elderly patients are recognizably biologically fit, with no overt degenerative disease or cognitive impairment. In these patients, the choice between dopamine agonists and levodopa should be discussed openly. The arguments put forward in this chapter may be put to the patient in an understandable form, giving patients some choice. This choice can sometimes be complicated by the publicity surrounding the introduction of new dopamine agonists. Patients and carers may be given the impression that a new 'wonder' drug has been developed for the disease, and so careful patient education is required. If levodopa is chosen, it is logical to maintain steady blood levels, using controlled-release preparations and the introduction of a COMT inhibitor, when wearing-off problems or nocturnal problems arise. We may see a trend to earlier use of the COMT inhibitor, since it is a logical adjunct to levodopa and a decarboxylase inhibitor. Clinical studies with entacapone are increasingly substantiating its efficacy and value. In a patient who is receiving a dopamine agonist, the logical step – when the response begins to wane – is to add levodopa and then a COMT inhibitor before considering the advanced possibility of either apomorphine or surgery. For a patient on levodopa and a COMT inhibitor, a dopamine agonist can be added at a late stage. The wider choice of dopamine agonists is helpful since each has its own particular strengths and evidence base. Increasingly, the dopamine agonists can be targeted at specific problems, such as considering pramipexole for a depressed patient and cabergoline for a patient with nocturnal problems. Pergolide and ropinirole are extremely effective all-round agents and very well tolerated. The choices and sequencing of drugs are probably the most crucial decisions that the clinician has to make in the management of PD, though increasing knowledge and availability of new studies may make these decisions gradually more simple. The promise of new agents, such as NMDA receptor antagonists, may well further revolutionize our management of PD. The disease is predominantly one of elderly people in whom the associated problems of dementia, depression, hallucinosis, bladder symptoms, swallowing difficulties, speech difficulties, constipation and orthostatic hypotension make decisions more complicated.

References

1. *British National Formulary*, No. 38. London: British Medical Association/Royal Pharmaceutical Society, 1999.
2. Quinn N. Drug treatment of Parkinson's disease. *Br. Med. J.* 1995; **310**: 575–9.
3. Playfer JR. Classical diseases revisited, Parkinson's disease. *Postgrad. Med. J.* 1997; **73**: 257–64.
4. Swift CG. Clinical pharmacology and therapeutics. In: Pathy MSJ. (ed.). *Principles and Practice of Geriatric Medicine*, 3rd edn. Chichester: John Wiley & Sons Ltd, 1998: 251–69.
5. Stephen PJ, Williamson J. Drug-induced parkinsonism in the elderly. *Lancet* 1984; **ii**: 1082–3.
6. Bhatia K, Brooks DJ, Burn DJ, *et al*. Guidelines for the management of Parkinson's disease. *Hosp. Med.* 1998, **59**: 469–80.
7. Koller WC, Silver DE, Lieberman A. An algorithm for the management of Parkinson's disease. *Neurology* 1994; **44** (suppl. 10): S1–52.
8. Clough CG. Parkinson's disease: management. *Lancet* 1991; **337**: 1324–7.
9. Manyam BC. Practical guidelines for management of Parkinson's disease. *J. Am. Board Family Pract.* 1997; **10**: 412–24.
10. Gibberd FB. The management of Parkinson's disease. *Practitioner* 1986; **230**: 139–46.
11. Cotzias GC, Wan Woert MH, Schiffer LM. Aromatic amino acids and modification of parkinsonism. *N. Engl. J. Med.* 1967; **276**: 374–9.
12. Diamond SG, Markham CH, Techiokas LJ. A double blind comparison of levodopa, Madopar and Sinemet in Parkinson's disease. *Ann. Neurol.* 1978; **3**: 263–7.
13. Quinn N. Parkinson's disease – recognition and differential diagnosis. *Br. Med. J.* 1995; **310**: 447–52.
14. Koller WC, Hubble JP. Levodopa therapy in Parkinson's disease. *Neurology* 1990; **40** (suppl. 3): 40–7.
15. Marsden CD, Parkes JD. Success and problems of long-term levodopa therapy in Parkinson's disease. *Lancet* 1977; **i**: 345–9.
16. Marsden CD, Parkes JD, Quinn N. Fluctuations of disability in Parkinson's disease; clinical aspects. In: Marsden CD, Fahn S (eds). *Movement Disorders*. London: Butterworths, 1982: 96–122.
17. Nutt JG, Woodward WR. Levodopa pharmacokinetics and pharmacodynamics in fluctuating parkinsonian patients. *Neurology* 1986; **36**: 739–44.

18. Chase TN, Mouradian MM, Engber TM. Motor response complications and the function of striatal efferent systems. *Neurology* 1993; **43** (suppl. 6): 523–7.

19. Marsden CD. Parkinson's disease. *Lancet* 1990; **335**: 948–52.

20. Pahwah R, Lyons K, McGuire D, *et al.* Comparison of standard carbidopa-levodopa and sustained release carbidopa-levodopa in Parkinson's disease: pharmacokinetic and quality of life measures. *Movement Disord.* 1997; **12**: 677–81.

21. Hardie RJ, Lees AJ, Stern GM. On-off fluctuations in Parkinson's disease: a clinical and neuropharmacological study. *Brain* 1984; **107**: 487–506.

22. Marsden CD, Parkes JD. 'On/off' effects in patients with Parkinson's disease on chronic levodopa therapy. *Lancet* 1976; i: 292–6.

23. Riley DC, Lang AE, The spectrum of levodopa-related fluctuations in Parkinson's disease. *Neurology* 1993; **43**: 1459–64.

24. Lees AJ. The on-off phenomenon. *J. Neurol. Neurosurg. Psychiatry* 1989; **52** (suppl.): 29–37.

25. Kurth MC, Tetrud JW, Tanner CM, *et al.* Double-blind, placebo-controlled, crossover study of duodenal infusion of levo-dopa/carbidopa in Parkinson's disease patients with on-off fluctuations. *Neurology* 1993;**43**: 1698–703.

26. Ogawa N, Edamatsu R, Mizukawa K, *et al.* Degeneration of dopaminergic neurons and free radicals; possible participation of levodopa. In: Narabayashi H, Nagatsu T, Yanagisawa N, *et al.* (eds). *Advances in Neurology*, Vol. 60: New York: Raven Press, 1993: 242–50.

27. Koller WC, Pahwa R. Treating motor fluctuations with controlled-release levodopa preparations. *Neurology* 1994; **44** (suppl. 6): 23–8.

28. Block G, Liss C, Reines S, Irr J, Nibbelink D and the CR first Study Group. Comparison of immediate-release and controlled release carbidopa/levodopa in Parkinson's disease. *Eur. Neurol.* 1997; **37**: 23–7.

29. Grandas F, Martinez-Martin P, Linazasoro G, on behalf of the STAR Multicentre Study Group. Quality of life in patients with Parkinson's disease who transfer from standard levodopa to Sinemet CR: the STAR study. *J. Neurol.* 1998; **245** (suppl. I): S31–3.

30. Obeso JA, Grandas F, Herrero MT, Horowski R. The role of pulsatile versus continuous dopamine receptor stimulation for functional recovery in Parkinson's disease. *Eur. J. Neurosci.* 1994; 6: 889–97.

31. Frankel JP, Kempster PA, Bovingdom M, *et al.* The effects of oral protein on the absorption of intraduodenal levodopa and performance. *J. Neurol. Neurosurg. Psychiatry* 1989; **52**: 1063–7.

32. Verhagen Metman L, Hoff J, Mouradian MM, *et al.* Fluctuations in plasma levodopa and motor responses with liquid and tablet levodopa/carbidopa. *Movement Disord.* 1994: **9**: 463–5.

33. Mannisto PT, Kaakkola S, Nissiene E, *et al.* Properties of novel, effective and highly selective inhibitors of catechol-O-methyltransferase. *Life Sci.* 1988; **43**: 1465–71.

34. Kaakkola S, Gardin A, Mannisto P. General properties and clinical possibilities of new selective inhibitors of catechol-O-methyltransferase. *Gen. Pharmacol.* 1994; **25**: 813–24.

35. Sawle GV, Burns DJ, Marrish PK, *et al.* The effect of entacapone (OR-611) on brain [18F]-6-L-fluradopa metabolism: implications for levodopa therapy of Parkinson's disease. *Neurology* 1994; **44**: 1292–7.

36. Entacapone safety. Update Report, Orion Corporation, Finland, 1998.

37. Ruottinen HM, Rinne UK. Effect of one month's treatment with peripherally acting catechol-O-methyltransferase inhibitor, entacapone on pharmacokinetics and

motor response to levo dopa in advanced Parkinson's disease patients. *Clin. Neuropharmacol.* 1996; **19**: 222–3.

38. Myllyla VV, Filomen Study Group. Long term safety of entacapone as an adjunct to levodopa in non-fluctuating and fluctuating patients with Parkinson's disease. *Movement Disord.* 1998; **13** (suppl. 2): 294.

39. Gordin A, Pentikainen P, Makimartti M, *et al.* Pharmacokinetics of the COMT inhibitor entacapone in liver failure and the effect of entacapone on liver function. *Neurology* 1998; **50** (suppl. 4): A387.

40. Nutt JG, Woodward WR, Beckner RM, *et al.* Effect of peripheral catechol-O-methyl transferase inhibition on the pharmacokinetics and pharmacodynamics of levodopa in parkinsonian patients. *Neurology* 1994; **44**: 913–19.

41. Rinne UK, Larsen JP, Siden A, *et al.* Entacapone enhances the response to levodopa in parkinsonian patients with motor fluctuations. *Neurology* 1998; **51**: 1309–14.

42. Parkinson Study Group. Entacapone improves motor fluctuations in levodopa-treated Parkinson's disease patients. *Ann. Neurol.* 1997; **42**: 747–55.

43. Kicburtz K. Entacapone improves motor fluctuations in levodopa-treated Parkinson's disease patients. Parkinson's disease Study Group. *Ann. Neurol.* 1998; **42**: 747–55.

44. Lyytinen J, Kaakkola S, Ahtila S, *et al.* Simultaneous MAO-B and COMT inhibition in L-dopa treated patients with Parkinson's disease. *Movement Disord.* 1997; **12**: 497–505.

45. Myllyla VV, Sontaniemi K, Maki-Ikola O, *et al.* Role of Selegiline in combination therapy of Parkinson's disease. *Neurology* 1996; **47** (suppl. 3): S200–9.

46. Tatton WG, Greenwood CE. Rescue of dying neurones; a new action for deprenyl in MPTP parkinsonism. *J. Neurol. Sci.* 1991; **30**: 666–72.

47. Parkinson Study Group Effect of deprenyl on the progression of disability in early Parkinson's disease. *N. Engl. J. Med.* 1989; **321**: 1364–71.

48. Olanow CW, Hauser RA, Gauger L, *et al.* The effect of deprenyl and levodopa on the progression of Parkinson's disease. *Ann. Neurol.* 1995; **38**: 771–7.

49. The Parkinson Study Group. Mortality in DATA TOP: a multicentre trial in early Parkinson's disease. *Ann. Neurol.* 1998; **43**: 318–25.

50. The Parkinson Study Group. Impact of deprenyl and tocopherol treatment on Parkinson's disease in DATATOP patients requiring levodopa. *Ann. Neurol.* 1996; **39**: 37–45.

51. Lees AJ, on behalf of the Parkinson's Disease Research Group of the United Kingdom. Comparison of therapeutic effects and mortality data of levodopa and levodopa combined with selegiline in patients with early, mild Parkinson's disease. *Br. Med. J.* 1995; **311**: 1602–7.

52. Olanow CW, Mytileneou C, Tatton WG. Current status of selegiline as a neuroprotective agent in Parkinson's disease. *Movement Disord.* 1998; **13** (suppl. 3): 55–8.

53. Olanow CW, Fahn S, Langston JW, Godbold J. Selegiline and mortality in Parkinson's disease. *Ann. Neurol.* 1996: **40**: 841–5.

54. Olanow CW. Selegiline: current perspectives on issues related to neuroprotection and mortality. *Neurology* 1996; **47** (suppl. 3): S210–16.

55. Ben-Schlomo Y, Churchyard A, Head J, *et al.* Investigations by Parkinson's Disease Research Group of the United Kingdom into excess mortality seen with combined levodopa and selegiline treatment in patients with early, mild Parkinson's disease; further results of a randomised trial and confidential inquiry. *Br. Med. J.* 1998; **316**: 1191–6.

56. Thorogood M, Armstrong B, Nichols T, Hollowell J. Mortality in people taking selegiline; observation study. *Br. Med. J.* 1998; **317**: 252–4.

57. Robertson D. Drugs in focus: Selegiline. *Prescribers J.* 1999; **39**: 31–8.
58. Richard IH, Kurlan R, Factor S, *et al.* Serotonin syndrome and the combined use of deprenyl and an antidepressant in Parkinson's disease. *Neurology* 1997; **48**: 1070–7.
59. Churchyard A, Mathias CJ, Bookongcheun P, Lees AJ. Autonomic effects of selegiline: possible cardiovascular toxicity in Parkinson's disease. *J. Neurol. Neurosurg. Psychiatry* 1997; **63**: 228–34.
60. Mahmood I. Selegiline. *Clin. Pharmacokinet.* 1997; **33**: 91–102.
61. Duvaisin RC. Cholinergic-anticholinergic antagonism in Parkinsonism. *Ann. Neurol.* 1967; **17**: 124–6.
62. Donnellan CA, Fook L, McDonald P, Playfer JR. Oxybutin and cognitive deficits in Parkinson's disease. *Br. Med. J.* 1997; **315**: 1363–4.
63. Dubois B, Dange F, Pilln B. Cholinergic dependent cognitive deficits in Parkinson's disease. *Ann. Neurol.* 1987; **22**: 26–30.
64. Quinn N. Drug treatment in Parkinson's disease. *Drugs* 1994; **28**: 236–62.
65. Timberlake WH, Vance MA. Four year treatment of patients with parkinsonism using amantadine alone or with levodopa. *Ann. Neurol.* 1978; **3**: 119–28.
66. Parkes JD, Zilkha KG, Calven DM, Knill Jones RP. Controlled trial of amantidine hydrochloride in Parkinson's disease. *Lancet* 1970; **i**: 259–62.
67. Verhagen Metman L, Del Dotto P, van den Munekhof P, Fang J, Mouradian MM, Chase TN. Amantadine as treatment for dyskinesias and motor fluctuations in Parkinson's disease. *Neurology* 1998; **50**: 1323–6.
68. Utti RJ, Rajput AH, Ahlskog JE, *et al.* Amantadine treatment is an independent predictor of improved survival in Parkinson's disease. *Neurology* 1996; **46**; 1551–6.
69. Strange PC. Dopamine receptors in the basal ganglion: relevance to Parkinson's disease. *Movement Disord.* 1992; **8**: 263–70.
70. Playfer JR. Dopamine agonists in the elderly. *Geriatr. Med.* 1994; **3**: 240–6.
71. Jenner PO. Is stimulation of D_1 and D_2 dopamine receptors important for optimum motor functioning in Parkinson's disease. *Eur. J. Neurol.* 1997; **4**: 50–1.
72. Jenner P. The rationale for the use of dopamine agonists in Parkinson's disease. *Neurology* 1995; **45** (suppl. 3): S6–12.
73. Chase TN, Engber TM, Mouradian MM. Contribution of dopaminergic and glutamatergic mechanisms to the pathogenesis of motor response complications in Parkinson's disease. *Adv. Neurol.* 1996; **69**: 497–501.
74. Lees AJ, Stern GM. Sustained bromocriptine therapy in previously untreated patients with Parkinson's disease. *J. Neurol. Neurosurg. Psychiatry* 1981; **44**: 1020–3.
75. Pal PK, Calne S, Samii A, Fleming JAE. A review of normal sleep and its disturbances in Parkinson's disease *Parkinsonism Rel. Disord.* 1995; **5**: 1–17.
76. Frucht S, Rogers JD, Greene PE, Gordon MF, Fahn S. Falling asleep at the wheel: motor vehicle mishaps in persons taking pramipexole and ropinirole. *Neurology* 1999; **52**: 1908–10.
77. Partinen M. Sleep disorder related to Parkinson's disease. *J. Neurol.* 1997; **244**: 1–6.
78. Playfer JR. Sleep disorders in Parkinson's disease. A review. Geriatric Medicine 2001 (in press).
79. Poewe W. Should treatment of Parkinson's disease be started with a dopamine agonist? *Neurology* 1998; **51** (suppl. 2): S21–4.
79. Marsden CD, Parkes, JD. Success and problems of long-term therapy in Parkinson's disease. *Lancet* 1997; **ii**: 345–9.
80. Stern M. Contemporary approaches to the pharmacotherapeutic management of Parkinson's disease: an overview. *Neurology* 1997; **49** (suppl. 1): 52–9.
81. Koller WC, Tolosa E. Current and emerging drug therapies in the management of Parkinson's disease. *Neurology* 1998; **50** (suppl. 6): S1–39.

82. Fahn S, Clarence-Smith KE, Chase TN. Parkinson's disease: neurodegenerative intervention – report of a workshop. *Movement Disord.* 1998; **13**: 759–67.
83. Parkinson's Disease Research Group in the United Kingdom. Comparisons of therapeutic effects of levodopa, levodopa and selegiline and bromocriptine in patients with early, mild Parkinson's disease three year interim report. *Br. Med. J.* 1993; **307**: 469–72.
84. Montastrue JL, Rascol O, Senard JM, Rascol A. A randomised controlled study comparing bromocriptine to which levodopa was later added, with levodopa alone in previously untreated patients with Parkinson's disease. A five year follow up. *J. Neurol. Neurosurg. Psychiatry* 1994; **57**: 1034–8.
85. Factor SA, Weiner WJ. Early combination therapy with bromocriptine and levodopa in Parkinson's disease. *Movement Disord.* 1993; **8**: 257–62.
86. Weiner WJ, Factor SA. Sanchez-Ramos JR, *et al.* Early combination therapy (bromocriptine and levodopa) does not prevent motor fluctuations in Parkinson's disease. *Neurology* 1993; **43**: 21–7.
87. Gimenez-Roldan S, Tolosa E, Burguera JA, Chacon J, Liano H, Forcadell F. Early combination of bromocriptine and levodopa in Parkinson's disease; a prospective randomized study of two parallel groups over a total follow up period of 44 months including an initial 8 month double-blind stage. *Clin. Neuropharmacol.* 1997; **20**: 67–76.
88. Przuntek H, Welzel D, Gerlach M, *et al.* Early institution of bromocriptine in Parkinson's disease inhibits the emergence of levodopa-associated motor side effects. Long-term results of the PRADO study. *J. Neural Transm.* 1996; **103**: 699–715.
89. Rinne UK. Early combination of bromocriptine and levodopa in the treatment of Parkinson's disease: a 5-year follow-up. *Neurology* 1987; **37**: 826–8.
90. Hely MA, Morris JGL, Reid WGL, *et al.* The Sydney multicentre study of Parkinson's disease: a randomised, prospective five year study comparing low dose bromocriptine with low dose levodopa-carbidopa. *J. Neurol. Neurosurg. Psychiatry* 1994; **57**: 903–10.
91. Clarke CE, Speller JM. Pergolide versus bromocriptine for levodopa-induced motor complications in Parkinson's disease (Cochrane Review). In: The Cochrane Library, Issue I Oxford: Update Software, 1999.
92. Pezolli G, Martignoni E, Pacchetti C, *et al.* Pergolide compared in bromocriptine in Parkinson's disease: a multicentre, cross-over, controlled study. *Movement Disord.* 1994; **9**: 431–6.
93. Vaamonde J, Luquin MR, Obeso JA. Subcutaneous lisuride infusion in Parkinson's disease: response to chronic administration in 34 patients. *Brain* 1991; **114**: 601–14.
94. Olanow CW, Fahn S, Muenter M. A multicentre double blind placebo controlled trial of Pergolide as an adjunct to Sinemet in Parkinson's disease. *Movement Disord.* 1994; **9**: 40–7.
95. Sharma JC, Ross IN. Value of pergolide in managing disability in Parkinson's disease. *Movement Disord.* 1998; **13** (suppl. 2): 252 (P4.149).
96. Sharma JC, Brotherhood J. Blood pressure and weight change in Parkinson's disease patients on therapy with levodopa and pergolide. *Movement Disord.* 1998; **13** (suppl. 2): 252 (P148).
97. Meara RJ, Cassidy TP, Dunn A, *et al.* How should pergolide treatment be initiated in elderly patients with Parkinson's disease? *Age Ageing* 1997; **26** (suppl. 1): 16.
98. Metcalf P, Sagar HJ. Rapid dose titration of pergolide is safe and effective in very elderly patients with Parkinson's disease. *Movement Disord.* 1998; **13** (suppl. 2): 293 (P5.052).
99. Hindle JV, Meara RJ, Sharma JC, *et al.* Prescribing pergolide in the elderly – an

open label study of Pergolide in elderly patients with Parkinson's disease. *Int. J. Geriatr. Psychopharmacol.* 1998; **1**: 78–81.

100. Fariello R, Carfagna N, Buonamici M, *et al.* Cabergoline: a long acting D2 agonist with antiparkinsonian properties: preclinical studies (abstract). *Ann. Neurol.* 1991; **30**: 258.

101. Lera G, Vaamonde J, Murazabal LM, *et al.* Carbergoline: a long-acting dopamine agonist in Parkinson's disease. *Ann. Neurol.* 1990; **28**: 593–4.

102. Strolin-Benedetti M, Cocchiara G, Battaglia K, *et al.* Pharmacokinetic and metabolic pattern of cabergoline, a long-acting dopamine agonist in healthy volunteers. Presented at the 10th International Symposium on Parkinson's Disease; 1991 October, Tokyo.

103. Steiger MJ, El-Debas T, Anderson T, Findley IJ, Marsden CD. Double blind study of the activity and tolerability of cabergoline versus placebo in parkinsonians with motor fluctuations. *J. Neurol.* 1996; **243**: 68–72.

104. Lieberman A, Imke S, Muenter M, *et al.* Multicentre study of cabergoline a long acting dopamine receptor agonist, in Parkinson's disease patients with fluctuating responses to levodopa/carbidopa. *Neurology* 1993; **43**: 1981–4.

105. Hutton JT, Koler WC, Ahlskog JE, *et al.* Multicentre placebo-controlled trial of cabergoline taken once daily in the treatment of Parkinson's disease. *Neurology* 1996; **46**: 1062–5.

106. Inzelberg R, Nisipeanu P, Rabey JM, *et al.* Double blind comparison of cabergoline and bromocriptine in Parkinson's disease patients with motor fluctuations. *Neurology* 1996; **47**: 785–8.

107. Rinne UK, Bracco F, Chouza C *et al.* and the PKDS009 Collaborative Study Group. Cabergoline in the treatment of early Parkinson's disease. Results of the first year of treatment in a double blind comparison of cabergoline and levodopa. *Neurology* 1997; **48**: 363–8.

108. Rinne UK, Bracco F, Chouza C *et al.* and the PDS009 Study Group. Early treatment of Parkinson's disease with cabergoline delays the onset of motor complications. Results of a double-blind levodopa controlled trial. *Drugs* 1998; **55** (suppl. 1): 23–30.

109. Rascol O, Brooks DJ, Korczyn AD, De Deyn PP, Clarke CE, Lang AE. A five year follow up study of the incidence of dyskinesia in patients with Parkinson's disease who were treated with ropinirole or levodopa. 056 Study Group. *N. Engl. J. Med.* 2000; **342**: 1484–91.

110 Calne D, Jenner P. *New Prospects in the Early Treatment of Parkinson's Disease.* SKB Publishers, 1999, London.

111. Sethi KD, O'Brien CF, Hammerstad JP *et al.* for the Ropinirole Study Group. Ropinirole for the treatment of early Parkinson's disease. *Arch. Neurol.* 1998; **55**: 1211–16.

112. Perez-Aharon J, Abbot RJ, Playfer JR, *et al.* Ropinirole: a placebo controlled study of efficacy as an adjunct therapy in parkinsonian patients not optimally controlled on L-dopa (abstract). *Neurology* 1994; **44** (suppl. 2): 244.

113. Brooks DJ, Abbott RJ, Lees AJ, *et al* A placebo-controlled evaluation of ropinirole, a novel D_2 agonist, as sole dopaminergic therapy in Parkinson's disease. *Clin. Neuropharmacol.* 1998; **21**: 101–7.

114. Mierau J, Schneider FJ, Ensinger HA, *et al.* Pramipexole binding and activation of cloned and expressed dopamine D_2 D_3 and D_4 receptors. *Eur. J. Pharmacol. Mol. Pharmacol.* 1995; **290**: 29–36.

115. Wright CE, Lasher Sisson T, Ichhpurani AK, *et al.* Steady-state pharmacokinetic properties of pramipexole in healthy volunteers. *Clin. Pharmacol.* 1997; **37**: 520–5.

116. Mohlo ES, Factor SA, Weiner WJ, *et al.* The use of pramipexole, a novel dopamine (DA) agonist in advanced Parkinson's disease. *J. Neural Transm.* 1995; **10** (suppl. 45): 225–30.

117. Lieberman A, Rdnhosky A, Korts D. Clinical evaluation of pramipexole in advanced Parkinson's disease: results of a double-blind, placebo-controlled, parallel-group study. *Neurology* 1997; **49**: 162–8.

118. Gutman M, and the International Pramipexole-Bromocriptine Study Group. Double-blind comparison of pramipexole and bromocriptine treatment with placebo in advanced Parkinson's disease. *Neurology* 1997; **49**: 1060–5.

119. Shannon KM, Bennett JP, Friedman JH. Efficacy of pramipexole, a novel dopamine agonist as monotherapy in mild to moderate Parkinson's disease. *Neurology* 1997; **49**: 724–8.

120. Hubble JF, Koller WC, Cutler NR, *et al.* Pramipexole in patients with early Parkinson's disease. *Clin. Neuropharmacol.* 1995; **18**: 338–47.

121. Parkinson Study Group. Safety and efficacy of pramipexole in early Parkinson's disease: a randomised dose-ranging study. *JAMA* 1997; **278**: 125–30.

122. Szegedi A, Hilbert A, Wetzel M, Kliester E, Gaebre W, Benkens O. Pramipexole, a dopamine agonist in major depression: antidepressant effects and tolerability in an open-label study with multi doses. *Clin. Neuropharmacol.* 1997; **20**: S36–45.

123. Corrigan M, Evans DG. Pramipexole. A dopamine agonist in the treatment of major depression. In-house study. Pharmacia & Upjohn, Clinical Research, 1997.

124. Pogarell O. A non-ergot dopamine agonist, pramipexole in the therapy of advanced Parkinson's disease: improvement of parkinsonian symptoms and treatment associated complications. A review of three studies. *Clin. Neuropharmacol.* 1997; **20**: S28–35.

125. Richardson C, Lees A J, Turner R. The use of apomorphine in Parkinson's disease. *Pharmaceutical J.* 1999; **262**: 264–6.

126. Frankel JP, Lees AJ, Kempster PA, Stern GM. Subcutaneous apomorphine in the treatment of Parkinson's disease. *J. Neurol. Neurosurg. Psychiatry* 1990; **53**: 96–101.

127. Kileedorfer B, Turjanski N, Ryan R, Lees AJ, Milroy C, Stern GM. Intranasal apomorphine in Parkinson's disease. *Neurology* 1991; **41**: 761–2.

128. Van Laar T, Jansen ENH, Essink AW, Neef C. Intranasal apomorphine in Parkinsonian 'on-off' fluctuations. *Arch. Neurol.* 1992; **49**: 482–4.

129. Hughes AJ, Bishop S, Lees AJ, Stern GM, Webester R, Bovingdon M. Rectal apomorphine in Parkinson's disease. *Lancet* 1991; **337**: 118.

130. Lees AJ, Richardson CL, Turner K. *Treatment of Parkinson's disease with apomorphine – Shared care guidelines.* 3rd edn. London: University College London Hospitals NHS Trust, 1999.

131. Stibe CMH, Kempster PA, Lees AJ, Stern GM. Subcutaneous apomorphine in parkinsonian on-off oscillations. *Lancet* 1988; **i**: 403–6.

132. Chaudhuri R. *Parkinson's Disease.* Mosley-Wolfe Medical Communications, 1999; 29–30.

Neurosurgery

T.R.K. Varma

Historical aspects

The past decade has seen a rapid, and somewhat phenomenal, expansion in the use of surgery to treat movement disorders. However, this field of neurosurgery is not new, and indeed has a long history during which there has been a gradual evolution towards the new techniques and methodology that are available today.

Early procedures involved open surgical techniques, and while many of these offered varying degrees of benefit they often had a high morbidity, especially with regard to the neurological deficits that they induced. The surgical procedures ranged from cortical excision[1] to section of spinal nerve roots[2]. Open surgery of the subcortical structures included transventricular resection of the caudate nucleus,[3] pedunculotomy[4] and open pallidotomy.[5] Spiegel and Wycis (1947) are widely credited with the introduction of stereotactic surgery into neurosurgery.[6-8] In the absence of satisfactory pharmacological treatment, the 1950s and 1960s saw the widespread introduction of stereotactic surgery in the treatment of Parkinson's disease (PD). Both thalamotomy and pallidotomy were carried out in large numbers, and while several patients undoubtedly benefited from surgery a combination of poor patient selection and limited technology resulted in a relatively high morbidity. The introduction of levodopa during the early 1960s saw a dramatic downturn in the use of stereotactic surgery for PD.

The recent revival in surgery of PD has been due to a combination of improvements in surgical techniques, and also to the recognition of the limitations of drug treatment. It is ironic that one of the best indications for pallidotomy is the treatment of levodopa-induced dyskinesia.

The introduction of computed tomography (CT) scanning during the 1970s, and magnetic resonance imaging (MRI) in the 1980s, provided a radical improvement in the visualization of the intracranial structures. Consequently, several existing stereotactic frames were modified while new frames were developed for use with these modern imaging modalities. Although these systems were initially used for tumour surgery, their usefulness in movement disorder surgery was soon recognized.[9] In recent years the introduction of advanced computer technology into stereotactic surgery has simplified the surgical procedures and aided in treatment planning.[10,11]

The use of implanted deep brain stimulators for the treatment of movement disorders[12–16] now provides an attractive alternative to the irreversible ablative techniques that were previously used.

Targets for surgery in PD

Better understanding of the pathophysiology of Parkinson's disease has helped identify the most appropriate anatomical targets for stereotactic surgery.

Thalamus

Hassler is credited with having carried out the first thalamotomy in 1954,[17] and since then the ventrolateral (VL) nucleus of the thalamus has been one of the most commonly used target sites in stereotactic surgery. Cells firing at the tremor frequency (tremor cells) can be recorded by microelectrodes in the ventralis intermedius (Vim) part of the ventrolateral nucleus in parkinsonian patients, and lesions or stimulators placed at this site give excellent control of tremor.[18,19] The anterior (VOA) part of the ventrolateral nucleus receives inputs from the basal ganglia, and lesions here are thought to reduce rigidity and bradykinesia, though the effects are rarely as dramatic as the abolition of tremor by lesions placed in Vim.

Globus pallidus

The observation by Cooper in 1953 that ligation of an accidentally damaged anterior choroidal artery during surgery resulted in a dramatic improvement in parkinsonian symptoms focussed attention on the pallidum as a target for surgery.[8,20] Leksell, in Sweden, identified the ventral and posterior part of Globus pallidus interna (Gpi) as the optimum site in the pallidum, and this procedure has been recently popularized by Laitinen and co-workers.[21]

In experimental and human PD there is increased activity in Gpi due to the reduced inhibitory drive from the corpus striatum and increased excitatory drive from the subthalamic nucleus (STN). Following pallidotomy, the interruption of activity in the motor region of Gpi should decrease the inhibitory influence on the motor thalamus.[15].

The most consistent and predictable effect of pallidotomy is the alleviation of contralateral levodopa-induced dyskinesia. There is also increased time in the 'on' state, and the reduction in dyskinesia allows an increase in levodopa intake.[22–27] While improvement in tremor[23,24,27,28] has been reported in various studies, the improvement in tremor is in the author's experience not as good as with thalamic surgery. Most studies have also shown 'off' state improvements in contralateral bradykinesia, with improvements in Unified Parkinson's Disease Rating Scale (UPDRS) motor scores and disability scores.[23,24] Improvements in axial symptoms and gait are, however, less predictable.[29] Some improvement in ipsilateral symptoms can be expected, though these are not always sustained.

Uncertainty remains as to the benefits of bilateral pallidotomy in comparison with the potential risks. Major cognitive and speech defects have been reported with bilateral lesions, though this can be avoided by chronic electrical stimulation in place of ablation.

Subthalamic nucleus

Experimental studies using the MPTP (1-methyl-4-phenyl-1,1,2,3,6-tetrahydropyridine) primate model has shown increased cellular activity in the STN in PD, and that lesioning or stimulation of the STN can reverse the cardinal motor symptoms of the disease.[30–32] However, surgeons were reluctant to lesion the STN in the human parkinsonian patient because of the possibility of inducing hemiballismus.[33,34] The Grenoble group was the first to report the results of bilateral electrical stimulation of the STN, and the dramatic improvement in parkinsonian symptoms and signs.[35–37] Since then, several groups have reported similar results and this remains one of the most significant advances in surgery for PD. STN stimulation has been shown to improve UPDRS motor scores, increase 'on' time and control tremor. While it has no direct effect on levodopa-induced dyskinesia, it has a secondary beneficial effect as a consequence of the reduction in levodopa intake.

There are a limited number of recent reports of similar benefits being obtained by thermal lesions in the STN without inducing hemiballismus, though further studies will be required before the safety of this approach is established.[38]

Indications and patient selection

While it is obvious to clinicians that current surgical techniques are not a cure for PD, patient and carer expectations are often unrealistic and careful, realistic counselling is required. Most patients would have already undergone a wide range of pharmacological treatment before being considered for surgery, and have either proved to be resistant to or intolerant of their medication. There is uncertainty as to the exact stage at which surgery should be considered, but it seems to provide little benefit to patients in the end stages of the disease. Careful discussion between the physicians and surgeon is needed in this matter, and as confidence in these relatively new techniques grows surgery will be offered at an earlier stage in the disease.

The diagnosis of Parkinson's disease should be conclusively established as the results of surgery for Parkinson's like or Parkinson's plus syndromes are generally poor.

Tremor, which is often resistant to drug therapy, responds consistently well to surgery[12,13,40,41] aimed at the Vim nucleus of the thalamus. As STN stimulation improves not only tremor but also other motor symptoms of PD, it is now the preferred treatment option in patients with both tremor and akinesia. However, in the few patients with tremor-dominant disease that has been stable for several years, thalamic surgery remains a reasonable option. Bilateral thalamotomy has a high morbidity,[41,42] and prior to the development of deep brain stimulation (DBS) treatment was usually aimed at improving symptoms unilaterally; however, with stimulation it is now possible to treat both sides effectively.

Pallidal surgery could be considered where drug-induced dyskinesia is the limiting factor in pharmacological treatment. Debate continues however as to the role of pallidal surgery as opposed to STN stimulation in the control of motor symptoms, and further studies will be required before this is resolved.

Where motor symptoms, gait dysfunction and postural instability predominate (with or without tremor), STN stimulation is currently the best surgical option

Surgery offers no benefit in cognitive and psychological symptoms of the disease, and the onset of dementia is a contraindication to surgery.[35–37]

Advanced age by itself is not a contraindication to surgery, though some studies have shown a poorer response to pallidotomy with advancing years.[29] Surgery however can involve a prolonged operation under local anaesthesia, and frail patients with intercurrent illnesses may have difficulty in tolerating the procedure. The presence of cognitive dysfunction makes intraoperative assessment difficult, and can increase morbidity. The presence of significant cardiovascular or respiratory disease is a relative contraindication to surgery.

The need for a team approach in patient selection and management cannot be over- emphasized. Most departments undertaking such surgery have a multidisciplinary team that includes neurosurgeons, physicians, neurophysiologists, nurse specialists and therapists to assess and manage patients before and after surgery.

Surgical techniques

Surgical techniques vary, but surgery is generally performed in three stages:

1. Radiological localization
2. Physiological localization
3. Ablation or stimulation

Radiological localization

This initially involves the fixation of a stereotactic localizer to the skull under local anaesthesia so that imaging can be performed under stereotactic conditions. In the past, ventriculography was the radiological technique used to identify reference points in the brain, but in most centres this has been replaced by CT or MRI. A short anaesthetic is sometimes administered to avoid patient movement during imaging. The position of the target site is calculated using measurements obtained from stereotactic atlases of the human brain, with reference to identifiable structures in the brain such as the anterior and posterior commissures. With good quality MRI it is now possible to visualize directly the pallidal and subthalamic targets, though the thalamic nuclei remain invisible and have to be located indirectly.

Computer software programmes are now available that facilitate the use of multiple image data sets and digitized atlases which help in the calculation of target coordinates.

Physiological localization

Despite modern imaging methods, the final localization of the target site has to be achieved using neurophysiological methods. These may include micro-electrode recordings, somatosensory evoked potentials, impedance measurement and electrical stimulation. Extensive neurophysiological localization can be prolonged: opponents consider them unnecessarily time-consuming with added risk, while proponents view them as essential for accurate localization.[19,43–45]

When radiological studies have been completed, the patient is returned to the operating theatre and the radiological localizer is replaced with the stereotactic frame. Under local anaesthesia a small opening is made in the skull and the stereotactic arc system is used to guide recording or stimulating electrodes to the chosen target. The final position of the target is decided on the physiological recordings and the patient's response to electrical stimulation of the target site. Unexpected or unwanted responses to stimulation will also warn the surgeon of erroneous positioning of the electrode, e.g. muscle contractions if the electrode is in the internal capsule.

When the target site has been identified there are currently two treatment options available:

- Ablation of the appropriate area by creating a thermal lesion has until recently been the standard method of treatment. A radiofrequency current is applied which heats the tip of the lesioning electrode and creates a thermal lesion in the tissue.
- In recent years, interest has focused on the use of chronic DBS using implanted electrodes as an alternative to ablation.

CHRONIC DBS

High-frequency stimulation of the target site has always been used as a method of identifying the targets during stereotactic surgery for movement disorders. Stimulation of the Vim nucleus at frequencies above 100 Hz was noted to arrest contralateral tremor, and that this effect was reversed as soon as stimulation was discontinued. Chronically implanted deep brain stimulators had been extensively used in the treatment of chronic pain,[46,47] but with publication of the first studies of the use of this technology in the treatment of movement disorders[12-14] there has been a massive resurgence in stereotactic surgery. This has been coincident with technical improvements in the electrodes and stimulators used for DBS.

The initial target localization is similar to that used for ablative surgery, but once the target has been identified the tracking electrode is replaced by an implantable quadripolar DBS electrode that is firmly anchored to the skull. It is then usual (though not always essential) that a trial of stimulation is carried out for a period of time by connecting the electrode to an external stimulator. When the surgeon and the patient are satisfied that stimulation is providing acceptable results, the system is internalized by connecting the electrode to a battery-powered pulse generator similar to a cardiac pacemaker placed subcutaneously in the infraclavicular fossa. The stimulator can be programmed, and stimulation parameters altered using an external programmer. The patient also has some control of the system using a hand-held programmer that can be used to alter the amplitude of the stimulation and to turn the device on or off.

DBS was initially used in the control of tremor by stimulation of the Vim nucleus of the thalamus,[12-14] but has subsequently been used as an alternative to pallidotomy by stimulation of the globus pallidus[48-50] and more recently with stimulation of the STN.[35,51,52]

Stimulation or ablation?

Since the introduction of DBS in the treatment of movement disorders there has been considerable debate as to its advantages and disadvantages over ablative procedures.

Ablative procedures have the advantage of being single, operative procedures not requiring frequent and long-term surgical follow-up. However, its irreversibility remains the major concern – especially if unwanted neurological sequelae result from the procedure. The morbidity of bilateral ablation is high, and as PD is most often a bilateral disease most patients will require bilateral treatment.

The reversibility of unwanted side effects by either removing or turning off the stimulator is seen as the major advantage with the use of DBS. There is, however, the need for long-term and frequent follow-up to maintain the system, and also the possibility of hardware failure. The hardware costs are also considerable, though this is offset by a reduction in long-term morbidity. There is some recent evidence that thalamic stimulation provides better long-term tremor control than thalamotomy.[53]

Other surgical procedures

At present, nigral and adrenal tissue transplants, gene therapy and the use of selective neurotrophic or neurotoxic agents remain experimental and are not in routine clinical use. However, these approaches hold hope in perhaps finding a surgical cure for PD.

Risks and morbidity of neurosurgery for PD

The mortality rate of stereotactic surgery is low (<1 per cent), and is usually the result of unexpected intracranial haemorrhage. Short periods of confusion sometimes occur, especially when the procedure has been prolonged. The incidence of wound infection is low but if it does occur it may be necessary to remove the implanted hardware. There is also a small risk of postoperative epilepsy.

Unexpected neurological deficits occur with varying frequency depending on the site of the lesion, and are often due to inaccurate localization of the target. Transient or permanent hemiparesis can be seen after thalamotomy or pallidotomy if the lesion encroaches on the internal capsule. The risks of cognitive dysfunction, speech deficits and dysphagia are higher after bilateral procedures (up to 18 per cent).[54]

The specific risks associated with pallidotomy include visual field loss (2.5–9 per cent),[19,48] hypophonia and cognitive deficits. These are again significantly higher with bilateral surgery. With DBS, side effects of stimulation can occur in up to 30 per cent of patients and include paraesthesia, dysarthria and ataxia. These are however often transient and can be reversed by altering the stimulation parameters.[14] Hardware-related complications include infection, electrode migration and battery depletion.

With increasing expertise and improving technology, the risks of modern stereotactic surgery for PD are low, and can offer considerable benefit in what is a severely disabling disease.

References

1. Bucy PC. Cortical extirpation in the treatment of involuntary movements. *Am. J. Surg.* 1948; **75**: 257–63.
2. Foerster OH Resection of the posterior spinal nerve roots in the treatment of gastric crises and spastic paralysis. *Proc. R. Soc. Med.* 1911; **3**: 226–54.
3. Meyers HR. Surgical procedure for postencephalitic tremor. *Arch. Neurol. Psych.* 1940; **44**: 455–9.
4. Cooper IS. Surgical treatment of parkinsonism. *Annu. Rev. Med.* 1965; **16**: 309–30.
5. Guiridi J, Lozano A. A brief history of pallidotomy. *Neurosurgery* 1997; **41**: 1169–80.
6. Spiegel EA. Development of stereoencephalotomy for extrapyramidal diseases. *J. Neurosurg.* 1966; **24**: 433–9.

7. Spiegel EA, Wycis HT, Marks M. Stereotactic apparatus for operations on the human brain. *Science* 1947; **106**: 349–50.
8. Redfern RM. History of stereotactic surgery for Parkinson's disease. *Br. J. Neurosurg.* 1989; **3**: 271–304.
9. Jeanmonod D, Thomas DGT. Application of CT-directed stereotaxy in the determination of neurosurgical targets in the diencephalon and cerebral hemisphere. *Br. J. Neurosurg.* 1989; **3**: 337–42.
10. Hardy TL, Smith JR, Brynildson LRD, *et al.* Magnetic resonance imaging and anatomic atlas mapping for thalamotomy. *Stereotact. Funct. Neurosurg.* 1992; **58**: 30–2.
11. Kall BA, Goerss SJ, Kelly PJ. A new multimodality correlative imaging technique for VOP/VIM (VL) thalamotomy procedures. *Stereotact. Funct. Neurosurg.* 1992; **58**: 45–51.
12. Benabid AL, Pollack P, Gervason C, *et al.* Long term suppression of tremor by chronic stimulation of the ventral intermediate thalamic nucleus. *Lancet* 1991; **337**: 403–6.
13. Blond S, Siegfried J. Thalamic stimulation for tremor and other movement disorders. *Acta Neurochir. Suppl.* 1991; **52**: 109–11.
14. Limousin P, Speelman JD, Gielen F, *et al.* Multicentre European study of thalamic stimulation in parkinsonian and essential tremor. *J. Neurol. Neurosurg. Psychiatry* 1999; **66**: 289–96.
15. Starr PA, Vitek JL, Bakay RA. Ablative surgery and deep brain stimulation for Parkinson's disease. *Neurosurgery* 1998; **43**: 989–1015.
16. Blond S, Caparros-Lefebvre D, Parker F, *et al.* Control of tremor and involuntary movements by chronic stimulation of the ventral intermediate thalamic nucleus. *J. Neurosurg.* 1992; **77**: 62–8.
17. Hassler R, Riechert T. Indikationen und Lokalisations-methode der gezielten Hirnoperationenen, *Nervenarzt* 1954; **25**: 441–7.
18. Lenz FA, Tasker RR, Kwan HC, *et al.* Selection of the optimal lesion site for the relief of Parkinsonian tremor on the basis of spectral analysis of neuronal firing patterns. *Appl. Neurophysiol.* 1987; **50**: 338–43.
19. Fukamachi A, Ohye C, Narabayashi J. Delineation of the thalamic nuclei with a microelectrode in stereotactic surgery for parkinsonism and cerebral palsy. *J. Neurosurg.* 1973; **39**: 214–25.
20. Cooper IS. Ligation of the anterior choroidal artery for involuntary movements in Parkinsonism. *Psychiatr. Q.* 1953; **27**: 317–19.
21. Laitinen LV, Bergenheim AT, Hariz MI. Leksells posteroventral pallidotomy in the treatment of Parkinson's disease. *J. Neurosurg.* 1992; **76**: 53–61.
22. Iacono RP, Shima F, Lonser RR, *et al.* The results, indications and physiology of posteroventral pallidotomy for patients with Parkinson's disease. *Neurosurgery* 1995; **36**: 1118–26.
23. Dogali M, Fazzini E, Kolodny E, *et al.* Stereotactic ventral pallidotomy for Parkinson's disease. *Neurology* 1995; **45**: 753–61.
24. Lozano AM, Lang AE, Galvez-Jimenez N, *et al.* Effects of Gpi pallidotomy on motor function in Parkinson's disease. *Lancet* 1995; **346**: 1383–7.
25. Sutton JP, Couldwell W, Lew MF, *et al.* Venteroposterior medial pallidotomy in patients with advanced Parkinson's disease. *Neurosurgery* 1995; **36**: 1112–17.
26. Scott R, Gregory R, Hines N, *et al.* Neuropsychological, neurological and functional outcome following pallidotomy for Parkinson's disease: a consecutive series of eight simultaneous bilateral and twelve unilateral procedures. *Brain* 1998; **121**: 659–75.

27. Lang AE, Lozano A, Montgomery E, *et al*. Posteromedial pallidotomy in advanced Parkinson's disease. *N. Engl. J. Med.* 1997; **337**: 1036–42.

28. Baron MS, Vitek JL, Bakay RA, *et al*. Treatment of advanced Parkinson's disease by posterior Gpi pallidotomy: 1- year results of a pilot study. *Ann. Neurol.* 1996; **40**: 355–66.

29. Starr PA, Vitek JL, Bakay RAE. Pallidotomy: Clinical results. In: Germano IM (ed.). *Neurosurgical Treatment of Movement Disorders*. Lebanon, New Hampshire: The American Association of Neurological Surgeons, 1998.

30. Aziz TZ, Peggs D, Sambrook MA, Crossman AR. Lesions of the subthalamic nucleus for the alleviation of 1-methyl-4-phenyl-1,2,3,6-tetrahydropyridine (MPTP) induced parkinsonism in the primate. *Movement Disord.* 1991; **6**: 288–92.

31. Benazzouz A, Gross C, Féger J, *et al*. Reversal of rigidity and improvement of motor performance by subthalamic high frequency stimulation in MPTP- treated monkeys. *Eur. J. Neurosci.* 1993; **5**: 382–9.

32. Bergman H, Wichmann T, DeLong MR. Reversal of experimental parkinsonism by lesions of the subthalamic nucleus. *Science* 1990; **249**: 1436–8.

33. Andy OJ, Jurko MF, Sias FR. Subthalamotomy in the treatment of Parkinsonian tremor. *J. Neurosurg.* 1983; **46**: 107–11.

34. Obeso J, Alvarez L, Macias RJ, *et al*. Lesion of the subthalamic nucleus (STN) in Parkinson's disease (abstract). *Neurology* 1997; **48** (Suppl.): A138.

35. Limousin P, Pollak P, Benazzouz A, *et al*. Effect on parkinsonian signs and symptoms of bilateral subthalamic nucleus stimulation. *Lancet* 1995; **345**: 91-5.

36. Moringlane JR, Ceballos-Baumann AO, Alesch F. Long term effect of electrostimulation of the subthalamic nucleus in bradykinetic-rigid Parkinson's disease. *Minimal. Invasive Surg.* 1998; **41**: 133–6.

37. Pollak P, Benabid AL, Limousin P, *et al*. Subthalamic nucleus stimulation alleviates akinesia and rigidity in parkinsonian patients. *Adv. Neurol.* 1996; **69**: 591–4.

38. Gill SS, Heywood P. Bilateral dorsolateral subthalamotomy for advanced Parkinson's disease (letter). *Lancet* 1997; **350**: 1224.

39. Tasker RR, Siqueira J, Hawrylyshyn P, Organ LW. What happened to VIM thalamotomy for Parkinson's disease? *Appl. Neurophysiol.* 1983; **46**: 68–83.

40. Matsumoto K, Shichijo F, Fukami T. Long term follow up review of cases of Parkinson's disease after unilateral or bilateral thalamotomy. *J. Neurosurg.* 1984; **60**: 1033–44.

41. Kelly PJ, Gillingham FJ. The long term results of stereotaxic surgery and L-Dopa therapy in patients with Parkinson's disease. *J. Neurosurg.* 1980; **53**: 332–7.

42. Forster A, Varma TRK, Latimer M, Cameron ID. Neurophysiological recordings during two stage thalamotomy. *Electroenceph. Clin. Neurophysiol.*; **87**: 101P.

43. Taren J, Guiot G, Derome P, *et al*. Hazards of stereotactic thalamectomy. Added safety factor in corroborating X-ray target localization with neurophysiological methods. *J. Neurosurg.* 1968; **29**: 173–82.

44. Favre J, Taha JM, Nguyen TT, *et al*. Pallidotomy: a survey of current practice in North America. *Neurosurgery* 1996; **39**: 883–92.

45. Hosobuchi Y. Subcortical electrical stimulation for control of intractable pain in humans. A report of 122 cases (1970–1984). *J. Neurosurg.* 1986; **64**: 543–53.

46. Gol A. Relief of pain by electrical stimulation of the septal area. *J. Neurol. Sci.* 1967; **5**: 115–20.

47. Bejjani B, Damier P, Arnulf I, *et al*. Pallidal stimulation for Parkinson's disease. Two targets? *Neurology* 1997; **49**: 1564–9.

48. Siegfried J, Lippitz B. Bilateral chronic stimulation ventroposterolateral pallidum:

a new therapeutic approach for alleviating all parkinsonian symptoms. *Neurosurgery* 1994; **35**: 1126–30.

49. Pahwa R, Wilkinson S, Smith D, *et al*. High frequency stimulation of the globus pallidus for the treatment of Parkinson's disease. *Neurology* 1997; **49**: 249–53.

50. Benabid AL, Pollak P, Gross C, *et al*. Acute and long term effects of subthalamic nucleus stimulation in Parkinson's disease. *Stereotact. Funct. Neurosurg.* 1994; **62**: 76–84.

51. Olanow CW, Germano IM, Brin MF, *et al*. Deep brain stimulation of the subthalamic nucleus for Parkinson's disease. *Movement Disord.* 1996; **11**: 598–9.

52. Tasker RR. Deep brain stimulation is preferable to thalamotomy for tremor suppression. *Surg. Neurol.* 1998; **49**: 145–53.

53. Osenbach RK, Burchiel KJ. In: Germano IM (ed.). *Neurosurgical Treatment of Movement Disorders*. Lebanon, New Hampshire: The American Association of Neurological Surgeons, 1998.

Complementary and alternative medicine

R.G. Brown

Introduction

Parkinson's disease (PD) is a progressive condition that has no known cure. Existing medical and surgical treatments are only partially effective in relieving the symptoms of PD, leaving all patients with the prospect of increasing disability and dependency. It is, therefore, little wonder that some patients seek extra help from outside the realms of conventional medicine, while at the same time waiting for improved treatments from within. Today, it is not necessary to look far for information about complementary and alternative approaches to health. From supermarket shelves to glossy magazines, material can be found promoting the health potential of vitamins, dietary supplements and herbal preparations; notice boards in public libraries advertise the services of aromatherapists and reflexologists; and the internet is awash with discussion groups and websites devoted to alternative and complementary health practices. Patients discuss among themselves the latest news, views and personal endorsements of a particular therapy. They are, therefore, far from underinformed – even if that information is often partial and of poor quality.

It is against this background that patients will often ask advice of their general practitioner or specialist, wanting to know whether or not they should be taking vitamin E, trying acupuncture, learning the Alexander technique or yoga. What should be said to patients in these circumstances? The purpose of this chapter is to consider what is known of the use of complementary approaches to health in those with PD, what evidence is currently available, and what hope there is for better information in the future.

Complementary and Alternative Medicine (CAM) covers a wide range of approaches that often have little in common, except that they lie outside the treatments and healthcare practices that form the basis of conventional western medicine. Whether they are seen as complementary or alternative is largely a matter of whether they are used instead of, or as an adjunct to, more conventional methods. In some therapies, for some conditions, the boundaries are blurring, although in the case of PD CAM approaches remain firmly on the medical fringe and beyond.

The use of CAM therapy by PD patients

To date, the only information available about the use of CAM in PD patients is the results from a survey carried out in the United Kingdom in 1997 by the Parkinson's Disease Society.[1] A mailing by the Society to its membership of around 25 000 people produced only 2274 replies. The low response rate, and the potential bias created by surveying only Parkinson's Disease Society members, means that the results should be interpreted with caution. However, in the absence of a more definitive study, the results provide the most detailed information yet.

The respondents' mean age was 61.5 ± 10.4 years, and the approximate duration of illness was 7.7 ± 6.1 years. As such, these patients are fairly typical of those seen in a specialist movement disorders clinic, although younger than those seen within a geriatric service. The severity of their parkinsonism can only be estimated, but in terms of disability [as measured by an Activities of Daily Living (ADL) scale[2]], the majority (51.4 per cent) had little or only mild restriction in normal activity. Of the remainder, most (30.9 per cent) had moderate disability, while only 17.9 per cent had severe disability or were totally dependent.

In terms of the use of CAM, just over one-third (34.9 per cent) were currently trying or had previously tried at least one therapy for problems related to their PD. The majority of these were aged <65 years, suggesting a bias for the younger patients in the use of complementary approaches to health – perhaps because of differences in attitude, or for reasons of finance. The latter may be particularly relevant, as 43 per cent of those trying a complementary therapy had paid £100 or more in the preceding year, with almost 10 per cent paying over £500.

The list of therapies covered in the survey, together with the proportion of the sample that had experience of them, is shown in Table 19.1. Most of the mainstream therapies are represented in the 'top 10', and this probably reflects their availability. One trend that emerged from the data was the change in choice of therapy as patients became more disabled. While yoga, relaxation therapy and meditation topped the list of the least disabled patients, aromatherapy and herbal medicine were likely to be chosen by the most disabled. There was no clear trend for therapy preference with increasing age.

Clearly, a survey such as this cannot provide either reliable or valid information about the possible efficacy of complementary medicine in general, or of any particular therapy. However, it is informative to consider the subjective 'consumer opinion' of the benefits of each therapy. The results for the ten most

Table 19.1 Parkinson's Disease Society of the United Kingdom: survey of the use of complementary and alternative medicine. Data are provided in rank order of the most commonly tried therapies

Therapy	Per cent of total sample (n = 2273)	Per cent of those with experience of CAM (n = 793)
Reflexology	9.3	27.0
Aromatherapy	9.2	26.7
Shiatsu/Massage	8.8	25.5
Relaxation/Meditation	8.5	24.7
Acupuncture/Acupressure	7.6	21.8
Yoga	6.7	19.4
Herbal medicine	6.5	18.9
Osteopathy/Chiropractic	6.5	18.9
Healing	6.3	18.3
Homeopathy	5.6	16.2
Alexander technique	3.2	9.3
Conductive eductation	2.8	8.1
Dietary therapy	2.7	7.8
Hypnotherapy	2.0	5.8
Tai Chi	1.7	4.9
Cranial osteopathy	1.3	3.8
Others (total)	1.0	2.9
Biofeedback	0.5	1.5
Feldenkrais	0.1	0.3

widely used therapies, each tried by at least 90 patients, are shown in Table 19.2. In terms of overall approval rating, yoga was the most positively endorsed, with two-thirds of patients feeling that they had obtained 'considerable' or 'extreme' benefit. As interesting as the degree of benefit was the nature of the benefit that respondents reported. Across all therapies, the main benefits reported related to psychological relaxation, stress relief, improved sense of 'well-being' and 'energy'. In terms of symptomatic relief, rigidity, stiffness and pain were the most commonly reported areas where people found benefit.

Table 19.2 Parkinson's Disease Society of the United Kingdom: survey of the use of complementary and alternative medicine. Subjective benefit of 10 most commonly used therapies, with rank order of satisfaction in square brackets. The remaining percentage is accounted for by complaints of negative or adverse outcome

Therapy	Considerable or extreme benefit (%)	Slight or no benefit (%)
Reflexology	36.6 [8]	62.6
Aromatherapy	41.4 [4]	57.9
Shiatsu/Massage	51.9 [2]	48.1
Relaxation/Meditation	41.1 [5]	58.9
Acupuncture/Acupressure	28.9 [9]	67.8
Yoga	66.5 [1]	33.5
Herbal medicine	36.7 [7]	62.0
Osteopathy/Chiropractic	39.8 [6]	55.9
Healing	42.8 [3]	57.2
Homeopathy	28.5 [10]	68.5

Although such a survey is of great interest, it fails to answer the most important questions, namely 'What therapies may be of value in the management of PD?', and 'for which particular features?' In this regard, only empirical evidence can provide the answers for patients and their doctors to make informed and rational decisions. Unfortunately, this evidence is almost non-existent, either in terms of demonstrating benefit or an absence of benefit. What is currently known on this subject will be discussed in the remainder of this chapter.

The 'evidence'

The cornerstone of modern evidence-based medicine is the randomized controlled trial (RCT). However, difficulties can arise in applying these methods to CAM. In part this can be due to the reluctance of some CAM practitioners to accept the validity of the RCT, or the ability to perform a controlled trial on what are seen as holistic and individualized therapies with belief systems or models that lie outside the field of conventional medicine. In addition, there is often an equal reluctance in conventional medical science to take on the challenge of evaluating CAM approaches.

Perhaps the easiest CAM therapies to rationalize and evaluate within a conventional medical model, are those that involve the ingestion or application of biologically active substance, as in the systems of traditional Chinese medicine and the Indian system or Ayurveda.[3] In Ayurveda, for example, treatment of the clinical entity closest to PD (*Kampavata*) is with the seeds of *Mucuna pruriens*, a concentrated natural source of levodopa . Another natural source of levodopa is the broad bean, *Vicia faba*, which can have significant antiparkinsonian effects.[4] However, while a clinical effect is probable, neither of these products has been tested formally against conventional synthetic levodopa to show that they are superior in efficacy, or produce fewer side effects. Of the other traditional approaches, Genghe[5] carried out an open trial of traditional Chinese medicine on 50 patients. He reported 'marked subjective improvement' in 30 per cent after 3 months of herbal treatment and acupuncture, while 22 per cent showed no benefit. While suggestive, such results constitute poor evidence by today's standards. Closer to home and western medicine, over-the-counter dietary supplements including antioxidant vitamins such as α-tocopherol (vitamin E)[6] and co-enzyme Q10[7] have received serious scientific attention for their potential neuroprotective properties. The DATATOP study is the largest example to date of a RCT for 'non-conventional' agents in the treatment of PD. In this case, the evidence of a significant effect of α-tocopherol was not found,[8] despite the promise of earlier open-label trials.[9] Such a finding highlights the importance of the RCT over open clinical trials, let alone subjective evaluation of efficacy.

Returning to the results of the Parkinson's Disease Society survey, it is interesting to note that herbal and dietary approaches lie somewhere down the list of preferred treatments, perhaps reflecting the patients desire for a non-pharmacological approach to their problems. Unfortunately, there is similarly scant evidence for the efficacy of more 'physical' approaches. In relation to massage – one of the more popular treatments – there is non-controlled evidence that it may be of value in the management of tremor.[10,11] Dance movement therapy has been shown to be superior to simple exercise in improving in movement initiation, at least within session.[12] The Alexander technique has also received support from a preliminary study by Stallibrass,[13] and is now the subject of a more rigorous evaluation.

What advice can we give to patients?

While encouraging, such results do little to satisfy the need for answers by both patients and their clinicians. Virtually none of the evidence available is adequate to advise patients either to try a therapy, or to avoid it. Patients are left with making choices on the basis of hear-say and hope. What practical advice *can* we give to patients at this stage? The following points are all important:

- Be aware that 'natural' herbal remedies may contain substances which interact with prescribed medications. Consult your doctor before taking.
- Be aware that some therapies may carry risk particularly if misused or poorly administered.

- Any CAM method tried should definitely be seen as a complement, and not as an alternative to conventional approaches.
- In the absence of empirical evidence, seek information from others who may have benefited form a particular approach.
- Look at the therapies available and choose one that seems to have at least face value in the problem at hand.
- Look at the range of therapies on offer, and choose one that fits your own personal likes and ideas about health.
- When choosing a practitioner, examine their qualifications and their expertise. If they are unfamiliar with PD, take the time to explain the disease and its problems as fully as you are able.
- Have a clear idea about what outcome you hope for, or expect.
- Have a realistic idea about how long any possible benefit might take to appear.
- Keep in mind the difference between feeling good during a treatment, and any more lasting benefit.
- Monitor progress, if any. Decide whether any improvement is worth the commitment of time and money already invested, and whether it is worth continuing.

Clearly, many patients with PD see a role for CAM approaches in the overall management of their condition. The clinician has a role in serving as an objective and impartial adviser to help patients make rational choices when considering CAM approaches. It is no more helpful for a clinician to recommend unreservedly a therapy in the absence of evidence, than it is for them to advise against it. Hopefully, in the future, more evidence will be available on which patients can base their decisions, and clinicians can base their advice.

References

1. Brown RG, and members of the Complementary Therapy Working Group. *The use of complementary therapy in Parkinson's disease: report on a survey of members of the Parkinson's Disease Society (UK)*. London: Parkinson's Disease Society, 1997.
2. Brown RG, MacCarthy B, Jahanshahi M, Marsden CD. Accuracy of self-reported disability in patients with parkinsonism. *Arch. Neurol.* 1989; **46**: 955–9.
3. Manyam BV, Sanchez-Ramos J. Traditional and complementary therapies in Parkinson's disease. In: Stern G (ed.). *Parkinson's Disease*. London: Raven, 1999: 565–74.
4. Vered Y, Rabey JM, Palevitch D, *et al*. Bioavailability of levodopa after consumption of *Vicia faba* seedlings by parkinsonian patients and control subjects. *Clin. Neuropharmacol.* 1994; **17**: 138–46.
5. Genghe L. Clinical analysis of Parkinson's disease treated by integration of traditional Chinese and western medicine. *J. Trad. Chinese Med.* 1995; **15**: 163–9.
6. de Rijk MC, Breteler MMB, den Breeijen JH, *et al*. Dietary antioxidants and Parkinson's disease: the Rotterdam Study. *Arch. Neurol.* 1997; **54**: 762–5.
7. Shults CW, Beal MF, Fontaine D, Nakano K, Haas RH. Absorption, tolerability, and effects on mitochondrial activity of oral coenzyme Q10 in parkinsonian patients. *Neurology* 1998; **50**: 793–5.

8. Koller W, Olanow CW, Rodnitzky R, *et al*. Effects of tocopherol and deprenyl on the progression of disability in early Parkinson's disease. *N. Engl. J. Med*. 1993; **328**: 176–83.

9. Fahn S. A pilot trial of high-dose alpha-tocopherol and ascorbate in early Parkinson's disease. *Ann. Neurol*. 1992; **32** (Suppl.): S128–32.

10. Steefel L. Massage therapy as an adjunct healing modality in Parkinson's disease. *Alt. Complement. Ther*. 1996; **2**: 377–82.

11. Miesler DW. Massage and Parkinson's disease. *Massage Therapy* 1996; **35**: 382.

12. Westbrook BK, McKibben H. Dance/movement therapy with groups of outpatients with Parkinson's disease. *Am. J. Dance Ther*. 1989; **11**: 27–38.

13. Stallibrass C. An evaluation of the Alexander technique for the management of disability in Parkinson's disease – a preliminary study. *Clin. Rehabil*. 1997; **11**: 8–12.

Part 5: Research in Parkinson's disease

Rehabilitation and physiotherapy

C. Chandler, D. Jones and R. Plant

Introduction

The research base of rehabilitation and physiotherapy in Parkinson's disease (PD) is minute in comparison with the overall literature on disease.[1] This view can be confirmed by a Medline search of the PD literature published in 1998: over 1000 articles would be identified of which <1 per cent relate to rehabilitation or physiotherapy. This relative poverty of evidence has severe implications for referral to the therapies, with only 27 per cent of a recent survey population being referred to a physiotherapist, and lower rates to other therapies.[2] In this chapter the recent evidence base for physiotherapy intervention in PD will be reviewed in the context of multiprofessional rehabilitation.

Defining rehabilitation

Rehabilitation is a complex concept of which many definitions exist. The Disability and Rehabilitation Open Learning Project, set up in response to the recognition that there was a need to develop multiprofessional education and training for professionals, defined rehabilitation as:

'an enabling process in which societies, communities, agencies and professionals meet the social, psychological, physical and economic needs of the disabled person through knowledge, skill, respect, understanding and agreement. The rehabilitative process includes an assessment of where the individual, community and carer(s) are, where they wish to be, and the contributions each must make to achieve ambitions and meet needs'.[3]

This definition emphasizes the handicap dimension of the International Classification of Impairments, Disabilities and Handicaps,[4] or the participation dimension under the draft ICIDH-2 International Classification of Functioning and Disability.[5] A similar emphasis was evident in the King's Fund[6] definition of rehabilitation as:

'a process aiming to restore personal autonomy in those aspects of daily living considered most relevant by patients or service users, and their family carers'.

However, the process of rehabilitation itself is linked to all levels in the classification. ICIDH-2[5] sees disablement as a complex interaction between the health condition, in this case PD, experienced at the level of impairment (the body), activity (daily tasks) and/or participation (life situations), and environmental and personal contextual factors. This framework provides a structure to examine the literature in relation to PD, to identify the individuals who may play a part in the rehabilitation process, the nature of interventions they may employ and for what reasons, and the appropriateness of the outcomes used to measure effect.

Effectiveness of rehabilitation

The King's Fund report entitled *Effective Practice in Rehabilitation. The Evidence of Systemic Reviews*[6] highlights problems with the definition of rehabilitation, defining the intervention, and the appropriate use of outcome measures in rehabilitation research. Positive findings in relation to stroke rehabilitation are likely to be important in relation to rehabilitation in PD. It points to the fact that 'effective rehabilitation may be achieved by the co-ordination of complex interventions addressing multiple risk factors, involving multiple professional disciplines and multiple phases of rehabilitation'.[6] Results providing no evidence of effectiveness applied particularly to single interventions, whilst uniprofessional reviews of speech and language therapy, occupational therapy and physiotherapy were largely equivocal. A review of the paramedical therapies and PD is currently being undertaken by the Movement Disorders Group of the Cochrane Collaboration.[7]

Interdisciplinary rehabilitation in PD

Ward[1] proposes that the management of PD has two main components: restoration and remediation. The use of drugs and surgery to ameliorate the physiological effects of the disease involves restoration at an impairment level. This also has the potential to modify activity, participation and personal contextual factors. Active processes of physical, psychological and social adjustment comprise remediation, which likewise may have effects on other dimensions of the ICIDH-2 classification. Rehabilitation provides a framework for both restoration and remediation, making it clear that it is an inherently multiprofessional process. Rehabilitation is largely undertaken within a coordinated, goal-oriented approach.[1,6]

The Romford Project[8] pioneered the concept of a patient-centred approach to diagnosis and management of PD. The essential features of the model were a multidisciplinary approach, involving patients and carers as part of the team, and a special focus on the telling and support at the time of diagnosis, and on the social and emotional consequences of the condition.[9] Patti et al.[10] evaluated a 4-week intensive, personalized, multidisciplinary inpatient rehabilitation programme using a range of outcome measures covering impairment and disability dimensions and illustrated improvements in functional performance. However, there was a trend for performance to return to baseline after 6 months, prompting a call for bi-annual top-up programmes. Health-related quality of life using the Nottingham Health Profile was the outcome chosen to evaluate a nurse-led multidisciplinary in-patient (5–10 days) neurological rehabilitation programme.[11] Post-treatment scores showed significant improvement, and further work was highlighted to examine longer-term effects.

The approach to interdisciplinary rehabilitation in PD employed by the Kingston Centre in Melbourne, Austrialia[12] is grounded in a shared knowledge base relating to the current understanding of the motor functions of the basal ganglia, and how these are affected by the condition. Guidelines are developed from the knowledge base from which strategies for overcoming everyday problems are formulated and used concurrently with medical treatment. Physiotherapists, occupational therapists, speech and language therapists, nurses, social workers and neuropsychologists work within a multidisciplinary team in an inter- and intradisciplinary capacity across healthcare settings.

Care pathway in PD

A project to evaluate the introduction of a multidisciplinary pathway of care, together with a care programme approach to an existing PD service based at a District General Hospital serving a population of 200 000 people, is currently being undertaken by Bilclough and colleagues.[13] A multidisciplinary pathway of care consists of patient-focused care specifying key events, tests and assessments, in a timely fashion to produce the best outcomes, within the resources available. The care programme approach encompasses an agreed assessment of health and social care needs, a negotiated programme of care, a review process and a key worker to coordinate the programme. A repeated measures design is being employed to compare a group of 50 people with PD and their carers who have received traditional services for more than 12 months with a matched group of newly referred people with PD and their carers. Outcome measures include service use, perceptions of users and professionals, together with a battery of impairment, disability and quality of life measures. Economic analysis will allow comparison of the cost of traditional versus managed care. Groups of service users have played a prominent part in the development of the new service. The two service user consultants on the project team also act as user researchers within the project.

Models of management

A commonly heard phrase from an older person with PD is, 'Well what would you expect at my age?' This question is well worth consideration within the context of rehabilitation. Whilst ageing is a complex biological process with heterogeneous effects, successful management of these changes by an individual can maintain a high quality of life. PD can be considered as a disease process superimposed on the trajectory of normal ageing. Due to the need for frequent pharmacological manipulation, medicalization of ageing may occur which can lead to an imposed dependency.[14]

Baltes [15] presents a meta-model of successful ageing which considers three processes that assist the adaptation to the challenges of ageing. These are selection, compensation and optimisation, and they seem equally relevant to the elderly person with PD. Selection involves a readjustment of the individual's expectations in response to, or in anticipation of, changes in function and abilities. Compensation again is a response to loss of function or ability, but in this case uses a different means to achieve the same goal and may require acquisition of new skills or means that are not pre-existing. Optimisation is more of a development process relating to existing goals or new goals to enrich or augment activity and participation in selected areas. Hence, successful ageing within the context of living with PD should be the outcome of choice for rehabilitation.

Turnbull[16] discusses three potential models of physiotherapy management in an attempt to develop a model that best fits the needs of people with PD. The cure model is appropriate for acute events which require an intensive period of rehabilitation followed by discharged, for example after a sports injury. Under the current PD model there is an assumption that medical management alone is needed initially to restore function. Physiotherapy is considered only when medication effects are reduced or become unpredictable with attendant loss of function. At this point established disability is likely to reduce the effect of therapy. A progressive model of physiotherapy management of PD is proposed which initiates a preventive treatment strategy on diagnosis, runs regular objective assessment to identify problem areas, targets treatment appropriately, and incorporates an on-going educational element for patients and carers. The progressive model enables the rehabilitation role, most commonly associated with physiotherapy intervention, to be combined with prevention, support, advice and health education.[17] The progressive model of physiotherapy management fits the model of PD care proposed by MacMahon and Thomas.[18] This four-stage clinical scale sets out criteria for inclusion at each stage, and also the range of services that individuals may require throughout the disease course. Under the model, multidisciplinary referral may be considered at any stage from Diagnosis, Maintenance, Complex to Palliative care. The work of a project to evaluate physiotherapy in PD has highlighted that, even in the practice of specialist physiotherapists working with people with PD, early referral is not occurring but is deemed highly desirable for successful practice.[19]

Historical context of physiotherapy in PD

Before the introduction of levodopa in the late 1960s, physiotherapy played an important part in the management of PD, related primarily to the prevention and treatment of musculoskeletal sequelae.[20] During the introduction of levodopa aggressive physiotherapy was employed to help individuals with established physical problems gain benefit from the new drug therapy.[21] Although some therapists were hopeful that traditional and newer neurophysiological treatment techniques could be adjunctive to levodopa therapy,[22] the dominance of the pharmacological approach subsequently marginalized

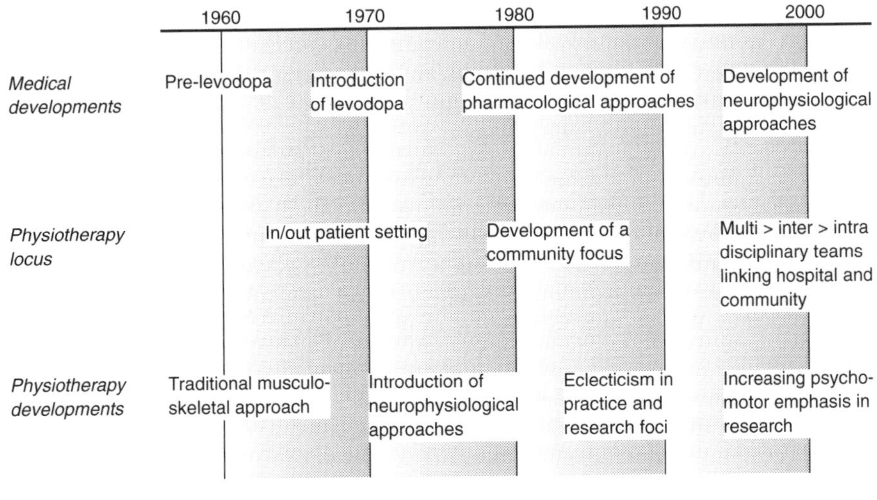

	1960	1970	1980	1990	2000
Medical developments	Pre-levodopa	Introduction of levodopa	Continued development of pharmacological approaches		Development of neurophysiological approaches
Physiotherapy locus		In/out patient setting	Development of a community focus		Multi > inter > intra disciplinary teams linking hospital and community
Physiotherapy developments	Traditional musculo-skeletal approach	Introduction of neurophysiological approaches	Eclecticism in practice and research foci		Increasing psycho-motor emphasis in research

Fig. 20.1   Medical and physiotherapy management time-line in Parkinson's disease.

physiotherapy input. However, there was renewed interest in the contribution of physiotherapy when the limitations and complications of long-term drug therapy were recognized.[23] The use of approaches developed largely in relation to other conditions is a feature of physiotherapy treatment in PD,[24] and has been mirrored in the wide range of research foci.[25] However, increasingly links are being made between the specific neurological deficits found in the condition and physiotherapy treatment approaches.[26] Acknowledgement of the diverse needs of the client group has led to an emphasis on multidisciplinary team work.[27] Figure 20.1 illustrates the relationship between developments in the medical and physiotherapy management of PD, together with changes in the locus and context of physiotherapy treatment.

Research into physiotherapy and PD

It is possible to map recent trials of physiotherapy and PD onto the historical context of management outlined in Fig. 20.1.

Conventional treatment approach

The conventional physiotherapy treatment approach is eclectic, combining techniques based on biomechanical, neurophysiological and motor learning principles. At its core are mobilising exercises designed to address movement, postural control, gait and balance.[28] Details of three trials that have evaluated a conventional approach to physiotherapy in PD are listed in Table 20.1.

Banks and Caird[29] taught an exercise regime in the home context aimed at encouraging trunk rotation and extension and lower-limb function, and used timed tests to assess before and after a 2-week period of exercising. Statistically significant improvements in walking, bed mobility and transfers were recorded. Comella et al.[30] employed a repetitive exercise treatment regime over 4 weeks, to be continued at home, to improve range of motion, endurance, balance, gait and dexterity in a randomized, single-blind, cross-over study. Following physiotherapy there was significant improvement in the Unified Parkinson's Disease Rating Scale (UPDRS) Activities of Daily Living (ADL) and motor scores, though these had returned to baseline at 6 months. Formisano et al.[31] evaluated a 4-month generalized physiotherapy regime in which active and passive movements were used to address posture, gait, dexterity and speech. Improvement was recorded on clinical rating scales and timed tests compared with control. In all three trials patients were encouraged to continue exercising after the trial had finished. Both Banks and Caird[29] and Comella et al.[30] acknowledged that at follow-up many patients had encountered difficulty in maintaining the regime. Formisano et al.[31] highlighted the need to monitor carryover of exercise activity and functional effects. MacKay-Lyons and Turnbull,[32] commenting on the work of Comella et al.,[30] highlighted the need for home exercise regimes to reflect individuals' goals and lifestyles, and to be based on a sound understanding of overall PD management.

Table 20.1 Details of three trials used to evaluate a conventional approach to physiotherapy in Parkinson's disease

Reference	Design	Number and stage	Treatment and timescale	Outcome(s)	Evidence of effect
Banks and Caird (1989)[29]	Pre- and post-test	n = 36 Hoehn and Yahr I–IV	Selected home exercise (20 min 2 × daily for 2 weeks)	Timed walking and transfer tests	Walking* Turning in bed* Lie to sit* Sit to stand*
Formisano et al. (1992)[31]	Experimental and control group	n = 33 Hoehn and Yahr II–III	Drug treatment plus group conventional exercise regime versus drug treatment only (1 h, 3 × weekly for 4 months)	Northwestern Disability University Scale (NUDS) Timed walking and dexterity tests	NUDS* Walking*
Comella et al. (1994)[30]	Randomized, single-blind, cross-over	n = 16 Hoehn and Yahr II–III	Progressive repetitive exercise regime (1 h, 3 × weekly for 4 weeks)	Unified Parkinson's Disease Rating Scale (UPDRS) (mentation, ADL and motor sections) Timed finger taps Geriatric Depression Scale	Total UPDRS* ADL UPDRS* Motor UPDRS*

*Statistically significant improvement.

Specific treatment approaches

A second group of studies of physiotherapy in PD have addressed specific problem areas encountered by the client group using targeted physiotherapy treatment approaches. The first part of Table 20.2 gives details of five studies that have evaluated the use of compensatory movement strategies and/or cues to improve motor performance in gross motor skills such as turning in bed, transfers and walking. Cues employed included cognitive prompts which are internally generated self-instruction, or external sensory cues of a visual or auditory nature. The second part of Table 20.2 gives details of two trials which have addressed specific musculoskeletal impairments with targeted physiotherapy programmes.

All five studies in the first part of Table 20.2 demonstrated the effectiveness of providing PD patients with a variety of cues to enhance motor performance. As with conventional studies, the issue for researchers in discussing the implications of their results for clinical practice is the carryover factor. Thaut et al.[33] reported that experimental group subjects were able to reproduce (without cueing) the fastest training cadence 24 h after the last training session. Morris et al.[34] reported that visual cues and attentional strategy training led to normalization of gait without visual cues for a 2-h follow-up period at least. However, secondary tasks and covert monitoring led to a reduction of stride length to baseline. The authors suggested that basal ganglia dysfunction may mitigate against movement automaticity, leaving patients reliant on their own focused attention and input from carers if appropriate. How realistic focused attention is as an ongoing strategy in everyday life[35,36] can be approached through the results of the studies by Kamsma et al.[26] and Dam et al.[28]

Kamsma et al.[26] followed their experimental group who had been taught to cue sequential compensatory movement strategies for one year, checking and retraining effective strategy performance at 1, 3, 6 and 12 months. Measurements were always higher than baseline prior to any retraining, indicating a learning effect throughout the study, and effectiveness increased after each retraining session. By contrast, there was a decline in overall performance in the control group. The effect of strategy training was found to be activity-specific, and did not generalize to other activities of daily living. Dam et al.[28] examined the effectiveness of a conventional physiotherapy regime against sensory-enhanced physiotherapy based on the use of cues. Immediately following each cycle of treatment, irrespective of type, significant functional improvements were recorded. However, the gains recorded for conventional therapy were short term, whilst individuals treated with sensory enhanced therapy maintained functional gains at 12 months.

The two studies in the base section of Table 20.2 address musculoskeletal impairments affecting the axial structures of the spine and thorax in PD, deficits which have the potential to affect balance, posture and respiratory function. In contrast to the studies in Table 20.1, very targeted exercise regimes have been developed and evaluated against specific outcome measures. The aerobic regime of Bridgewater and Sharpe[37] incorporated specific trunk-strengthening exercises into the warm-up phase. Schenkman et al.[38] used exercises designed to improve mobility and coordination of spinal movement, focusing on relaxation to counteract rigidity rather than specific strengthening and stretching. Both studies suggest that trunkal impairments can be remedied by specific physiotherapy regimes, but acknowledge that there is a need to investigate the potential of such programmes to impact on performance of everyday activities.

Individualized approach

The individualized approach is based on a client-centred holistic model. Central to this approach is the exploration with the individual of their problems and needs in the context of their everyday lives and ambitions. A trial in which this approach was used is illustrated in Table 20.3. In this study,[39] physiotherapy intervention was offered to a randomly allocated group. Assessments of both the intervention and control groups were undertaken at 3-monthly intervals.

The quantitative assessments demonstrated that there were no significant differences between the control and intervention groups at the start of the study, and that the sample population did indeed represent the spectrum from diagnosis to late stage of the disease. No significant treatment effects were demonstrated using these scales. However, qualitative analysis of the detailed physiotherapy records and assessments revealed clear effects. Individual needs were being addressed often enhancing the independence of the person, their safety and reducing the burden on carers for those at a later stage of the disease trajectory. This seemingly contradictory outcome is explained, firstly by the individualized nature of the physiotherapeutic input targeted towards the specific needs and ambitions of the individual which would tend to mask group effects; and secondly by the relative insensitivity of many of the quantitative outcome measures to short-term changes in the face of a long-term progressive disorder.[39,40] Outcome measures need to relate back to the aims of rehabilitation which may be very specific to the individual and quite different across a group.

Contextual studies

There is a large body of research in areas which impact on the physiotherapy management on PD, for example on the management of chronic illness in the nursing literature, or more specifically on the management of falls in PD. Patients with PD are at risk of falls, and physiotherapists have found falls diaries to be a useful management tool.[41] The work of Stack and Ashburn[42] has highlighted the ways that people with PD talk about their experience of falls and fall events (near misses), and the association between depression and anxiety and an increased risk of falling.[43] The first of these studies points to the importance of clinicians finding out where falls occur and addressing the situation specifically, checking the safety of turning and addressing

Table 20.2 Details of trials used to evaluate specific approaches to physiotherapy in Parkinson's disease

Reference	Design	Number and stage	Treatment and timescale	Outcome(s)	Evidence of effect
Compensatory movement strategies and cueing					
Kamsma et al. (1995)[26]	Experimental and control group	n = 38 Hoehn and Yahr II–IV	Compensatory movement strategy training programme (learning phase 3 months, consolidation phase 9 months) versus non-specific group exercise programme (45 min, 1 × weekly; 36 sessions over 1 year)	Video recording of gross motor skills Gait parameters UPDRS ADL and motor sections Subjective Well-being in the Elderly Exit questionnaire	Improved performance and use of alternative movement strategies in everyday life Higher applicability of strategy training High rating of both programmes
Thaut et al. (1996)[33]	Experimental with two control groups	n = 37 Hoehn and Yahr II–III	Rhythmic auditory stimulation in home-based gait training programme (3 weeks) versus no gait training or internally self-paced training	Gait parameters EMG	Velocity* Cadence* Stride length* EMG anterior tibialis and vastus lateralis*
Morris et al. (1996)[34]	Experimental	Total n = 54 Three studies	Visual cues versus attentional strategies (20 min of repeated 10-m walks with set stride length)	Computerized stride analysis (spatial and temporal)	Normal stride length elicited by both sets of cues and both maintain normal gait for at least 2 h

Reference	Design	Number and stage	Treatment and timescale	Outcome(s)	Evidence of effect
Dam et al. (1996)[28]	Matched groups	$n = 40$ Hoehn and Yahr II–V	Conventional versus sensory enhanced physiotherapy (1–2 h, 5 × weekly for 4 weeks, 3 cycles with 3-month breaks)	Northwestern University Disability Scale (subscores for walking – GAIT – and dressing, eating, feeding and hygiene – DEFH)	Sensory-enhanced physiotherapy GAIT score* DEFH score*
Nieuwboer et al. (1997)[36]	Case study	$n = 1$	External cues to overcome freezing (30–45 min, 1–2 × daily for 3 weeks)	Number of freezing episodes during obstacle course	Reduction in freezing episodes
Secondary musculoskeletal/respiratory problems					
Bridgewater and Sharpe (1997)[37]	Experimental and control group	$n = 26$ Hoehn and Yahr I–III	Aerobic exercise group with trunk muscle training (2 × weekly for 12 weeks) versus control group attending four interest talks	Isostation B200 dynamometer Webster Disability Rating Scale Northwestern University Disability Scale Human Activity Profile	Improved isometric torque production and velocity against resistance
Schenkman et al. (1998)[38]	Randomized control	$n = 51$ Hoehn and Yahr II–III	Spinal flexibility exercises (3 × weekly for 10 weeks) versus no specific exercise	Functional axial rotation Functional reach Timed supine to stand	Functional axial rotation* Functional reach*

*Statistically significant improvement.

Table 20.3 Evaluation of an individualized approach to physiotherapy in Parkinson's disease

Reference	Design	Number and stage	Treatment and treatment length	Outcome(s)	Evidence of effects
Chandler and Plant (1999)[39]	Randomized control	$n = 67$ Langton–Hewer stages 1–4	Individualized assessment Intervention focused on individual strategies including specific treatment, advice and education	Detailed physiotherapy assessment FIM NEADL UPDRS motor section Timed walk 9-hole peg test Semi-structured interview SF36 PDQ39 Qualitative analysis of enhanced physiotherapy records	No significant treatment effects were shown using the standardized scales. Enhanced physiotherapy records showed clear effectiveness on a case-by-case basis.

prevention through saving strategies. The second study suggests the need to address the management of depression and anxiety in PD, particularly those who fall regularly.

Best practice physiotherapy in PD

A study of best practice physiotherapy in PD[44] comprised a Delphi survey of specialist physiotherapists (n = 49) and case studies of best practice sites (n = 9). Results of the Delphi survey identified that, even within the practice of specialist physiotherapists, provision for people with PD was variable. A working definition of the purpose of physiotherapy in PD – to maximize functional ability and minimize secondary complications through movement rehabilitation within a context of education and support for the whole person – was constructed following high levels of consensus about the reasons for physiotherapy in the condition. Specialist physiotherapists deemed an eclectic treatment approach to be most effective, with effects most appropriately measured in relation to the specified aims of treatment and principally in relation to function.

Case study data were gathered from interviews with physiotherapists, managers, team members, patients and carers, together with a documentary analysis of patients' notes. Triangulation of this data with the Delphi survey results allowed the articulation of three frameworks against which to examine physiotherapy in PD. The first is a service framework which proposes a context for practice incorporating external, internal and individual features. External features such as long-term management and contact on diagnosis relate to the setting up of the service; internal features such as communication and keyworking relate to teamwork; and individual features such as jointly agreed goals and standardized assessment relate to the physiotherapy–patient relationship. A theoretical framework relates physiotherapy input to all parts of the old International Classification of Impairments, Disabilities and Handicaps (ICIDH) impairment-disability-handicap continuum[4], recognizing that other pathologies may be present, that management is optimal when carried out within the context of a multidisciplinary team and that the patient and carer must be included in the team. In addition, a practice framework has been proposed which relates the core areas of physiotherapy in PD – gait, balance, posture and transfers – to service provision, purpose, treatment, assessment and training.[45,46]

Summary

As rehabilitation is an inherently multifactorial and multiprofessional activity,[6] it is a weakness that much of the research base consists of studies involving single interventions and single professions. The interpretation of a review of physiotherapy in the rehabilitation of stroke[47] also holds true of physiotherapy in PD. Whilst complex, the evidence suggests that patients benefit from physiotherapy; the optimal type remains unclear; and evaluation is problematic given the complexity of the condition, and its management and methodological and measurement shortcomings. It is hoped that the three frameworks articulated within the study of best practice[45] relating to service, theory and practice will provide a basis on which to site existing work and plan future research on the effectiveness of physiotherapy in PD.

References

1. Ward C. Rehabilitation in Parkinson's disease. *Rev. Clin. Gerontol.* 1992; **2**: 254–68.
2. Yarrow S. Members' 1998 survey of the Parkinson's Disease Society of the United Kingdom. In: Percival R, Hobson P (eds). *Parkinson's Disease: Studies in Psychological and Social Care.* Leicester: The British Psychological Society, 1999: 79–92.
3. Baker M, Fardell J, Jones B. *Disability and Rehabilitation: Survey of education needs of health and social service professionals. Full report: The case for action.* London: The Disability & Rehabilitation Open Learning Project, 1997.
4. World Health Organization. *International classification of impairments, disabilities and handicaps (ICIDH).* Geneva: World Health Organization, 1980.
5. World Health Organization. *ICIDH-2: International classification of functioning and disability. Beta-2 draft, Full version.* Geneva: World Health Organization, 1999.
6. Sinclair A, Dickinson E. *Effective Practice in Rehabilitation: The Evidence of Systematic Reviews.* London: King's Fund, 1998.
7. Deane K, Jones D, Ellis-Hill C, Clarke C, Playford D, Ben-Shlomo Y. Physiotherapy for patients with Parkinson's disease – a comparison of physiotherapy techniques for patients with Parkinson's disease. (Submitted.) The Cochrane Library, 1999. Update software, 2000. www.update-software.com/clibhome.
8. Oxtoby M, Findley L, Kelson N, *et al. A strategy for the management of Parkinson's disease and for the long-term support of patients and their carers.* London: Parkinson's Disease Society, 1988.
9. Oxtoby M. The Romford Project: action research in a time of rapid change. In: Percival R, Hobson P (eds). *Parkinson's Disease: Studies in Psychological and Social Care.* Leicester: The British Psychological Society, 1999: 285–92.
10. Patti F, Reggio A, Nicoletti F, Sellaroli T, Deiniti G, Nicoletti F. Effects of rehabilitation therapy on Parkinsonians' disability and functional independence. *J. Neurol. Rehab.* 1996; **10**: 223–31.
11. Sitzia J, Haddrell V, Rice-Oxley M. Evaluation of a nurse-led multidisciplinary neurological rehabilitation programme using the Nottingham Health Profile. *Clin. Rehab.* 1998; **12**: 389–94.
12. Iansek R. Interdisciplinary Rehabilitation in Parkinson's Disease. In: Stern G (ed.). *Advances in Neurology,* Vol 80. Philadelphia: Lippincott Williams & Wilkins, 1999: 555–9.
13. Bilclough J. Managed care: evaluating the impact of a multidisciplinary pathway of care and the care programme approach in Parkinson's disease. *The Science and Practice of Multidisciplinary Care in Parkinson's Disease and Parkinsonism.* London, 1999; 22–3.
14. Gignac M, Cott C. A conceptual model of independence and dependence for adults with chronic physical illness and disability. *Soc. Sci. Med.* 1998; **47**: 739–53.

15. Baltes MM. Successful ageing. In: Ebrahim S, Kalache A (eds). *Epidemiology in Old Age*. London: BMJ Publishing Group, 1996: 162–8.
16. Turnbull G (ed.). *Physical Therapy Management of Parkinson's Disease*. New York: Churchill Livingstone Inc., 1992.
17. De Souza L. *Physiotherapy. Multiple Sclerosis: Approaches to Management*. London: Chapman & Hall, 1990.
18. McMahon D, Thomas S. Practical approach to quality of life in Parkinson's disease. *J. Neurol*. 1998; **245** (Suppl. 11): S19–22.
19. Plant R, Jones D, Ashburn A, Lovgreen B, Kinnear E, Handford F. Evaluation of physiotherapy in Parkinson's disease: Project update. *The Science and Practice of Multidisciplinary Care in Parkinson's Disease and Parkinsonism*. London, 1999; 21.
20. Doshay LJ. Method and value of physiotherapy in Parkinson's disease. *N. Engl. J. Med*. 1962; **266**: 878–80.
21. Stern P, McDowell F, Miller J, Robinson M. Levodopa and physical therapy in treatment of patients with Parkinson's disease. *Arch. Phys. Med. Rehab*. 1970; **51**: 273–7.
22. Irwin-Carruthers SH. An approach to physiotherapy for the patient with Parkinson's disease. *Physiotherapy* 1971; **March**: 5–7.
23. Franklyn S, Imms FJ, Stern G. *Physiotherapy and Parkinson's disease: an evaluation of four treatment regimes*. London: Parkinson's Disease Society, 1985.
24. Yekutiel MP. A clinical trial of the re-education of movement in patients with Parkinson's disease. *Clin. Rehab*. 1991; **5**: 207–14.
25. Jones D. *Research into Physiotherapy and Parkinson's Disease: the Physiotherapist*. London: Parkinson's Disease Society, 1997.
26. Kamsma YPT, Brouwer WH, Lakke JPWF. Training of compensational strategies for impaired gross motor skills in Parkinson's disease. *Physiotherapy Theory and Practice* 1995; **11**: 209–29.
27. Morris M, Iansek R. *Parkinson's disease: a team approach*. Cheltenham, Australia: Southern Healthcare Network, 1997.
28. Dam M, Tonin P, Casson S, *et al*. Effects of conventional and sensory-enhanced physiotherapy on disability of Parkinson's disease patients. In: Battistin L, Scarlato G, Caraceni T, Ruggieri S (eds). *Advances in Neurology*, Vol. 69. Philadelphia: Lippincott-Raven, 1996: 551–5.
29. Banks M, Caird F. Physiotherapy benefits patients with Parkinson's disease. *Clin. Rehab*. 1989; **3**: 11–16.
30. Comella CL, Stebbins GT, Brown-Toms N, Goetz CG. Physical therapy and Parkinson's disease. *Neurology* 1994; **44**: 376–8.
31. Formisano R, Pratesi L, Modarelli FT, Bonifati V, Meco G. Rehabilitation in Parkinson's disease. *Scand. J. Rehab. Med*. 1992; **24**: 157–60.
32. MacKay-Lyons M, Turnbull G. Physical therapy in Parkinson's disease. *Neurology* 1995; **45**: 205.
33. Thaut M, McIntosh G, Rice R, Miller R, Rathbun J, Brault J. Rhythmic auditory stimulation in gait training for Parkinson's disease patients. *Movement Disord*. 1996; **11**: 193–200.
34. Morris M, Iansek R, Matyas T, Summers J. Stride length regulation in Parkinson's disease. Normalization strategies and underlying mechanisms. *Brain* 1996; **119**: 551–68.
35. Playford D. Is using a cue the clue to the treatment of freezing in Parkinson's disease? *Physiother. Res. Int*. 1997; **2**: 133–4.
36. Nieuwboer A, Feys P, Weerdt WD, Dom R. Is using a cue the clue to the treatment of freezing in Parkinson's disease? *Physiother. Res. Int*. 1997; **2**: 125–34.

37. Bridgewater K, Sharpe M. Trunk muscle training and early Parkinson's disease. *Physiother. Theory Pract.* 1997; **13**: 139–53.
38. Schenkman M, Cutson T, Kuchibhatla M, *et al.* Exercise to improve spinal flexibility and function for people with Parkinson's disease: a randomized, controlled trial. *J. Am. Geriatr. Soc.* 1998; **46**: 1207–16.
39. Chandler C, Plant R. A Targeted physiotherapy service for people with Parkinson's disease from diagnosis to end stage: a pilot study. In: Percival R, Hobson P (eds). *Parkinson's Disease: Studies in Psychological and Social Care.* London: BPS Books, 1999: 256–69.
40. Hobson P, Holden A, Meara J. Measuring the impact of Parkinson's disease with the Parkinson's Disease Quality of Life questionnaire. *Age Ageing* 1999; **28**: 341–6.
41. Yekutiel MP. Patients' fall records as an aid in designing and assessing therapy in Parkinsonism. *Disab. Rehab.* 1993; **15**: 189–93.
42. Stack E, Ashburn A. Fall events described by people with Parkinson's disease: implications for clinical interviewing and the research agenda. *Physiother. Res. Int.* 1999; **4**: 190–200.
43. Ashburn A, Stack E, Pickering R, Ward C. Depression and anxiety experienced by fallers and non-fallers among a community sample of people with Parkinson's disease and controls. *Physiotherapy* 1998; **84**: 165.
44. Jones D, Plant R, Lovgreen B, Ashburn A, Handford F, Kinnear E. Best practice physiotherapy in Parkinson's disease. *J. Neurol. Rehab. Neural Repair* 1999; **13**: 73.
45. Ashburn A, Jones D, Lovgreen B, Plant R. Physiotherapy and Parkinson's disease; evaluating best practice. *Physiotherapy* 2000; **86**: 32.
46. Plant R, Jones D, Ashburn A, Lovgreen B, Handford F, Kinnear E. Physiotherapy for people with Parkinson's disease: UK Best Practice. Newcastle upon Tyne. Institute of Rehabilitation, 2000.
47. Ashburn A, Partridge C, De Souza L. Physiotherapy in the rehabilitation of stroke: a review. *Clin. Rehab.* 1993; **7**: 337–45.

Prospects for research in elderly patients with Parkinson's disease

21

J.C. Sharma

Introduction

As demographic changes lead to an increase in the number of patients with Parkinson's disease (PD), there is an increasing need for evidence-based diagnosis and management of idiopathic PD in the elderly. There are major opportunities for research in elderly PD patients in the following areas:

- diagnosis and clinical symptoms;
- disability and neuropsychiatric features;
- drug and non-pharmacological management; and
- surgical management

Diagnosis and clinical symptoms

A significant error in the diagnostic accuracy of PD has been demonstrated when neuropathological criteria are correlated with clinical features. This has led to the development of Parkinson's Disease Society brain bank diagnostic criteria for PD. When applied to a community sample of parkinsonism, mean age 76 years, only 53 per cent patients qualified to be diagnosed as having idiopathic PD.[1] A number of patients with parkinsonism may not meet these criteria but are partially responsive to levodopa. It is questionable whether these patients be denied the benefit of dopaminergic therapy for the limited duration just because they do not meet the diagnostic criteria. In addition, it should be considered whether a positive Babinski response in an elderly patient excludes PD, or simply reflects the coexistence of cerebrovascular disease or some other corticospinal pathology in older patients. Since imaging with PET (positron emission tomography) and SPECT (single photon emission computed tomography),[2] growth hormone release with clonidine,[3] and even magnetic resonance imaging[4] are unlikely to be available or even useful as a routine diagnostic tools, clinical diagnostic criteria need to be developed for application to elderly patients.

A number of questions should be asked in this respect. Why does tremor-predominant PD behave differently? Has it a less aggressive course and less cognitive impairment, and is this due to a difference in nigrostriatal pathophysiology as compared with akinetic, rigid patients? Does the presence of tremor have a protective effect, or is it that the akinetic rigid syndrome includes patients who have other pathological diagnoses such as multisystem atrophy and progressive supranuclear palsy.[5] Do the presenting symptoms and their progression in elderly PD patients differ from those in young-onset patients? Are a number of the symptoms that occur commonly in elderly PD (e.g. constipation, bladder symptoms, cognitive impairment, imbalance and falls and sleep disorders) due to ageing, or are they a consequence of parkinsonian pathology? How can the influence of ageing be differentiated from PD, and would a better understanding lead to more rewarding management? The evidence in the literature on the natural history of PD in the elderly and many of the above issues is remarkably sparse, despite a vast clinical experience of the condition among elderly care physicians.

Disability and neuropsychiatric features

Elderly PD patients seem to suffer from a higher functional disability for each stage of PD compared with younger patients. The reasons for this are unclear. Is it due to an ageing effect or is it related to co-morbidity? Moreover, what is the impact of coexistent pathology on treatment strategy for PD? Today, an increasing number of elderly patients are resident in care homes, and the prevalence of PD and related morbidity in these homes should be closely monitored. How well such homes are managed also warrants close scrutiny.

Prevalence of depression in PD has been difficult to assess, partly due to lack of sensitive tests to detect depression in elderly PD patients, and this explains the variance in the prevalence of reported depression.[6] It is unclear whether depression is related to disease severity or is secondary to abnormalities of neurochemical pathways, and independent of nigrostriatal pathways. It is also unclear whether depression would improve with dopaminergic intervention alone, or whether it would require anti-depressant therapy. Moreover, if the latter situation were true, then would such therapy lead to an improvement in quality of life – which should be the ultimate goal of intervention as the increased mortality in older PD patients cannot be influenced.[7] Among the other neuropsychiatric problems, the most common and distressing are hallucinations and cognitive impairment. Why the elderly are more prone to these is unclear, the possibility being that the elderly do not have a mono-aminergic neurodegeneration, as is the case in the young patients.[8]

Pharmacological and non-pharmacological management

Since the first description of deficiency of dopamine in nigrostriatal tissues in PD, an improved understanding of dopaminergic pathways and receptors has resulted in an improved control of the condition's symptoms. Identification of the subsets of dopamine receptors has enabled therapy to be targeted and to provide a greater benefit – and possibly also to delay disease progression by neuroprotection. Regrettably, however, very few pharmacological studies have recruited patients aged over 75 years.[9]

A literature search for clinical trials evaluating newer dopamine agonists and catechol-O-methyltransferase (COMT) inhibitors reveals a similar picture (Table 21.1). The double-blind or controlled studies of dopamine agonists pergolide, ropinirole, cabergoline and pramipexole as monotherapy, or as adjunct to levodopa, have been conducted in patients with a mean age of 60–67 years, with one study evaluating cabergoline in recruited patients aged up to 81 years. The COMT inhibitor entacapone is rapidly gaining a place in the therapy of PD (tolcapone is currently not available in Europe), although COMT inhibitor studies have also been limited to the age of 52–65 years. The reason why so few clinical trials recruit very old patients is unclear, but may possibly reflect either the clinical practice of the researchers or the reluctance of older patients to participate in such investigations. The contentious study which revealed a possible increased mortality using selegiline as an adjunct therapy to levodopa included centres run by geriatricians, and the inclusion of these older patients may have confounded the mortality data.[21] It was recommended, however, that selegiline should be avoided in advanced disease and in those with dementia and falls. Since many elderly patients fall into these categories, the question should perhaps be asked whether elderly patients should avoid selegiline. All these studies raise questions about the applicability of results to older patients, and based on current evidence it is doubtful whether selegiline, dopamine agonists and COMT inhibitors could be used with the confidence in elderly PD patients. A lack of research conducted in very elderly patients is the most likely reason for reluctance among geriatricians to use these drugs in such cases. It unlikely that placebo-controlled clinical trials will be repeated specifically in elderly PD patients, and a compromise must be accepted by performing observational studies such as those demonstrating the efficacy of pergolide as an adjunct therapy in the elderly.[23,24] Whilst these observational studies have limitations, they do

Table 21.1 Details of some published pharmacological trials in Parkinson's disease

Reference	Subject	Mean (± SD) age (years)	Conclusion
Olanow et al. (1994)[11]	Pergolide adjunct to levodopa	63 ± 8	Pergolide is an effective agent
Kulisevsky et al. (1998)[12]	Pergolide versus levodopa	63	Pergolide effective as monotherapy
Rascol et al. (1998)[13]	Ropinirole versus levodopa	63 ± 9	Ropinirole as effective in mild but less in advanced disease
Adler et al. (1998)[14]	Ropinirole versus placebo in early PD	65 ± 9	Ropinirole is effective as monotherapy
Steiger et al. (1996)[15]	Cabergoline versus placebo. As monotherapy	61 ± 8	Cabergoline better than placebo
Hutton et al. (1996)[16]	Cabergoline versus placebo as adjunct therapy	63 ± 8	Cabergoline better than placebo
Parkinson Study Group (1997)[17]	Pramipexole as monotherapy, early disease	62 ± 11	Pramipexole effective as monotherapy
Lieberman et al. (1997)[18]	Pramipexole as adjunct therapy	63	Pramipexole effective
Inzelberg et al. (1996)[19]	Cabergoline versus bromocriptine	71 ± 8 (30–75)	Cabergoline effective as bromocriptine
Baas et al. (1997)[20]	Tolcapone adjunct to levodopa	62 ± 10	Tolcapone prolongs 'on' time
Rinne et al. (1998)[21]	Entacapone adjunct to levodopa	62 ± 7	Entacapone has long-term benefit to reduce 'off' phase

provide some evidence for clinical practice. Another observational study[24] revealed that selegiline, in contrast to the UKPDRG study,[11] did not increase mortality in patients aged over 80 years, whereas the younger patients had a higher mortality. Thus, the role of selegiline, and its safety in elderly patients with different stages of PD remains uncertain.

Levodopa

In the treatment of PD, levodopa may cause nigrostriatal cell death and motor complications, and it is recommended that it should be avoided in the early stages of PD, when dopamine agonists may have a neuroprotective effect.[25] However, it is not clear whether elderly patients with mild and moderately severe PD should always be treated with levodopa or whether a rapid titration of dopamine agonists produce an equally effective result, without adverse effects. Moreover, it is also unclear whether such a strategy would be safe and the long-term levodopa syndrome be averted. The complexities of managing advanced disease in the elderly remain a challenge, notably with regard to what constitutes the best treatment strategy in this group. Although a dopamine agonist such as pergolide appears to prevent deterioration of PD with continuing dopaminergic stimulation,[23] there is a fall in body weight and blood pressure with disease progression, the reasons for which are not clear and require further investigation.

Traditionally, geriatricians have a better access to rehabilitation facilities. The role of rehabilitation in PD is in need of investigation in order to study its interaction with drug therapy and its influence on disability. How this can be measured, and whether this influence is independent of, or additive to, drug therapy is not clear. Also not clear is whether rehabilitation techniques can contribute in advanced PD, and whether they can prevent falls. These are but few of the many pertinent questions that require answers in order to achieve an optimum treatment strategy for elderly PD patients.

Surgical management

Surgical treatment of PD patients is proving to be successful to alleviate disabling symptoms related to PD or dyskinesia. Lesional (pallidotomy, thalamotomy) or deep brain stimulation procedures have been studied in younger patients, while only a few studies have included patients aged over 65 years. The reasons for not studying elderly PD might be a reluctance by the patients and higher operative risk, or simply that the early experimentation of new techniques has been conducted in younger patients. The mean age of patients for pallidotomy or pallidal stimulation has been about 50–55 years. There is some evidence that the higher age (62 years versus 52, i.e. not really old!) is associated with residual cognitive impairment following surgery,[26] though how this relates to the 'older' elderly patients is not clear. Since the effect of pallidal stimulation lasts for 2 years[27] and perhaps more, it would seem that elderly patients should not be denied its benefits. Indeed, it may be that they achieve more benefit because of the more complex problems in advanced disease. It is possible that stimulation techniques are more suitable to the elderly because of their reversibility and less invasive nature. However, answers to these questions can only be obtained from experience with older patients, who should be encouraged to accept (and the surgeons coerced to perform) these procedures. A multicentre register of these procedures may provide evidence of their benefit to the elderly.

Each clinician who provides care to elderly PD patients can help to expand the knowledge base and ultimately improve evidence-based practice, to the benefit of this patient group.

References

1. Meara J, Bhowmick BK, Hobson P. Accuracy of diagnosis in patients with presumed Parkinson's disease. *Age Ageing* 1999; **28**: 99–102.
2. Amer HB, Grosset D. SPECT imaging in the diagnosing and staging of parkinsonism. *CNS* 1999; **2**: 9–13.
3. Kimber JR, Watson I, Mathias CJ. Distinction of idiopathic Parkinson's disease from multi-system atropy by stimulation of growth hormone release with clonidine. *Lancet* 1997; **349**: 1877–81.
4. Schrag A, Kingsley D, Phatouros C, Mathias CJ, Lees AJ, Daniel SE, Quinn NP. Clinical usefulness of magnetic resonance imaging in multiple system atrophy. *J. Neurol. Neurosurg. Psychiatry* 1998; **65**: 65–71.
5. Rajput AH, Pahawa R, Pahwa P, Rajput A. Prognostic significance of onset mode in Parkinsonism. *Neurology* 1993; **43**: 829–30.
6. Meara J, Mitchelmore E, Hobson P. Use of GDS-15 geriatric depression scale as a screening instrument for depressive symptomatology in patients with Parkinson's disease and their carers in the community. *Age Ageing* 1999; **28**: 35–8.
7. Ben-Shlomo Y. The epidemiology of Parkinson's disease. *Baillière's Clin. Neurol.* 1997; **6**: 55–68.
8. Rakshi JS, Uema T, Ito K, *et al*. Frontal, midbrain and striatal dopaminergic function in early and advanced Parkinson's disease. *Brain* 1999; **122**: 1637–50.
9. Mitchell SL, Sullivan EA, Lipsitz LA. Exclusion of elderly subjects from clinical trials for Parkinson's disease. *Arch. Neurol.* 1997; **54**: 1393–8.
10. Olanow CW, Fahn S, Muenter M, *et al*. A multicentre double blind, placebo controlled trial of pergolide as an adjunct to Sinemet in Parkinson's disease. *Movement Disord*. 1994; **9**: 40–7.
11. Kulisevsky J, Lopez-Villegas D, Garcia-Sanchez C, *et al*. A six-month study of pergolide and levodopa in de novo Parkinson's disease patients. *Clin. Neuropharmacol.* 1998; **21**: 358–62.
12. Rascol O, Brookes DJ, Brunt ER, *et al* on behalf of the 056 study group. Ropinirole in the treatment of early Parkinson's disease; a 6-month interim report of a 5-year levodopa controlled study. *Movement Disord*. 1998; **13**: 39–45.
13. Adler CH, Sethi KD, Hauser RA, *et al*. For the Ropinirole study group. Ropinirole for the treatment of early Parkinson's disease. *Neurology* 1997; **49**: 393–9.
14. Steiger MJ, El-Debas T, Anderson T, *et al*. Double blind study of the activity and tolerability of cabergoline versus placebo in parkinsonians with motor fluctuations. *J. Neurol.* 1996; **243**: 68–72.
15. Hutton JT, Koller WC, Ahlskog JE, *et al*. Multicentre placebo controlled trial of cabergoline taken once daily in the treatment of Parkinson's disease. *Neurology* 1996; **46**: 1062–5.
16. Parkinson study group. Safety and efficacy of pramipexole in early Parkinson's disease. A randomised dose-ranging study. *JAMA* 1997; **278**: 125–30.

17. Lieberman A, Ranhosky A, Korts D. Clinical evaluation of pramipexole in advanced Parkinson's disease: results of a double-blind, placebo-controlled, parallel-group study. *Neurology* 1997; **49**: 162–8.

18. Inzelberg R, Nisipeanu P, Rabey JM, *et al.* Double-blind comparison of cabergoline and bromocriptine in Parkinson's disease patients with motor fluctuations. *Neurology* 1996; **47**: 785–8.

19. Bass H, Beiske AG, Ghika J, *et al.* On behalf of the study investigators. Catechol-O-methyltransferase inhibition with tolcapone reduces the wearing off phenomenon and levodopa requirements in fluctuating parkinsonian patients. *J. Neurol. Neurosurg. Psychiatry* 1997; **63**: 421–8.

20. Rinne UK, Larsen JP, Siden A, Worm-Peterson J, and the Nomecomt study group. Entacapone enhances the levodopa response in parkinsonian patients with motor fluctuations. *Neurology* 1998; **51**: 1309–14.

21. Investigation by Parkinson's disease research Group of United Kingdom into excess mortality seen with combined levodopa and selegiline treatment in patients with early, mild Parkinson's disease: further results of randomised trial and confidential inquiry. *Br. Med. J.* 1998; **316**: 1191–6.

22. Hindle J, Meara J, Sharma JC, *et al.* Prescribing pergolide in the elderly – an open label study of pergolide in the elderly patients with Parkinson's disease. *Int. J. Geriatr. Psychopharmacol.* 1998; **1**: 78–81.

23. Sharma JC, Ross IN. Long term role of pergolide as an adjunct therapy in Parkinson's disease: influence on disability, blood pressure, weight and levodopa syndrome. *Parkinsonism Rel. Disord.* 1999; **5**: 111–14.

24. Thorogood M, Armstrong B, Nichols T, Hollowell J. Mortality in people taking selegiline: observational study. *Br. Med. J.*1998; **317**: 252–4.

25. Monastruc JL, Rascol O, Senard JM. Treatment of Parkinson's disease should begin with a dopamine agonist. *Movement Disord.* 1999; **14**: 725–30.

26. Vingerhoets G, van der Linden C, Lannoo E, Vandewalle V, Caemaert J, Wolters M, Van den Abbeele D. Cognitive outcome after unilateral pallidal stimulation in Parkinson's disease. *J. Neurol. Neurosurg. Psychiatry* 1999; **66**: 297–304.

27. Ghikha J, Villemure JG, Fankhauser H, Favre J, Assal G, Ghikha-Schmid F. Efficiency and safety of bilateral contemporaneous pallidal stimulation (deep brain stimulation) in levodopa responsive patients with Parkinson's disease with severe motor fluctuation: a 2-year follow-up review. *J. Neurosurg.* 1998; **89**: 713–18.

Appendix 1

Useful texts

Wade D. *Measurement in Neurological Rehabilitation*. Oxford: Oxford Medical Publications, Oxford University Press, 1996.
This book is a useful resource for standard measures in the management of people with disability arising from neurological conditions.

Burns A, Lawlor B, Craig S. *Assessment scales in old age psychiatry*. London: Martin Dunitz, 1999.
This is a new compendium of over 150 scales used in mental disorders of the elderly.

Hodges JR. *Cognitive Assessment for Clinicians*. Oxford: Oxford Medical Publications, Oxford University Press, 1996.
This small book reviews neuropsychological assessment and explains the principles behind the tests.

A brief review of some commonly used rating scales and references

DIAGNOSIS

United Kingdom Parkinson's Disease Society Brain Bank Clinical Diagnostic Criteria. These are well-validated criteria used for research, trials and database. They may be difficult to apply clinically especially early in the disease, as they require evidence of progression and levodopa responsiveness. The presence of mixed pathology in elderly patients (e.g. vascular lesions giving an extensor plantar response) may lead to exclusion.

- Hughes AJ, Daniel SE, Kilford L, Lees AJ. Accuracy of clinical diagnosis of idiopathic Parkinson's disease: a clinicopathological study of 100 cases. *J. Neurol. Neurosurg. Psychiatry* 1992; **55**: 181–4.

Calne Clinical Diagnostic Criteria. These criteria are based on the presence of extrapyramidal signs and asymmetry. They are easy to apply clinically, producing categories of possible, probable and clinically definite PD. Postural instability is included as a criteria but in the elderly this may be due to a variety of causes.

- Calne D, Snow BJ, Lee C. Criteria for diagnosing Parkinson's disease. *Ann. Neurol.* 1992; **32**: 125–7.

DISEASE SEVERITY

Hoehn and Yahr (1967). This is a basic 5-point scale used in many studies, but is of little day-to-day clinical use. Mixes pathology, with impairments and disabilities and should no longer be used.

- Hoehn MM, Yahr MD. Parkinsonism: onset, progression and mortality. *Neurology* 1967; **17**: 427–42.

Webster (1968)[2]. This was previously widely used. It has 10 sections with a maximum score of 3 for each. There is no differential weighting for different symptoms, e.g. seborrhoea and loss of self-care have equal scores. There is no scoring for dyskinesia.
Webster DD. Critical analysis of the disability in Parkinson's disease. *Modern Treatment* 1968; **5**: 257–82.

Unified Parkinson's Disease Rating Scale – UPDRS (1987)[3]. Widely used in research, and some sections useful clinically. Includes sections on mental function, daily activities, motor function and side effects. Useful for monitoring progress, but time-consuming. Selective use of sections (e.g. motor function) can be useful.

- Fahn S, Elton R. Members of the UPDRS development committee. In: Fahn S, Marsden CD, Calne DB, Goldstein M (eds). *Recent Developments in Parkinson's Disease. Vol. 2.* Florham Park, NJ: Macmillan Health Care Information 1987; 153–63, 293–304.

Parkinson's Aware in Primary Care. A new model for staging disease management reviewing care needs in diagnostic, maintenance, complex and palliative stages. Easy to follow, and useful particularly at primary and secondary care interface.

- The Primary Care Task Force for the Parkinson's Disease Society (UK). Parkinson's Disease Aware in Primary Care, 1999. Parkinson's Disease Society, 215 Vauxhall Bridge Road, London SW1V 1EJ, UK.

SIDE EFFECTS OF MEDICATION

Complications of therapy section of UPDRS.
Abnormal involuntary movement scale (AIMS). Good validity and reliability. Not widely used.
Chien CP, Jung K, Ross-Townsend A. Methodological approach to the measurement of tardive dyskinesia: piezoelectric recording and concurrent validity tests on five clinical scales. In: Fann WE, Smith RC, Davis JM, Domino EF (eds). *Tardive Dyskinesia; Research and Treatment.* New York: Spectrum, 1980; 233–66.

ACTIVITIES OF DAILY LIVING

UPDRS – See above.

Barthel ADL Index (1965). A generic scale in common use in geriatric medicine. Widely used and well-validated.

- Wade DT, Collin C. The Barthel ADL index: a standard measurement of physical disability? *Int. Disability Studies* 1989; **10**: 64–7.

Nottingham extended ADL. Little published information or validation. Can be used as a postal questionnaire.

- Nouri FM, Lincoln NB. An extended activities of daily living scale for stroke patients. *Clin. Rehab.* 1987; **1**: 301–5.

Schwab and England – Used as part of the UPDRS, giving a percentage disability. Subjective, and of little clinical use.

- Schwab RS, England AC. Projection technique for evaluating surgery in Parkinson's disease. In: Gillingham FJ, Donalson MC (eds). *Third Symposium on Parkinson's Disease*. Edinburgh: Livingstone, 1969; 152–7.

COGNITION

Mini mental test score of Folstein – MMSE. Used as a screening tool. Usefulness in following progress in dementia in doubt. No frontal lobe functions assessed.

- Folstein MF, Folstein SE, McHugh PR. 'Mini Mental State': a practical method of grading the cognitive state of patients for the clinician. *J. Psychiatr. Res.* 1975; **12**: 189–98.

Cambridge examination for mental disorders (CAMDEX) Cognitive section- revised (CAMCOG-R). A well-validated tool for screening for cognitive dysfunction, which is more sensitive to early change than MMSE. Revised format now includes more frontal assessment.
Roth M, Huppert F, Mountjoy C, Tym E. *The Cambridge Examination for Mental Disorders – Revised*. Cambridge University Press, 1999.
Rivermead Behavioural memory test. This is a test of everyday cognitive tasks. It is easy to apply and widely used. It can be administered repeatedly using parallel versions.

- Wilson BA, Cockburn J, Baddeley AD. *The Rivermead behavioural memory test*. Titchfield, Hants: Thames Valley Test Company.

Frontal assessment battery (FAB). A simple and well-validated 10-minute bedside frontal lobe screen.

- To be published shortly. Litvan I, Dubois B.

Clock drawing test. A simple test of frontal and temperoparietal function. Scored using the Schulman scale. Not validated in PD.
Shulman K, Shedletsky R, Silver I. The challenge of time. Clock drawing and cognitive function in the elderly. *Int. J. Geriatr. Psychiatry* 1986; **1**: 135–40.

DEPRESSION

Geriatric depression scale (GDS-15). This is a well-validated and widely used scale for depressive symptoms. Validated for use in PD.

- Yesavage JA, Brink TL. Development and validation of a geriatric depression screening scale: a preliminary report. *J. Psychiatr. Res.* 1983; **17**: 37–49.

Other scales, including the **Hamilton, Beck** depression inventory and **The Hospital Anxiety and Depression Scale** can be used, but are not as well validated in the elderly and in PD.

CARERS

Caregiver strain index. Increasingly used, well-validated measure specifically designed to measure strain in the carer.

- Robinson BC. Validation of a caregiver strain index. *J. Gerontol.* 1983; **38**: 344–8.

QUALITY OF LIFE

Parkinson's disease quality of life questionnaire (PDQL). An easy-to-use 37-point scale specific for PD. Well-validated, and used in longitudinal cohort study.

- De Boer AGEM, Wilker W, Speelman JD, de Haes JCJM. Quality of life in patients with Parkinson's disease: development of a questionnaire. *J. Neurol. Neurosurg. Psychiatry* 1996; **61**: 70–4.

Parkinson's disease questionnaire (PDQ-39). Easy to use, disease-specific scale. Responsive to disease severity, and good longitudinal validation.

- Jenkinson C, Peto V, Fitzpatrick R, Greenhall R, Hyman N. Self reported functioning and well-being in patients with Parkinson's disease: comparison of the short form health survey (SF-36) and the Parkinson's disease questionnaire (PDQ-39). *Age Ageing* 1995; **24**: 505–9.

Appendix 2

- The Parkinson's Disease Society of the United Kingdom, 215 Vauxhall Bridge Road, London, SW1V 1EJ, UK. Tel: 020 7931 8080; Fax: 020 7233 9908; E-Mail mailbox@pdsuk.demon.co.uk www\parkinsons.org.uk
- British Geriatrics Society Special Interest Group in Parkinson's Disease. www.parkinsons-bgs-sig.org.uk or www.bgs.org.uk
- British Geriatrics Society, Admark House, 31 St Johns Square, London EC1M 4DN, UK. Tel: 020 7608 1369: Fax 020 7608 1041
- PSP Europe Association, Wappenham, Towchester, Northants, NN12 85Q, UK. Tel: 01327 860299; Fax: 01327 860923. (Progressive supranuclear palsy)
- The Autonomic Disorders Association, Sarah Matheson Trust, St Mary's Hospital, Praed Street, London, W2 1NY, UK. Tel: 01718 861520; Fax: 01718 861540
- International Tremor Foundation, Disablement Services Centre, Harold Wood Hospital, Romford, Essex. RM3 0BE, UK. Tel: 0170 8378050; Fax: 0170 837 8032; Web-site. www.essentialtremor.org
- The Stroke Association, Stroke House, Whitecross Street, London EC1Y 8JJ, UK. Tel: 0171 566 0300; Fax: 0171 490 2686
- The Movement Disorder Society, 611 East Wells Street, Milwaukee, W1 53202, USA. Tel: +1-414-276-2145; Fax: +1-414-276-2146; E-mail info@movementdisorders.org web-site www.movementdisorders.org
- DVLA Swansea, SA99 1BN, UK. Medical Unit. Tel: 01792 783686
- Mobility Advice and Vehicle Information Centre (MAVIS), Department of Transport, TRRL, Crowthorne, Berks. RG11 6AU, UK.
- Neurosciences on the net – links to many sites and journals. www.neuroguide.com
- WEMOVE – Worldwide Education and Awareness for Movement Disorders. www.wemove.org

Index

Note: page numbers in *italics* refer to tables, page numbers in **bold** refer to figures.

reboxitine 121
records, patient-held 247
referral 223, 226, 329
reflex amplitude 194
reflux oesophagitis 144
rehabilitation
　care pathway 331–2
　definition 329–30
　effectiveness 330
　interdisciplinary 250–69, 331
　　definition 251–2
　　examples 267–8, *268*
　　ingredients for 255–8, *256*
　　need for 254
　　practice 260–7, **261–2**
　　regular reviews 254
　　services 254–5
　　staff members 256–8, *256*
　　strategies/theory 259–60
　　terminology and concepts
　　　252–4, *253*
　models of management
　　332–3
　multidisciplinary 250–1, 252
　research into 329–42, 349
　see also specific therapies
Rehabilitation Unit, Bath 260
rehearsal strategies 265–6
remacemide 300
remediation 331
repetitive transcranial magnetic
　stimulation (rTMS) 122
research
　in physiotherapy 329–42
　prospects for 345–50
　　diagnosis and clinical
　　　symptoms 345–6
　　disability and
　　　neuropsychiatric
　　　features 346–7
　　pharmacological
　　　management 347–49
　　rehabilitation 349
　　surgical management
　　　349–50
　in rehabilitation 329–42
　support for 80
resection, transventricular of
　the caudate nucleus 309
'restoration' 331
retropulsion test 195
Richer P 6
rigidity 43, 47, 193
riluzole 300
rimitorole 290
risk factors
　for DIP 66
　global variation in 32–3
　for IPD 67, 78
　see also aetiology
risperidone 126
rivastigmine 126
road traffic accidents 200–1, 202
Roman GC 33
Romford Project 331
ropinirole
　characteristics 283–4, 297, 302
　research into 347, *348*
　side effects 206–7, 297
Royal College of General

Practitioners 239–40
Royal College of Nurses 273

Sacks O 8
Schenkman M 337, *339*
schizophrenia 128
secondary care
　health economics of 229
　role of the PDNS 224, 233
　relationships and roles **223**
　structure 216, 218
secondary causes of
　parkinsonism 43, *44*,
　　66–8
'See Saw' study 289–90
selective
　　neurotrophic/neurotoxic
　　　agents 315
selective serotonin re-uptake
　　inhibitors (SSRIs)
　for anxiety management 122
　for depression management
　　120, 121
　and DIP 66
　drug interactions 292
　movement disorders
　　associated with 129
selegiline
　characteristics 284, 291–2
　for depression management
　　in PD 120
　drug interactions 292
　formulations 292
　research into 347, 348, *348*
　side effects 168, 292
　withdrawal 292
self-care 218
self-feeding 144
self-modification, and
　　swallowing problems
　　145
self-rated reports
　on ADL 83
　on depression 93–4
　on mood 83
　practical issues 85
　on quality of life 89, 90–1
senile gait disorder 186
sensory assessment 82
sequences, breaking up 266,
　266
serotinergic activity, and
　　hallucinosis 123, 125
serotonin and noradrenaline re-
　　uptake inhibitors
　　(SNRIs) 121
serotonin syndrome 120
service commissioning
　GPs 231, 235–6, 247–8
　in the NHS 230–3
　　reviewing current services
　　　232–3, *232*
　service demands 230–1
service organization 215–36
　carer's needs 234
　commissioning services in
　　the NHS 230–3
　comprehensive 234–6
　　care management 235
　　example 235–6

　steering groups 235
　team work 235
　diagnosis 221
　health economics 215–16,
　　228–30, *229*
　health outcome measures
　　233–4
　incidence of PD 222
　medical care 222–3
　needs assessment 218–19
　palliative care 227
　prevalence of PD 222
　quality 233
　role of the PDNS 224
　self-care 218
　services and structures
　　216–18
　treatment 225–6
sexual dysfunction 122–3, 171,
　178, 275–6
'shaking palsy' 3, 5, 6
shared care 245
Sharpe M 336, *339*
Short Form-36 (SF36) 84, 90
Shy GM 166
Shy-Drager syndrome (SDS) 62,
　165, 176, 179
　see also multiple system
　　atrophy
sialorrhoea 170–1
Sickness Impact Scale (SIP) 90
sign-and-symptom test items
　81–2
simultaneous tasks, avoidance
　145, 264
Sindepar study 291
Sinemet 287
single gene defects 20–1, 36
single limb stance 195
single photon emission
　　tomography (SPECT) 55,
　　109, 221, 346
sleep disorders
　daytime sleepiness 206–7,
　　209, 294, 297, 298
　drug-related 206–7, *209*, 292,
　　294, 297, 298
　impact 92
　interdisciplinary
　　management 268, *268*
　linked to PD depression 118
　in MSA 64
　of REM sleep 64
smoking, protective effects
　22–3, 36, 116
social environmental issues 84,
　89, *90*, 148–9, *148*
　see also handicap
social models of disability 253
Social Services 230, 234, 235,
　236, 251, 255
social workers 258
sodium valproate 66
spastic catch 47
spasticity 47
Special Interest Groups of the
　British Diabetic
　Association 149
specialist services 92–4, 243
　see also specific services